THE HOLISTIC PEDIATRICIAN

THE
HOLISTIC
PEDIATRICIAN

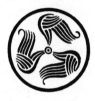

A Parent's Comprehensive Guide to Safe and Effective
Therapies for the 25 Most Common Childhood Ailments

Kathi J. Kemper, M.D., M.P.H.

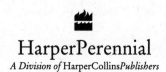

HarperPerennial
A Division of HarperCollins*Publishers*

This book is intended to educate parents about a variety of approaches to children's health care needs. This book should not be a substitute for the personal care and treatment of a qualified physician, but rather should be used in conjunction with a physician's care, in order to consider the full range of health care options available to your child. The author and publisher expressly disclaim responsibility for any adverse effects resulting from the information contained herein.

HarperCollins books may be purchased for educational, business, or sales promotional use. For information please write: Special Markets Department, HarperCollins Publishers, Inc., 10 East 53rd Street, New York, NY 10022.

FIRST EDITION

Designed by Nancy Singer

Library of Congress Cataloging-in-Publication Data

Kemper, Kathi J.
    The holistic pediatrician: a parent's comprehensive guide to safe and effective therapies for the 25 most common childhood ailments/Kathi Kemper.—1st ed.
        p.   cm.
    Includes bibliographical references and index.
    ISBN 0-06-095177-X
    1. Pediatrics—Popular works.   2. Holistic medicine.   3. Children—Diseases—Alternative treatment.   I. Title.
    RJ61.K325   1996
    618.92—dc20   95-48456

96 97 98 99 00 ❖/RRD 10 9 8 7 6 5 4 3 2 1

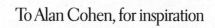

To Alan Cohen, for inspiration

CONTENTS

FOREWORD

The Holistic Pediatrician by Kathi Kemper is a comprehensive guide to medical care presenting the best of both mainstream and alternative medicine to parents. As a pediatrician, I recognize that far too often, patients are frustrated by the seemingly "either-or" mentality demonstrated by both mainstream medical practitioners and alternative healers. They are often not aware that the current split between so-called alternative therapy and mainstream medicine is actually a political and economic battle going back hundreds of years. This book, for the first time, in language that parents can understand, presents a comprehensive view of the child's health from many different medical traditions, including conventional medicine, Chinese medicines, homeopathy, herbal remedies, and mind-body healing techniques.

The Holistic Pediatrician is a practical manual meant to be used on a regular basis by parents. In the chapter on cough, for example, the first issue that Dr. Kemper addresses is the warning signs that show something serious is going on, requiring urgent medical attention. She then presents a thorough discussion of the common causes of cough, including how parents can prevent and treat coughs. She begins with the typical conventional medical approach to the diagnosis and treatment of a cough in a manner that any parent can understand and learn from.

She then looks at the symptom of cough-ing from a completely holistic point of view. She brilliantly blends together a rich variety of medical traditions, including medicine, vitamin therapies, nutrition, homeopathy, and mind-body integration techniques. In one chapter, a parent can learn how antibiotics can help to treat bronchitis as well as how to unlock the healing power of the mind as a useful adjunct to conventional treatments. Dr. Kemper presents proved folk and herbal remedies for coughs that are often safer and more effective than conventional medications. Every parent who has stayed up all night with a coughing child needs to read this chapter.

Dr. Kemper skillfully blends the best of Western medicine, Chinese medicine, and alternative therapies in creating a holistic approach to your child's health. The book is unique and invaluable, since too often these medical traditions portray themselves as being incompatible with each other. Conventional doctors often accuse naturopathic or homeopathic physicians of being frauds, pushing worthless remedies to gullible patients who, if they improve, only do so because they believe in the otherwise worthless cure. Alternative physicians conversely portray conventional physicians as narrow-minded and arrogant, caring only about the treatment of superficial symptoms. Medical consumers often feel caught in the middle, having to choose either antibiotics and vaccinations or good nutrition, visualization and massage. This is because competing physicians too commonly focus on one medical strategy to the exclusion of others. Only the patient is the loser in such medical turf battles.

Thomas Edison predicted that one day physicians would not prescribe medicines but would be interested primarily in diet and the cause and prevention of disease. Yet from the most ancient times, healers have used medicines and surgery to treat specific problems. The great Greek physician Hippocrates was one of the first to recognize that we need to incorporate both strategies in treating patients. Modern medicine seems to have forgotten that wise physicians of all medical traditions have understood the dual role of the healer as nurturing the spirit as well as treating specific symptoms.

The split between Western medicine and alternative therapies represents these two theoretically complementary approaches to good health. Conventional physicians focus heavily on the use of specific medications and surgeries for specific problems. For example, one third of a typical pediatrician's day is spent treating ear infections. Conversely, alternative therapies focus on issues of spiritual health, nutrition, and allergies, using treatment modalities such as natural herbs and massage. Visits to alternative physicians and healers are longer and involve more talking, listening, and education than the typical physician visit.

To a great measure, the amazing successes of modern medicine have led to unrealistic expectations of what it can accomplish. Vaccines, antibiotics, and modern surgical techniques have led to virtual disappearance of once commonplace occurrences such as polio, meningitis, and hearing loss from recurrent ear infections. Medical success stories include organ transplants, heart valve replacements, and greatly improved maternal and infant survival rates after delivery. These extraordinary successes have caused alternative therapies to seem ineffective in comparison.

Yet, as Dr. Kemper points out, many problems that affect children must be addressed from a holistic point of view. Allergies, recurrent ear infections, attention deficit disorder, or serious chronic diseases often respond best to many different medical strategies. Dr. Kemper defines holistic medicine as "addressing the well-being and optimal functioning of the child in the context of family, culture, and community. Holistic practitioners see the whole child — body, mind, emotions, spirit, and relationship with others."

It would seem simple common sense to take the best of different medical traditions in planning our children's health. A child who has pneumonia or an ear infection needs antibiotics. A child with appendicitis or a hernia needs a surgeon. Children with chronic abdominal pain or irritable bowel syndrome might see an herbalist or a Chinese medical doctor. Those with chronic pain could perhaps see an acupuncturist. General Practitioners such as myself should be well versed in nutrition, exercise, massage therapy, folk and home remedies, and herbal treatments as part of providing the best medical care. Dr. Kemper's book provides the information parents need in designing a holistic medical program for their child. In reading this book, we learn what different therapies have to offer, as well as how to choose a practitioner.

It is important to recognize that the medical traditions Dr. Kemper draws from have impressive pedigrees and have established success in treating illness and promoting health for hundreds of years or, in the case of Chinese medicine, thousands of years. It is only because of the bitter feud which started 150 years ago that we see such an irrational division between conventional and alternative medicine today. At that time, conventional doctors had little to offer except bloodletting, blistering the skin, and large doses of poisons such as mercury. Although Native Americans and some country women treated patients with herbs, no university-trained physicians at the time would have anything to do with them, and in those days doctors did, in fact, poison patients in an effort to cure them.

Most of today's so-called alternative therapies were born as a reaction to the treatments of conventional doctors. Homeopathy, for example, was founded by the German physician Samuel Hahnemann. He was one of the first to set up a system for purifying and testing the effects of drugs. He emphasized nutrition and exercise and pioneered modern concepts such as the use of specific remedies for specific diseases and vaccinations. By the mid–1800s, homeopathy dominated medicine with successes in the treatment of malaria, cholera, and yellow fever. So great was Hahnemann's fame that his statue in Washington, D.C., simply says Hahnemann to identify it.

Numerous other alternative medical therapies developed in the 1800s. Chiropractic medicine, osteopathy, and naturopathy developed during this time. An active popular health movement repealed all medical licensing laws, to allow, as they said, "every man to be his own doctor." Physicians started to pay attention and learn from country women and Native American healers who were skilled in the use of herbs. In fact, most of modern medications are based on the study of traditional herbal remedies.

Predictably enough, there ensued a long and bitter battle between the conventional physicians of the time and these alternative practitioners, especially the homeopaths. Rival medical schools were built, and fierce medical licensing battles were fought. By 1900, with the advent of new therapies, including the use of narcotics for pain control and anesthetic agents for surgery, conventional medicine had regained its preeminence. By 1950, with discoveries of antibi-

otics, vaccinations, vitamins, and life-giving hormones, medical technology seemed to have the answers to human problems. By 1970 the Surgeon General declared infectious diseases to be no longer an important problem. By 1980 heart transplant surgeon Denton Cooley said of efforts to prevent heart disease, "It [the prevention of heart disease] all sounds good, but from a practical standpoint it has not paid off." This resulted in today's climate in which few states even permit naturopaths to be licensed physicians.

Today, of course, mainstream medicine recognizes the value of vitamins, antioxidants, and diet in preventing heart disease and has acknowledged that heart transplants are in fact of limited use in extending the human life span. These therapies were promoted by naturopaths for decades and once dismissed as useless placebos. Other alternative medical therapies are becoming routine in the treatment of problems as diverse as AIDS and attention deficit disorder.

Dr. Kemper's book is a giant step toward the reunification of these competing medical systems. This book can be read at several levels, form a simple "how to" manual for late night emergencies to in-depth discussions of every important aspect of common childhood ailments. Her writing is clear and logical. Clinical problems are illustrated with excellent case histories, which provide invaluable psychological insights to corresponding medical conditions. Every parent will identify with at least one of the case histories presented. This book makes entire shelves of child health books obsolete. *The Holistic Pediatrician* is required reading for every parent who wants the best for his or her child's health.

Melvin L. Morse, M.D.
Associate Professor of Pediatrics
University of Washington

ACKNOWLEDGMENTS
AND THANKS

No great work is accomplished in isolation. This was never more apparent to me than in the preparation of this book. I am deeply grateful to many people who supported me during this process. Direct contributions which vastly improved the quality of this effort were made by:

The librarians who performed amazing feats in locating all of the references: Ellen Howard at Harborview Medical Center, Mike Scully, Bob Hollowell, and Chris Saraidaridis at Swedish Medical Center;

Research assistance, organizational and secretarial support: Katherine Dawson, Brenda Nissley, Nicolette Vajtay, Julie West, Ann Marchand and Yvonne Koshi;

The many parents and health care professionals who reviewed early drafts: Kari Kemper (who read every chapter and helped with all the Latin derivations), Ken Kemper (copy editor extraordinaire), Paula Bock, Peter Donovan, Ellen Kleiner, Ursula Martens, Diane Wade, Drs. Nancy Rudner (friend, nurse practitioner, public health advocate and mother), Howard Bauchner, Carol Berkowitz, Cora Breuner, Robin Cole, Ellen Crain, Nancy Danoff, Bob Davis, Mark Del Beccaro, Julie Francis, Frances Glascoe, Jane Gloor, Neal Halfon, David Heimbach, Robert Jacobson, Eileen Klein, Paula Lozano, Ed Marcuse, Tom Newman, Jack Pascoe, Lee Pachter, Fred Rivara, Michael Rothenberg, David Springer, Barbara Starfield, and Jim Taylor.

Dr. Melvin Morse—supporter and way-shower;

Dr. Barton Schmitt—a truly holistic, inspirational pediatrician;

Dr. Michael Tuggy and Dr. Dedra Buchwald for the illustrations;

Friends and colleagues: Dr. Dedra Buchwald, who discussed the title with her friends at the gym; Dr. Kathleen Hanlon, who believed in me and made me take days off; Roxanne Springwater, ARNP, who remembered me and my dogs; Toni Weschler, MPH — always 9 months ahead in the writing process;

All of the general pediatricians at the University of Washington who helped me stretch my wings, especially Drs. Al Novack and Abe Bergman;

Dr. Joe Scardapane and the Family Medicine faculty and residents at Swedish Medical Center in Seattle, who gave me time, space, and office equipment, and who served as guinea pigs for the early drafts.

Editors: Diane Reverend who suggested adding the stories; Janet Goldstein who came up with the title; Betsy Thorpe who supported and encouraged me in the nitty gritty editing and paring down; and Meaghan Dowling who picked it up in the middle and carried it through to the end.

My friends and family in the Seattle Course in Miracles whose love and support sustained me through everything.

INTRODUCTION

"We heard you were open to holistic medicine, and we wanted you to see our daughter, Shelly," Lisa and Larry Bradshaw began. "She's had asthma since she was 9 months old, and she just isn't getting over it. We don't like the idea of giving her drugs every day, but we don't want her to be sick either. We've treated our own health problems with Chinese herbs and homeopathic remedies, but we aren't sure what's safe for a 2-year-old like Shelly. Can you help?"

Lisa and Larry are typical of the growing number of parents who have sought and used alternative therapies for themselves and who want to provide the safest, most effective care for their children. Although there has been a veritable explosion in the number of books on holistic medicine, few are aimed at children's health issues. Several that do focus on children are limited to a particular therapy such as herbs, homeopathy, or acupuncture. None integrates the best of modern medical science with proven therapies from herbal medicine, homeopathy, and other healing techniques in a truly holistic approach to common childhood illnesses. However, most parents want to know about ALL their options, not just one or two approaches.

This book was written to educate and empower you to exercise your options in taking care of your child's health care needs. Despite all the recent talk about health care reform and managed care, the fact is that parents are the primary providers of their children's health care. Parents manage their children's home environment, diet, and medical care. Mothers characteristically cope with most minor illnesses using home or folk remedies, and ask for advice from relatives and friends before seeking help from a health care professional. Parents are generally very competent in caring for their children's illnesses. Parents today are well-educated consumers of a variety of goods and services. Although formal medical education can be long and arduous, most parents can easily learn enough to be excellent consumers of pediatric health care. In my practice, I see parents as the primary providers of health care and myself as their coach.

Who needs another book on holistic medicine? Parents do! A 1993 study in the *New England Journal of Medicine* reported that nearly one out of every three American adults used alternative medical therapies in 1990.[1] Many parents also seek alternative care for their children.[2] When given an option between a non-drug home remedy and a drug, nearly 85% of parents prefer the home remedy.[3] Parents most likely to seek alternative care are those whose children suffer from a serious, chronic disease such as rheumatoid arthritis, and those for whom traditional medical care has not been of much help, such as children suffering from recurrent ear infections or allergies.[4] Parents want the best for their children—safe, effective, personal care which is low in cost and side effects. Most parents who seek holistic care are intelligent and well-educated, and most take their children to regular medical doctors in addition to other types of health care providers.

What is holistic medicine? Holistic medicine has as many definitions as there are people. At times it seems that the term is used more as a marketing tool than as a description of a distinct approach to health care. Here's my definition:

Holistic medicine addresses the well-being and optimal functioning of the child in the context of family, culture, and community. Holistic practitioners see the whole child — body, mind, emotions, spirit, and relationships with others. From a variety of potential treatments, holistic practitioners choose those that are best suited to the individual child and family.

One of the most holistic doctors I've ever met is Dr. David Heimbach, a burn surgeon at Harborview Medical Center in Seattle. You might wonder if a surgeon could really be holistic. Dr. Heimbach has assembled a team of surgeons, nurses, physical and occupational therapists, pediatricians, nutritionists, social workers, and psychologists to help meet the needs of children who have suffered severe burns. When he takes care of a burned child, he looks not only at the burn, but at the whole child and the child's family. He makes sure that the out-of-state families have a place to stay in Seattle while their child is being treated, and has implemented a fund to help pay for their housing. He asks about the child's school, friends, and church. On one occasion, he even made arrangements for a seriously burned child to be visited in the hospital by his puppy. (Yes, hygiene was maintained, and the visit was a rousing success for both boy and puppy.) The psychologists on the team use hypnosis to help children cope with the pain of the initial burn and the subsequent surgeries. Nutritionists help ensure that children are not only getting enough calories, but also additional vitamins and minerals to hasten healing. For children whose families are far away, Dr. Heimbach asks for volunteers from the community to play with, read to, and hold injured children. Yes, even surgeons in major academic medical centers can be holistic physicians.

On the other hand, practitioners who believe that all ailments can be traced to allergies, yeast infections, or vitamin deficiencies are no more holistic than those who believe that all illness is due to germs. These practitioners may call themselves holistic, but in fact, they are ideologues with good marketing skills. Not all unconventional therapies are holistic, nor is mainstream medical practice necessarily NOT holistic. A single therapy, be it medication, surgery, nutrition, supplements, herbs, exercise, or massage is not holistic unless it is done in the context of the whole child and the child's family, culture, and community.

I try to avoid the terms "alternative" and "unconventional" medicine, despite their widespread use, because they are very difficult to define. One's definition of "alternative" depends very much on what one considers mainstream. For many Americans, Chinese medicine is an alternative. But for Chinese-Americans, it is mainstream. Other so-called alternatives, such as chiropractic, are as American as apple pie. Hypnosis and acupuncture used to be considered unconventional, but they are now used in major medical centers across America. Rather than try to define mainstream, alternative, and unconventional medicine, we'll look at the therapies themselves [Chapter 1] and how they can complement each other.

Illness versus disease. Disease is an abnormal condition in the body. Illness is one's *experience* of abnormal or sub-optimal functioning. You can have a disease such as cancer for weeks or months before symptoms develop and you feel ill. In general we cure disease and heal illness.

Healing versus curing. In this book, curing means the elimination of symptoms or signs of a disease. For example, a child is cured of pneumonia when the fever and the cough are gone, and signs of infection are gone from the X ray. There are no cures yet for many illnesses which affect children. The symptoms of cystic fibrosis may be minimized, but the underlying disease will not be eradicated until we come up with genetic therapies. Yet, even children with chronic or genetic diseases such as cystic fibrosis can be considered healed if they feel happy, loved, and function as well as they'd like. Being healed is

an emotional/mental/spiritual state. Being cured is a physical phenomenon. We can compare the cure rates of different therapies, but we cannot accurately measure healing. When I describe the effectiveness of different therapies, I am talking about the effectiveness of those therapies in curing, not healing.

ABOUT THE AUTHOR

I am a pediatrician, a medical doctor specializing in the care of children. My medical training has spanned many years at several institutions — the University of North Carolina (MD degree and Masters Degree in Public Health, specializing in maternal and child health), the University of Wisconsin (internship and residency in pediatrics), and Yale University (fellowship training in pediatric research). In 1988, I joined the faculty of the University of Washington, where I taught medical students and pediatric residents how to be good pediatricians. In 1994 I joined the staff of Swedish Medical Center in Seattle, helping to train family doctors in pediatrics. I have had over 30 scientific articles and chapters published in medical journals such as the *New England Journal of Medicine* and the *Journal of the American Medical Association.* On one hand, my research has pointed out the costs and hazards of unnecessary medical treatment; on the other hand, I have tried to increase physicians' awareness of the psychological and social factors in a family which affect children's health. Throughout my training, I have learned and been stimulated to do research the most by my patients and their families.

Even before starting my formal medical education, I became interested in holistic medicine. My undergraduate work in Psychology at the University of Chicago included a research project examining the relationship between psychological stress and insulin doses in diabetics. During medical school I was able to take extra training in hypnosis, biofeedback, and nutrition. My residency program allowed me to study medical acupuncture with Dr. Joseph Helms through the UCLA Extension Course. I have also enjoyed the opportunity to study Therapeutic Touch with its founders, Dr. Dolores Krieger and Ms. Dora Kunz. My colleagues in the American Holistic Medical Association have continued to keep me informed about nutritional advances, homeopathy, and exercise. To all of these teachers and mentors, I am thankful.

The book is organized for you to read selectively. You do not need to read it from cover to cover. I suggest that you read the first and second chapters, and then skip to the chapters that are pertinent for your child. By reading the first chapter first, you will be better able to understand all of the rest of the chapters. Chapter 1, "The Therapeutic Mountain," describes a new paradigm for understanding the relationship between different types of therapies, describes the therapies, the professionals who recommend them, and how to select a practitioner for your child. Chapter 2, "Trust Me, I'm a Doctor," describes how you can evaluate claims that different treatments are effective for your child. Appendix A describes additional resources for parents interested in more information about particular therapies or practitioners. Appendix B provides detailed descriptions of how to prepare and give different remedies to your child.

Note on organization: To maintain a consistent, systematic, comprehensive approach, all of the chapters on a particular illness and condition are organized the same way, outlined in Chapter One. If you want a quick summary of how I approach a particular condition, flip to the end of the chapter, "What I Recommend."

Note on gender: To avoid using cumbersome phrases such as he/she and him/her, I have alternated males and females throughout the book. All of the case stories are composite descriptions; to preserve confidentiality, fictitious names, gender, and ethnicity are used.

1

THE THERAPEUTIC
MOUNTAIN

*"I've taken my child to so many doctors, I've lost count," Helen began. "The
pediatrician put him on antibiotics for his ear infections, but the medicines
gave him diarrhea and a yeast infection. The chiropractor said that adjusting
his neck would help, but I didn't like him getting so many X rays. The natur-
opath recommended some herbs and vitamins, but my insurance wouldn't
pay for them. None of these doctors thought the other ones did any good;
they all seemed more interested in promoting their own particular therapy
than in working with each other to help my child. I'm frustrated and confused. How can the best, the safest and most effective of all available treatments be combined for my child's well-being?"*

Helen's story epitomizes many families'
complaints about the health care system.
Different kinds of practitioners have different
theories, rely on different treatments, and
often compete rather than cooperate with one
another. It doesn't have to be this way. Rather
than being therapy-centered, polarized, and
competitive, healing can be child-centered,
integrated, cooperative, and holistic.

The bedrock underlying all true healing
activities is compassion for the patient.
Whether the health care provider is a physician, nurse, acupuncturist, herbalist, or parent, concern for the patient's well-being is the
first prerequisite for healing. Ideally, both
professionals and parents lay aside their concerns about themselves when faced with an
ill child. The focus should be on relieving the
child's pain and fear and restoring a sense of
well-being rather than on the particular therapy used to achieve that goal.

The truth of this fundamental belief about
healing was brought home to me recently
during a conversation with my favorite mas-

sage therapist, Masaji. Masaji is an unassuming yet remarkable Japanese man who practices *shiatsu*, the ancient Japanese therapy that combines acupuncture theory with advanced techniques of massage. When the Prime Minister of Japan was in town for an economic summit, he called on Masaji to provide relief from the stresses of international meetings. Many of Masaji's clients are, like me, regular medical doctors who also teach at university hospitals.

While Masaji kneaded the tiny muscles of my feet, we talked about the nature of healing and the differences between Eastern and Western approaches. He described the Eastern philosophy of healing as the attempt to restore harmony and balance to the entire system. The Western approach looks at the chain of cause and effect, trying to fight or change the underlying cause in order to relieve the symptoms or effects. The Eastern approach draws on the right-brain functions of seeing patterns, looking at the global picture, relying on intuition and a sense of subtle energies and interactions. The Western approach relies more on left-brain, logical, linear, reductionist thinking. Masaji spoke with admiration about the power of Western medicine to cure serious infections, overwhelming burns and trauma, and many kinds of cancer. Yet I pointed out that many local physicians who achieve these impressive cures seek his services to address their own symptoms related to stress, the meeting place of the mind and body.

Most Western physicians are hardpressed to explain how acupuncture and other Eastern therapies actually work. Being pragmatists, many of us agree that such techniques effectively treat problems ranging from pain to addictions to morning sickness. We didn't know how aspirin worked for the first one hundred years that we used it, but that didn't keep us from relying on it for treating fever and pain. Although American medical schools don't yet train physicians in Eastern healing, more and more physicians refer patients for acupuncture therapy.

As we talked, Masaji and I realized that Eastern and Western medicine are two sides of the one coin of healing. Just as the right and left sides of the brain are both necessary for optimal functioning, the two kinds of healing complement and enhance one another. Despite vast differences in philosophy and history, both have important roles to play in addressing humanity's ills.

In addition to the traditional models of Eastern and Western medicine, there are many other healing traditions. Massage, herbal medicine, ritual, and prayer have been used around the world since ancient times. Chiropractic and osteopathy are nineteenth-century American inventions. The use of vitamins and nutritional supplements to prevent and cure illness is largely a twentieth-century phenomenon. Regardless of their historical origins, all of these techniques share the primary goal of healing.

I have spent many years thinking about the different kinds of healing techniques, appalled at the gulf that frequently exists between different practitioners. I wanted to find a way to bridge the gap between those with different backgrounds, to put the patient back in the center of the picture, and to create a paradigm or model in which all therapies could be seen as related and complementary to one another, on common ground in pursuit of the highest and best for their patients. The image that emerged is the Therapeutic Mountain.

The mountain is an archetypal symbol of a high goal, achieved with dedication, preparation, persistence, and hard work. Such is the nature of healing. The goal is the well-being of the patient. Regardless of background, the professional therapist must be

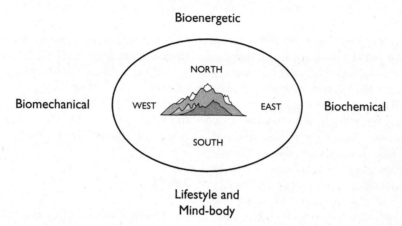

Therapeutic Mountain

Bioenergetic

Biomechanical

NORTH

WEST   EAST

SOUTH

Biochemical

Lifestyle and
Mind-body

dedicated to this goal, undergo years of training, and continue to learn from and listen to each patient, refining and enhancing his or her skills.

There are many sides to a mountain and many ways to reach the top. For the sake of simplicity, we will picture all of the primary healing modalities as occurring on one of four sides of the Therapeutic Mountain.

THERAPEUTIC MOUNTAIN

1. East Side: Biochemical Therapies

2. South Side: Lifestyle and Mind-Body Therapies

3. West Side: Biomechanical Therapies

4. North Side: Bioenergetic Therapies

Therapies on each side of the mountain are grouped together because of their functional, not their historical or philosophical similarities. Let's look at each side of the Therapeutic Mountain in more detail.

EAST SIDE OF THE THERAPEUTIC MOUNTAIN: BIOCHEMICAL THERAPIES

All of the therapies on the east side of the Therapeutic Mountain share a common mechanism of action: biochemistry. The three primary techniques of this side of the mountain are:

- Medications
- Herbs
- Nutritional Supplements

Each molecule of a therapeutic compound—whether it is a medication, an herb, or a vitamin—interacts with tiny molecules far smaller than even a single cell.

Medications

When most of us think of medical therapy, the first thing that comes to mind is taking medication. Today, most medicines are chemically synthesized, but originally many were derived from plants (herbs).

Amoxicillin is a good example. The most

common medicine used to treat children with ear infections, amoxicillin is a modern version of penicillin. In 1928, a Scottish microbiologist, Alexander Fleming, noticed that a blue *Penicillium* mold growing on his laboratory cultures was killing the bacteria. Just as he was about to throw the ruined cultures away, he realized that the mold's deadly effect on the bacteria might have therapeutic importance. He was right. Penicillin, derived from the *Penicillium* mold, has saved millions of lives. Synthesizing medications such as penicillin and amoxicillin ensures their purity and strength, and children can take a simple pill, syrup or injection to get well rather than ingesting the mold from which it was derived.

Medications are lifesaving when it comes to acute, severe illnesses such as shock, meningitis, and septicemia. They are also highly effective in managing certain chronic illnesses such as diabetes, in reducing pain, and in curing previously fatal diseases such as childhood leukemia. However, medications are practically useless in curing many common childhood illnesses such as colds. Even used properly, medications have side effects. Penicillin and amoxicillin commonly cause stomach aches, diarrhea, and diaper rashes; for 1 in 10,000 children they cause a severe, life-threatening allergic reaction.

Prescription medications are powerful, often dangerous, and are therefore highly regulated. Though many medications can be purchased by parents over the counter, prescription medication is available only with a physician's order. M.D.'s (Doctors of Medicine), D.O.'s (Doctors of Osteopathy), and dentists are fully licensed to prescribe medications. Nurse-Practitioners have Master's Degrees, and they are licensed to prescribe many common medications. Physician's Assistants (P.A.'s) prescribe only under a physician's supervision. Only a handful of states license Naturopathic Doctors (N.D.'s);

most allow naturopaths to prescribe from a list of certain antibiotics but do not allow them to prescribe other kinds of medication. Other health care providers are not licensed to prescribe regulated medications.

Always ask about the risks, benefits, side effects, and alternatives to prescription medications. Many pharmacies carry drug information sheets that describe specific medications and their effects in detail.

Herbs

Herbal, botanical, or phyto-therapy* medicines have been used around the world since ancient times to prevent and cure disease. Herbal medicines contain a complex mixture of chemical ingredients. Some people feel Nature combined the ingredients in plants for good reason, more wisely than a chemist distilling out a single active ingredient. For many herbal remedies, the active ingredient has not yet been identified, extracted, or synthesized in a laboratory. For example, chamomile tea (prescribed by Peter Rabbit's mother) is used around the world to soothe distressed babies and children. Its therapeutic effect does not depend on a single ingredient but on a complex mixture of chemicals, which has not been duplicated in any lab.

Regardless of whether you take the chemically isolated active ingredient (medication) or an herbal compound, herbs and medicines work basically the same way, biochemically. Medication is more highly purified, and herbs contain more of the original natural ingredients, but their effectiveness is based on the same chemical principles.

Herbs tend to be both more subtle and

Phyto means plant.

more variable in their effects than medications. Because herbs are natural products, their potency and purity vary. Mercury and lead contaminate some imported herbal remedies. Even commonly used natural products such as chamomile and tea tree oil trigger allergic reactions in some people.[1,2] Many herbs are toxic if used improperly. Adult-sized doses of the Chinese herbal medicine *Jin Bu Huan* led to the near-fatal poisoning of three children in 1993. Currently, herbal products are not regulated by the Food and Drug Administration the same way medications are, so standardization and quality control are variable. This doesn't matter very much if you're treating a stomach ache with peppermint tea, but it could cause problems if you are using more potent herbs or use adult-sized doses for a child. *You cannot assume that a product is safe simply because it is natural.*

Family members, friends, folk healers, shamans, medicine men, chiropractors, naturopaths, Ayurvedic physicians, practitioners of traditional Chinese medicine, and even some medical doctors recommend herbal remedies. No special degree is required to prescribe or advise about herbs. Herbs are not a panacea, however. Beware of anyone who claims that herbs can cure everything that ails your child. That is no more holistic than claiming that medications cure everything.

Nutritional Supplements

Vitamins and minerals are essential for maintaining health. A deficiency of any of the essential vitamins or minerals causes illness. Vitamin C deficiency plagued early long distance sailors with scurvy. British sailors recognized and effectively prevented scurvy by bringing along a supply of vitamin C–rich limes—hence their nickname Limeys.

Normally the body's needs for vitamins and minerals can be met adequately with a healthy diet emphasizing fruits, vegetables, and whole grains.

Nutritional supplements, including foods such as garlic extracts, are also recommended as treatments for a variety of ailments. Vitamin C can reduce the duration of common cold symptoms. Extra vitamins A, D, E, and K are required by children with the genetic disease cystic fibrosis. Children who require daily seizure medicine may also need nutritional supplements to counteract some of the medication's effects. Toddlers who drink more than three or four glasses of cow's milk a day often need extra iron. Supplements may also be useful for children who do not eat a balanced, healthy diet such as teenagers who avoid vitamin A–rich vegetables.

It's almost impossible to overdose on vitamin-rich foods. However, as with medicine, vitamins and minerals can have dangerous side effects. Although vitamin A is important for normal vision, too much can cause problems in the brain, liver, bones, and skin. Excessive vitamin C causes diarrhea. Iron overdoses can be fatal. Garlic poultices cause burnlike irritations if left on delicate skin too long. Nature designed us to be in balance. When we take super-high doses of any one substance, we run the risk of upsetting the balance. Some vitamins can also trigger allergic reactions. The vitamin E cream in some cosmetics actually *causes* a skin rash in some sensitive folks.[3]

As with herbal remedies, no particular license is required to recommend nutritional supplements, and there are a lot of deceptive claims (pro and con) about the need for supplements. Unfortunately, there is little standardization in nutrition education and far too little research on optimal use of supplements in children. Medical doctors and osteopaths receive more training than in the past, but most rely on trained nutritionists or dietitians to help children who have complex nutritional needs. Naturopaths and chiropractors also receive nutrition education, but it may not be specifically geared to children's needs. Be sure to ask your health care practitioner about his or her training in pediatric nutrition because it is a specialized field.

SOUTH SIDE OF THE THERAPEUTIC MOUNTAIN: LIFESTYLE AND MIND-BODY THERAPIES

All of the therapies on the south side of the Therapeutic Mountain have such common-sense benefits that we sometimes forget how potent they are. The techniques of this side of the mountain are integral to healing traditions worldwide. They are:

- Nutrition
- Exercise
- Environment
- Mind-Body

All of these factors are primarily regulated by the child and family with occasional professional advice. Nutrition, exercise, environment, and mind-body interactions are a part of daily life. As components of lifestyle, they are under our control but paradoxically take more effort to change than using a biochemical therapy such as medications, herbs, or vitamins. For example, it's harder to transform a fast-food diet into a healthy whole foods regimen than to take vitamins. It's more challenging to develop and maintain an exercise program than to take high-blood-pressure medicine or diet pills. Despite the challenges involved in changing lifestyle and habits, parents who

are interested in their child's life-long health make the effort to learn about and use these therapies.

Nutrition

"You are what you eat." Proper nutrition is the backbone of a healthy lifestyle. Children's nutritional needs change as they develop. Newborn babies need mothers' milk, not fruits and vegetables. Young children increase their food vocabulary one food at a time and gradually adopt their families' eating habits. By the time children reach adolescence, the nutritional patterns for a lifetime have been established.

Nutritional therapy is especially important for children suffering from chronic conditions (such as cystic fibrosis and cancer) and for children recovering from major trauma (such as injuries and burns). For everyday problems (such as constipation), you can easily treat your child with extra servings of fruit and bran muffins. Children with special health care needs or suspected food allergies need the help of a trained nutritionist.

Anyone, regardless of training, can offer nutritional advice. Be a smart consumer of nutritional advice. When someone recommends a particular diet (macrobiotic, low fat, etc.), ask about the data showing that it has proved helpful in a child like yours. Children can grow perfectly well on vegetarian diets, but I have seen several young children who were growing and developing poorly because their parents had been erroneously advised to put them on a low-fat diet before they'd completed their infant growth spurt. (See Chapter 2 for more advice on evaluating health claims.) Check your sources before making radical changes in your child's diet. *What is helpful for adults may not be helpful for children.*

You can help your child heal and prevent future problems by modifying your own lifestyle. Avoiding cigarette smoke is a crucial element of therapy for childhood asthma, allergies, colds, and ear infections. Parental smoking, excessive drinking, and drug use have obvious adverse effects. These habits almost always start during adolescence and are often learned from the child's primary role models—parents. Save your child the later struggle of overcoming an addiction by quitting these habits yourself NOW.

Exercise

A proper balance of exercise and rest is basic to maintaining health and is an important element of healing when we become ill. Exercise releases the body's own antidepressants and painkillers. Exercise improves circulation, lung function, and brain functioning. Whether it is organized soccer or a backyard game, exercise is good for children. Other habits, such as excessive time in front of the television, promote a sedentary lifestyle and compete with more active pursuits. Developing a routine of regular physical activity during childhood is an antidote to the national epidemic of "couch potatoitis."

Exercise therapy includes everything from strengthening muscles and joints after an injury to yoga breathing exercises to help with asthma. Exercise can help children deal with stress, lift layers of depression, and build self-esteem. Outside the specialized area of sports medicine, training in exercise therapy for children is limited. A therapeutic exercise program should be tailor-made for each individual child.

Most children suffering from a short-term illness such as a cold, flu, ear infection, or diarrhea will rest more and exercise less. Rest is as important as exercise in allowing the

body's energy to be redirected to healing. Do not push your child to romp and play when he's acutely ill.

Environment

Children are extraordinarily sensitive to their physical and emotional environments. Unhealthy environments, burdened with pollution, noise, and violence, are leading causes of illness in children. When trying to help heal a child, paying attention to the environment pays off. Environmental activism is simply health care on a larger scale. Specific examples of environmental therapies for children are:

- Air filters to remove airborne allergens
- Tepid baths to reduce the itching of chicken pox or eczema
- Phototherapy (special waves of sunlight) to reduce newborn jaundice
- White noise to soothe a colicky baby
- Ice packs to minimize swelling of a sprained ankle
- Mist tents for croup

Never underestimate the therapeutic value of the smell of home cooking or the presence of the child's favorite blanket or stuffed animal! As with herbal and nutritional therapies, no formal degrees or licenses are required to make recommendations about environmental therapy. Much of the wisdom about environmental therapies is simply based on experience or common sense. However, more research is being done in this area all the time. A recent study in an intensive care unit indicates that aromatherapy, using oil of lavender, improves the mood and decreases the anxiety of seriously ill adults.[4]

Mind-Body

Mind-body therapies encompass a range of techniques from behavior management to self-hypnosis and professional psychological counseling. Perhaps the most well-known technique for relaxing the mind is the Relaxation Response, described by the Harvard physician Dr. Herbert Benson. Around the world, the Relaxation Response and other meditative techniques are used to calm the mind and emotions of patients with high blood pressure, cancer, and other chronic illnesses.

Even infants learn to calm themselves, primarily by sucking on their hands or a pacifier. Older children can learn more complex techniques to calm themselves. Relaxation therapies have beneficial effects on conditions ranging from asthma to chronic diarrhea. They can also improve concentration for tests and sports.

Despite its popular image as a stage technique to get hapless victims to embarrass themselves, *hypnosis* is a safe, effective therapy used with thousands of children. It has been endorsed by the American Psychiatric Association, the American Psychological Association, and the American Dental Association. It is widely used by pediatricians, pediatric psychologists, and behavioral therapists to assist children confronted by pain, chronic headaches, and behavioral problems such as bedwetting. Hypnosis is simply a state of focused, concentrated attention. Lamaze breathing to reduce the pain of childbirth is one type of hypnosis. Parents and children can learn to use hypnotic techniques to improve health and to manage the discomfort of medical procedures such as injections and sutures. These techniques can be as simple as focusing on breathing, becoming absorbed in a story or fantasy, or counting sheep. (See Appendix A for more resources on hypnosis.)

Remember mood rings? By turning a deep blue when your hands were relaxed and warm, they gave you *biofeedback* that blood flow was increased to your fingers. Every moment, children regulate temperature, heart rate, breathing, muscle tone, and millions of other functions that are not part of conscious awareness. If they receive help in focusing on one of these processes and get feedback about it, they can begin consciously to regulate that function. For example, children can learn to increase and decrease the temperature in their fingers if they are given feedback by a machine in the form of sound or lights. This technique can be very helpful in reducing the frequency and severity of migraine headaches. Biofeedback is also helpful in severe, chronic constipation in which bowel function has been abnormal for so long that the child needs to learn again how to sense and respond to the body's signals.

Biofeedback is generally practiced by psychologists, but formal training and licensure are not required. Before taking your child to a therapist for biofeedback, ask for and check references to other parents whose children were treated. (See Appendix A for more sources of information on biofeedback.) Also ask about fees and how much of the cost your insurance might be expected to cover.

Meditative practices such as focusing on the breath or a word can result in profound states of relaxation. Relaxation is helpful in just about any kind of healing endeavor. Studies in adults have shown that meditation can help lower blood pressure and reduce ulcer symptoms. There have been fewer studies in children. There are no particular licensure requirements for teaching meditation techniques. Almost every town has one or more centers that teach meditation. Choose whatever kind fits with your personal beliefs and is convenient.

Many types of therapists provide *counseling* and *psychotherapy* to parents and their children. Treatment by counselors, support groups, behavioral therapists, psychologists, and psychiatrists can be helpful in addressing the thoughts and emotions that affect children's health. Like adults, children experience stress and negative emotions that challenge their health. Children whose parents are going through a divorce, for example, are prone to behavior problems, school problems, sleep problems, stomach aches, and headaches. Children who suffer from chronic illnesses such as cancer or asthma or who depend on wheelchairs to get around can benefit from support groups of similarly affected peers. Such groups offer kids the opportunity to share strategies for managing their common problems. (See Appendix A for more information on national parent support groups.)

If you seek professional assistance because of a serious behavioral or psychological problem, please ask about the therapist's training in pediatrics and family issues; ask for and check references.

WEST SIDE OF THE THERAPEUTIC MOUNTAIN: BIOMECHANICAL THERAPIES

All of the therapies on the west side of the Therapeutic Mountain are biomechanical in nature. Whereas the therapies on the east side work biochemically, the therapies on the west side affect larger tissues and organs by stimulating, realigning, moving, or removing them. The three primary techniques on this side of the mountain are:

- Massage and Physical Therapy
- Spinal Manipulation (Chiropractic and Osteopathic adjustments)
- Surgery

Massage and Physical Therapy

Massage is an ancient healing technique. Parents practice informal massage when they encourage burps by rubbing or patting babies' backs. Formal massage techniques range from Swedish massage to Rolfing, deep tissue massage, and physical therapy to rehabilitate muscles and joints after an injury. The various massage techniques all contribute to relaxation and well-being by stimulating blood flow, calming nervous impulses, and stretching and relaxing the tendons and ligaments that hold the bones and joints together. Massaging one part of the body can help draw attention away from another painful part of the body, reducing discomfort. The close personal interaction during massage also enhances the bond between parents and children.

Many massage therapists use oils to help reduce friction between the therapist's hands and the patient's body. Oil lubricates the skin and makes massage more comfortable. By adding aromatic oils to the base oil (usually some sort of vegetable oil), the massage can have even more benefit. In my family, our parents massaged Vicks Vaporub or Mentholatum into our necks and chests when we had colds. The camphor and eucalyptus oil helped unclog our noses while the massage itself comforted and reassured us that we were loved and cared for, no matter how miserable we felt. Professional massage therapists must be licensed, but licensing requirements vary by state.

Physical therapists do massage as well as exercise and other therapies to help strengthen, relax, and heal muscles, tendons, and connective tissues.

Spinal Manipulation

Chiropractic therapy was invented by an Iowa grocer, Daniel Palmer, in 1895. Palmer believed that all human ailments were due to misalignment (subluxation) of the spine and that therefore all ailments could be cured by manually realigning the spine. Today there are two main types of chiropractors—those who still believe that manipulating the spine can cure all ills and those who make more limited claims and also recommend nutrition and exercise therapies as well as spinal manipulation. Chiropractic treatment is used by about 10% of American adults and 5% of children.

Scientific studies have documented the effectiveness of chiropractic treatment in helping adults with back and neck pain. However, studies of the effectiveness of chiropractic manipulation in treating children are practically nonexistent. Children rarely experience back pain; when they do, serious diseases such as spinal infections and cancer must be considered. Reliance on repeated X rays to document spinal changes puts children at risk from exposure to excessive radiation.

Chiropractors are licensed to practice in all fifty states. Most insurance covers chiropractic treatments. Chiropractors are not specially trained to recognize or treat serious childhood illnesses, and they are not licensed to prescribe medications or to perform surgery. They may be very helpful if your child has a wrenched back or stiff neck, but be wary about claims to cure serious problems such as diabetes or infections.

Osteopathic manipulation was invented by the American Dr. Andrew Taylor Still in the late 1800s. Still believed that manipulating the spine and other joints would improve the circulation and lead to more balanced functioning of the nervous system. Although Still rejected the use of all drugs (including homeopathic remedies), his descendants have adopted a more holistic approach. Some osteopaths do not perform spinal or joint manipulation, while others have expanded the scope of therapy to include manipulation of the cranium (head) and sacrum (pelvis). No scientific studies have been performed to evaluate the effectiveness of this type of treatment for children. Osteopathic physicians (D.O.'s—Doctors of Osteopathy) are licensed in all fifty states and have the same prescriptive and practice privileges as medical doctors (M.D.'s).

There are very few studies on the effectiveness of spinal manipulation in treating childhood ailments. Throughout this book, spinal manipulation is discussed only when there are claims that it is effective *and* research studies have evaluated those claims.

Surgery

Surgery has been practiced since ancient times. Lancing a boil is a surgical procedure as is repairing a hernia or removing an inflamed appendix. Surgeons set fractures, remove brain tumors, perform skin grafts, and deliver babies. Modern techniques have made surgery far safer than it was fifty years ago. Simple surgical procedures (such as the placement of ear tubes in children with recurrent ear infections) can be done on an outpatient basis. Surgeons undergo at least five years of training after completing medical (or osteopathic) school. Becoming board-certified in pediatric surgery requires at least two years of additional training. Before you agree to a nonemergency surgical procedure for your child, ask for a second opinion. Some insurance companies now require a second opinion anyway. Ask the surgeon about his or her credentials, alternatives to surgical treatment, and references to parents of children who have undergone the procedure recommended for your child.

NORTH SIDE OF THE THERAPEUTIC MOUNTAIN: BIOENERGETIC THERAPIES

All of the therapies on the fourth side of the Mountain are based on the principle of an invisible energy or spirit that animates, flows through, and surrounds the body. The aim of all of these techniques is to restore a harmonious balance of energy, which in turn improves the functioning of molecules, cells, tissues, and organs.

Some people think that the therapies on the fourth side of the Mountain are invalid because they are not based on the known laws of chemistry and physics that govern everyday life. Despite their enigmatic nature, these therapies do have demonstrated effectiveness in diverse circumstances. Acupuncture, for example, is effective in reducing pain in racehorses. Prayer effectively enhances plant growth. Homeopathy is effective in reducing diarrhea among infants too young to understand the power of suggestion. These therapies work—at least for some children, some of the time. We just don't know how they work or the best way to elicit their effects on a consistent basis. The four types of therapy on this side of the mountain are:

- Acupuncture
- Therapeutic Touch, Healing Touch, Laying On of Hands, Reiki, and Qi Gong
- Prayer and Ritual
- Homeopathy

Acupuncture

Acupuncture has been practiced in China for over 2,000 years. It is based on the theory that illness is caused by an imbalance in the body's flow of energy, called *Qi* or *Chi*. Treatment is aimed at restoring balance of the yin and yang (negative and positive aspects of *Qi*) along the twelve meridians or vessels that carry *Qi* throughout the body. In classical acupuncture, the points along the meridians are stimulated by needles or heat (moxibustion), but they can also be stimu-

lated with vigorous massage (*shiatsu*), tiny hammers, lasers, or electrical currents.

Like surgeons' knives, acupuncture needles actually penetrate the body. But unlike surgery, in which healing is effected through rearranging tissues, in acupuncture treatment the needles' purpose is to restore proper energy flow. Most of the scientific studies of acupuncture's effectiveness have been performed on adults. These studies indicate that acupuncture can be helpful in the treatment of surgical pain, morning sickness, and chronic allergies. Acupuncture treatment releases endorphins, the body's own painkilling chemicals.

Acupuncture treatment is complex. Proper training is extensive. The Chinese, Japanese, and Koreans all have somewhat different styles of acupuncture, but there are no studies suggesting substantial differences in their effects. Choose a therapist who has a title, L.Ac.(Licensed Acupuncturist) or Dipl.Ac. (Diplomate of Acupuncture from the National Commission for the Certification of Acupuncturists). If your child's physician practices acupuncture, ask whether he or she belongs to the American Academy of Medical Acupuncture. Traditional Chinese doctors carry the title O.M.D. (Oriental Medical Doctor), indicating additional training in herbal medicine. These initials do *not* indicate that the practitioner has any training as an M.D. Be sure that your acupuncture therapist uses disposable needles to reduce your child's risk of acquiring AIDS or hepatitis. Insurance reimbursement and licensing requirements for acupuncture therapy vary from state to state. For more information on acupuncture, see Appendix A.

Therapeutic Touch, Healing Touch, Laying On of Hands, Reiki, Qi Gong

The practice of healing by transmitting energy from the therapist's hands to the patient's body has been around since the beginning of time. The formal technique Therapeutic Touch was developed by Dr. Dolores Krieger, a professor at the New York University School of Nursing. This technique develops the intuitive senses, enabling practitioners to sense blockages in the energy flow in and around the patient and to help correct the energy flow. Therapeutic Touch is akin to massage, but its practitioners do not actually touch the body; rather, they work in the energy fields surrounding it. Laying on of hands, the Chinese technique known as *Qi Gong*, Reiki, and Healing Touch are all variations on this same theme. Therapeutic Touch has undergone scientific study and has proved useful in the treatment of pain, high blood pressure, anxiety, headache and wound healing in adults. Therapeutic Touch is practiced primarily by nurses. It has been taught and is practiced in over eighty countries around the world. Although formal training is available, certification and licensure are not required to practice Therapeutic Touch. Spend some time asking your prospective practitioner about his or her philosophy of healing, references, and experiences in working with children. Although I am particularly interested in and use Therapeutic Touch in my practice, there are very few research studies evaluating its effectiveness in children (so far); thus, it is not discussed in most of the chapters of this book. For more information on Therapeutic Touch and how to find a trained practitioner, see Appendix A.

Prayer and Ritual

Healing prayer seeks to direct the Unseen Power (God, Spirit, Great Absolute) toward healing the visible condition of the patient. Prayer forms an invisible connection between the patient and the Universal Energy or Spirit, thus restoring balance, wholeness, and health. Prayer and spiritual rituals are as old

as the human race. Effective prayer does not require formal training or licensure. One does not need to practice a particular religion. Prayer has proved effective for numerous conditions in numerous studies. Unfortunately, prayer does not *cure* in every case, but sincere prayer often brings a sense of peace and genuine *healing* to both the person praying and the patient.

There are several studies on the effectiveness of prayer in healing adults but very few studies in children. Thus, in this book, I do not discuss prayer in every chapter. By the time you read this book, many more studies (hopefully!) will be under way to evaluate the effectiveness of prayer in helping children with common ailments. Despite the current lack of scientific evidence, I recommend prayer as a therapy for all kinds of conditions in children whose family beliefs include this spiritual tradition.

Homeopathy

Homeopathy was founded by a German physicist and chemist, Samuel Hahnemann, at the end of the eighteenth century. This was an era when the other main type of medical practice (called allopathy by Hahnemann) had little to offer patients except bleeding, sweating, and purging. Given the allopathic alternatives at the time, homeopathy was definitely a safer treatment! In the intervening years, homeopathy has remained largely unchanged, whereas allopathic medicine has developed advanced diagnostic and surgical techniques, antibiotics, and effective treatments for cancer and other killer diseases. Although homeopathy is disparaged by most American physicians, it is widely used in India and Europe.

Homeopathy is based on two principles. The first principle is *like cures like*. Hahnemann said that a substance which produces symptoms in a healthy person cures those same symptoms in a sick person. For example, *belladonna* causes flushing, fever, and a rapid heart rate. Thus, it would be the remedy of choice for a child with a sudden onset of fever, flushing, and a fast heartbeat. The theory behind this principle is that the body will tend to react to the remedy, fighting the symptoms it provokes and thereby fighting the symptoms the body is experiencing. By paying careful attention to the whole range of the child's experience, the homeopathic practitioner matches the remedy that comes closest to causing those symptoms and therefore curing them. Homeopathic practitioners are very interested in the entire constellation of symptoms the child experiences; they ask a lot of questions and don't rely much on laboratory tests.

The second principle has to do with the bioenergetic or vibrational aspects of homeopathic remedies. It is *the more dilute the remedy, the more potent it is*. Homeopathic remedies are diluted anywhere from 1:10 to 1 in billions. The theory states that the 1:10 remedies are not as powerful as the 1:1,000,000 remedies. During each dilution, the compound is vigorously shaken or succussed, which is thought to further increase its potency. Of course, this principle violates our current concepts of chemistry and physics, which is why homeopathy is disparaged by most medical doctors. Nevertheless, scientific studies have demonstrated homeopathy's effectiveness in treating hay fever and childhood diarrhea.

Legally, homeopathy can only be practiced by health professionals who are licensed to prescribe medications. In most states this means that homeopathic practice is legally limited to M.D.'s, D.O.'s, dentists, nurse-practitioners, naturopaths, and chiropractors. Despite these legal regulations, many people without formal pediatric training prescribe homeopathic remedies, and remedies can be purchased through mail order catalogs and at many health food stores. Be aware that there is no uniformity in the training standards for homeopathic practice. Although the remedies themselves are probably safe, the danger is that an untrained practitioner may not recognize that your child is seriously ill and in need of other types of therapy. (See Appendix A for more information about homeopathy.)

The four sides of the Therapeutic Mountain cover the gamut of healing techniques. No one technique—no matter how organic or high tech, ancient or modern—is a panacea. Some problems are best treated with therapies from one side of the mountain and some respond better to others. The challenge for parents is to figure out what kind of therapy and practitioner will be most helpful for their child's problem. Although practitioners often draw upon an array of therapies, they are usually best trained in and most familiar with only a few.

PRACTITIONERS

Medical doctors (M.D.'s) and *osteopathic doctors* (D.O.'s) prescribe medicine, give advice about lifestyle, do counseling about child behavior, growth, development, nutrition, and safety and perform surgery. Osteopaths are also trained in performing spinal manipulation. With a few notable exceptions, most do not give advice about herbal medicine, meditation, or any of the bioenergetic therapies. However, more and more medical schools are offering courses on holistic medicine, and increasing numbers of practicing physicians are referring their patients to alternative and complementary practitioners.[5, 6, 7]

To become an M.D. or a D.O., physicians must complete a college degree, medical school, and one to five years of additional residency training. After completing years of training at approved institutions, a physician is eligible to take a grueling set of examinations to become board-certified. Pediatricians are required to recertify every seven years to ensure up-to-date knowledge and practice. If you want to be sure your doctor has met these standards of training, ask if he or she is board-certified in family medicine or pediatrics. If your child's physician practices a specialty (e.g., cardiology or allergy medicine), ask if he or she is board-certified in that specialty.

Most important, you need to be able to trust your child's physician. Get a recommendation from someone you trust, such as a co-worker, relative, or friend. Even if someone is highly trained and competent, you may not "click" or be on the same wavelength of values and style. Ask questions. Don't be afraid to let a physician know that you are interviewing a number of physicians to find the best one for your family. You probably spent at least a few weekends shopping for your last automobile; the choice of your child's physician is at least as important as your choice of cars. For more information on contacting a holistic physician, see Appendix A.

Naturopathy as a separate healing tradition was born in Germany in the early twentieth century, although its roots in the health spa movement go back considerably farther. Early naturopaths emphasized the importance of mineral baths, steam baths, and fasts. The founder of the modern movement, Benedict Lust, strongly believed in the body's own regenerative powers and decried the use of coffee, white flour, sugar, tobacco, and alcohol. Naturopathic physicians complete a four-year curriculum covering a wide range of therapies: herbal and homeopathic remedies, nutrition, exercise, environment, massage, and spinal manipulation. Not all naturopaths use all of these therapies. They reject the use of surgery and medications except as a last resort. Only eight states currently license naturopaths. (See Appendix A for more information.)

Traditional Chinese Medicine is one of the most ancient and holistic of all healing systems. The theory on which it is based—the flow and balance of *Qi* or energy in the body—is not intuitively obvious to most Westerners. Yet numerous studies have shown the effectiveness of Chinese herbs and acupuncture treatments. Other traditional Chinese therapies include diet, exercise (such as *Tai Chi*), meditation, massage, spinal manipulation, *Qi Gong* (transfer of healing energy from the practitioner to the patient), and bone setting.

Ayurvedic medicine is an ancient system of medicine from India that has been recently popularized by Dr. Deepak Chopra. The theory behind Ayurvedic medicine is similar to that of traditional Chinese medicine: balancing the flow of the body's life force or life energy—*prana* as it is known in the Ayurvedic tradition. Ayurvedic therapies include herbs, proper nutrition, meditation, environmental changes (aromatherapy and sound therapy), and massage.

PAYING FOR HOLISTIC HEALTH CARE

The systems for financing health care are changing rapidly. Many therapies are not covered by insurance, even with a medical doctor's prescription. This means you could end up paying "out of pocket" for these therapies. Be sure to talk with your child's health care provider about payment and insurance coverage right up front. Be sure to ask not only about professional fees but also about the cost and coverage for treatments and devices that the provider might recommend (such as vitamins, herbs, psychotherapy, or biofeedback devices). Check your insurance policy and call your agent about coverage for specific services or treatments before you start a course of therapy for your child. Get the agent's statement about coverage in writing in case there are any questions later.

GENERAL ADVICE

Practitioners work best when they know the complete story about your child. If you seek care from more than one practitioner, let everyone know what kind of care your child is receiving and from whom. Ask the different practitioners if they are willing to cooperate with each other and send each other copies of their records and recommendations. You can contact your state department of licensing regarding regulations for the various kinds of health professionals in your state. Ask questions. Ask for references. Doubt

claims about panaceas. If something sounds too good to be true, it probably is. How do you know what to believe? That's what Chapter 2 is all about.

ADDITIONAL READING

Alternative Therapies in Health and Medicine, a bimonthly journal published by InnoVision Communications
Alternative and Complementary Therapies, a bimonthly journal published by Mary Ann Liebert, Inc.
Complementary Therapies in Medicine, a quarterly journal published by Bell & Bain Ltd.
The Journal of Alternative and Complementary Medicine, a quarterly journal published by Mary Ann Liebert, Inc.

2

"TRUST ME,
I'M A DOCTOR"

*"Doctor Kemper, I read somewhere that there was this boy in California who
had cancer, and that he was cured with bee pollen. My cousin's son was just
diagnosed with cancer. Do you think he should take bee pollen, too?" So
began a recent conversation with friend and patient Toni Lozano.*

When a child is ill, we all want to help. In general, we prefer remedies that are natural, safe, good for the environment, and in harmony with our beliefs about ourselves and the world. Stories about dramatic cures are inspiring and give us hope that we, too, can overcome the painful challenges of a child's illness.

"I know that I can't trust everything I read," Toni continued. *"There are so many claims out there about certain foods or whatever being bad for you and other foods or vitamins being good for you. It's everywhere—magazines, billboards, TV, radio talk shows, friends, and neighbors. And they're all saying different things. Sometimes I feel overwhelmed, and I don't know who to trust. How do I know what really works and what is safe for my family?"*

Several years ago, a colleague gave me an aphorism I adore. I immediately put it on my office door, and it has hung there ever since:

"In God we trust; everyone else must have data."

This is the era of the skeptic. Given scandals such as Watergate and the graceless falls of spiritual leaders and athletic heroes, many of us have lost faith in traditional authority figures. Before trusting their child to a surgeon's knife, many well-informed parents ask for a list of potential alternative treatments, possible side effects, evidence of effectiveness from recent studies, and a second opinion. When it comes to your child's health, skepticism is your right as a loving and prudent parent.

"In God we trust. . . "

On the other hand, most of us do have faith in something or someone. Many have complete faith in their own doctor, though they distrust others. Some believe in the power of prayer. If you have complete faith in something, you don't need any evidence to know what to do. You follow your faith. Faith alone can be one of the most healing powers on earth. I have seen miraculous healings based on faith.

More and more hospitals now allow and encourage various types of spiritual healers (such as Native American medicine men) to visit patients and perform healing rituals. Numerous scientific studies have demonstrated the healing power of prayer. Prayer is effective whether the seeker is Christian, Jewish, Muslim, Buddhist, or Hindu—the words and the form don't matter. It is the faith and the intent that count.

On the other hand, I have also witnessed the suffering of children whose parents slavishly adhered to religious doctrines. One child died of meningitis because the parents saw the illness as a test of their faith rather than seeking "worldly" antibiotics. Another child suffered for days from a low blood count following a serious injury because the parents refused a transfusion. Children have been bruised and battered, permanently scarred, and brain damaged because parents felt they needed to "beat the devil" out of them. These parents forgot to put their children's needs and well-being ahead of their own need to follow their rigid interpretation of religious doctrine.

Our cultural beliefs, our sense of who we are, our connectedness to family and community, and the meaning we assign to health and illness are vital factors in the healing process. In many Eastern cultures, illness is seen as a lack of balance within a person or between a person and the environment. Western culture looks at disease in terms of cause and effect (e.g., germs cause illness). It is impossible for science to prove whether Eastern or Western philosophies are more "true." But science can

compare the effectiveness of different kinds of therapies in curing children with different kinds of disease.

We all have values that guide our judgments about what is best for our children. Some believe that natural methods are better than chemicals. Some believe in vitamin C, and others believe in chicken soup.

Toni believed in natural remedies, but she wasn't sure if bee pollen was powerful enough for a disease like cancer. She wondered if natural methods are always better.

Given equal effectiveness and safety, we'd all choose natural therapies over artificial ones. But keep in mind that many modern conveniences such as central heating, hot running water, and jet airplanes are not natural. The lowest infant mortality rates in the world are found in the industrially advanced nations. There are some lifesaving advantages to modern medicine. On the other hand, many times physicians and families take the easy way out and choose a drug when a change in nutrition, exercise, or environment would do more good in the long run. We all have to balance our values, priorities, and resources when choosing therapies.

THE OLD PARADIGM: THEORY, TRADITION, AND PERSONAL EXPERIENCE

Prior to this century, medicine was largely an art rather than a science. Medical practice was based on tradition and theory. Unfortunately, practices based on theory alone, while they may be well intentioned, can be disastrous for the patient. For example, the practice of bloodletting using leeches was based on the reasonable-sounding theory that it would rid the body of evil humors. It is now believed that excessive bloodletting is what ultimately killed the first U.S. President, George Washington. Many therapies that sound good in theory turn out to be at best ineffective and at worst dangerous in actual practice.

Despite spectacular advances in medicine, much of health care continues to be based on tradition. Health care practitioners, like all human beings, tend to do things the way they were taught. Is it wrong to recommend things based on tradition and experience? Not necessarily. Some traditions are simple common sense, and experience can be our greatest teacher.

On the other hand, some traditions based on short-term successes turn out to be hazardous or costly. Though it is a traditional herbal remedy for coughs, coltsfoot has recently been shown to be a liver toxin and carcinogen (cancer-causing) and is no longer regarded as safe. Even ten years after scientific evaluations indicated that aggressively treating healthy jaundiced babies was probably unnecessary, physicians continued to order phototherapy. Why? In part because of tradition and in part because we doctors feared that if we broke with tradition and anything bad happened, we would be held liable. Leaving traditions behind can be scary.

Finally, our own experience shapes our attitudes and recommendations. Recently a prominent pediatrician related the story of a teenage patient who had severely smelly feet. The pediatrician had counseled him extensively about hygiene to no avail. One day the boy showed up for a routine physical exam, and the physician braced himself for the overwhelming aroma before entering the exam room. To his surprise, the foot odor was completely gone. He began to congratulate the boy on his hygiene, but the boy told him it had nothing to do with washing his socks. "Zinc," he said. "I started taking some of my mom's zinc supplements and the smell went away." The pediatrician was dubious. The boy said he, too, thought it was just a fluke, so he stopped the zinc. Within a few days the odor returned, so he resumed the

zinc. On the basis of this experience, this physician now recommends zinc supplements to his patients with smelly feet. While zinc is probably safe in low doses, there are no studies demonstrating its effectiveness in treating foot odor. It may not affect other boys the same way. The boy may have adopted other healthy habits, diet, or exercise changes at the same time. Even impressive experiences such as that of the boy with smelly feet are not necessarily a solid scientific foundation for making treatment suggestions to others.

THE NEW PARADIGM: EVIDENCE-BASED MEDICINE

If you're like most people, you care less about theory and tradition than about how well a treatment actually works. *Evidence based medicine* means that you look at the scientific evidence that a treatment is effective rather than relying on tradition, theory, or anecdotal experience when making a medical decision. This way of thinking is a paradigm shift away from relying on theory, tradition, and personal experience. Evidence-based medicine relies on several *levels of evidence* to evaluate the effectiveness of therapies. Let's look at these different levels of evidence.

The Lowest Form of Evidence: The Anecdote or Case Report

"Child with fatal cancer cured with coffee enema!"

"Ancient Amazon ointment reverses ravages of acne!"

When doctors tell these stories, they usually begin, "I had a patient once who . . . ." This is the kind of claim that caught Toni's eye and impressed my colleague with the power of zinc. We're intrigued by the possibility of instant or miraculous cures. The more exotic, mysterious, or organic the treatment, the greater is the appeal. Those who market "the cure" may cite impressive and rational-sounding philosophical theories to support their claims.

These stories are called *anecdotes* in the popular press and *case reports* in scientific journals. They usually take the form of a hopelessly ill child who is cured with a wondrous or unexpected therapy. Anecdotes grab our attention, pique our curiosity, and give us hope. In the typical anecdote there is insufficient information to tell if the child in the story is similar to your child or if the illness is really like your child's illness. It is also difficult to tell what other therapies the child may have been receiving and exactly what is in the miracle cure.

Be very wary of people marketing miracle cures by phone or mail. Unfortunately, many are available only with a substantial outlay of cash up front. Although case reports may be intriguing, they do **not** provide a sufficient basis for recommending a certain therapy for any but the most desperate parents who have exhausted all proven remedies.

The Case Series: A Collection of Anecdotes

"We treated 100 feverish children with Brand X, and they all felt better within hours."

"I have used vitamin C with my patients for years, and they've all done very well."

A *case series* is simply a collection of anecdotes. Although the numbers make the claim sound scientific, a case series is also weak evidence that a treatment works. Consider the first claim—children treated with Brand X felt better within hours. Why did they have a fever? What other therapies were they given? Would they have gotten bet-

ter regardless of what kind of therapy they received or if they didn't receive any therapy? Case series provide promising leads for scientists to test. But a collection of hopeful anecdotes is *not* sufficient grounds for saying that a therapy has proven effectiveness.

Variations on the Theme of Case Series: The Twenty-first Doctor

"I took my child to twenty doctors, and none of them could figure out what was the matter with him. Nothing they recommended worked, and they pronounced him incurable. Just when I was about to give up, I took him to Doctor Jones. He put my baby on these food supplements, and now he's like a different child. Now he's active and full of life. I'm sure glad we took him to Dr. Jones. Maybe you should take your son to him, too. Or maybe you just want to try these supplements. . . ."

This scenario is the prototype for "the twenty-first doctor syndrome." It is really just a variation on the anecdote or case report. The story starts off with a difficult illness, resistant to the ministrations of numerous healers. The parent is frustrated and about to give up but tries one last doctor or therapy. The story is usually told by someone who is genuinely convinced that the final treatment caused the cure.

In some cases, it does take one unique healer or one unique treatment to cure a child. However, in many more cases, the marvelous cure is the result of the parents' own strong hope and faith or the illness having finally run its course (such as the infant who outgrows colic at the same time she starts eating solids). Was the child about to get better anyway? Perhaps. Does this make the cure less remarkable or less true? Of course not. These stories remind us that the human mind and spirit are among the most powerful healing tools available. But bear in mind that the visible trigger (the doctor or the diet) for this particular cure may not be the key to healing for your child.

"Well, this is all very disappointing," Toni complained. *"If I can't trust friends' stories, and if I can't trust doctor's anecdotes, how do I know who to trust? My husband says that all this holistic stuff is nothing but a placebo anyway. Just what is a placebo?"*

The Placebo Effect: A Psycho-Neuro-Immunologic Modulator?

Anecdotes about miraculous cures, stories about spontaneous remission, and the twenty-first doctor syndrome all raise the issue of the *placebo effect*. A placebo is an inert or inactive substance, such as water or sugar pills. The word *placebo* comes from the Latin *placere,* "to please." Placebos were originally devised to satisfy demanding patients who did not need or would not benefit from real medicine. A placebo can be anything—a word, pill, diet, exercise, or operation. For example, a patient takes the inert sugar pill, believing it will help him, and he is healed.

You might think that placebos work only for the weak-minded and suggestible, but you would be wrong. The placebo effect occurs in about 20 to 30 percent of *all* patients with every imaginable disease. It benefits the gifted as well as the gullible. It can reverse real disease as well as overcome imaginary symptoms. It illustrates the amazing capacity of the power of the mind to bring about healing.

Recently I have begun telling my medical students and residents that we should replace the word *placebo* with the phrase *Psycho-Neuro-Immunologic Modulator,* or PNIM. Why should we use such a cumbersome phrase? Because many people associate the word *placebo* with something that is worthless. But placebos are far from inactive. After many years of research, we know that there are direct connections between the mind (Psycho-), the nervous system (Neuro-), and the immune system (Immuno-). In themselves placebos may be nothing, but by modulating the psycho-neuro-immunologic system, they release a powerful healing force that can effectively cure real diseases.

Although placebos are effective in helping some children sometimes, they do not always cure everyone. An active ingredient is sometimes necessary to kill the bacteria or restore balance to the system. The difficulty in scientific research is in figuring out how much better the proposed therapy is than a placebo.

"Well," Toni said, *"as good as placebos may be, I want something better for my family. What kinds of studies prove a treatment is better than a placebo?"*

Comparative Studies

"American children who are not immunized have the same rate of polio as those who are immunized."

"Children who are breast-fed are smarter than those who are fed formula."

These kinds of claims compare one group of patients to another. Such studies look very scientific, and they are a big improvement over case studies, but they can also be misleading. What would you think of the first example if I told you that the rate of polio was nearly zero for both groups? The risk of polio for any child in the United States is very small now because of the success of the polio vaccine. What about breast-feeding and IQ? IQ scores are generally a few points higher among infants who are breast-fed than among formula-fed infants. However, American babies who are breast-fed generally also have parents with higher IQs and better education. Is the higher IQ due to the breast milk, the intelligence genes of the parents, or the environment?

Sometimes this type of comparative study is the best that can be done in the situation. A scientist can't tell one hundred new mothers, "Now you fifty are going to breast-feed for at least four months, and you other fifty are going to feed your baby nothing but formula for the first four months. At the end of that time, we'll measure your babies and see how smart they are." You just can't make people have certain health habits. You can't enforce what they eat or how much they exercise or whether or not they smoke. It's likely that the people who practice one healthy habit are healthier in other ways too. All of this makes it challenging to figure out exactly what's making children healthy (or sick). Many factors must be taken into account before you can conclude that the one thing you're interested in is the thing that matters.

"Well," Toni continued, "what do you think about using remedies on children that have been proved to work in adults?"

Children Are Not Sophisticated Rodents or Small Adults

"Rats who are fed only 80 percent of their needed calories live twice as long."

"Herbal remedy kills bacteria in test tubes."

"Cold medicines reduce symptoms in adults."

What's good for other animals isn't necessarily what's best for human beings. Calves thrive on cow's milk, while human infants do best with their own mother's milk. What happens in isolation in a test tube bears little resemblance to what happens inside a complex human being. Therapies that work in adults don't necessarily work in babies and young children. For example, cold medicines

reduce adults' symptoms but are useless in infants. Unless a therapy has been proved useful in humans, I don't recommend it. If it has been proved useful in adults, it's worth testing in children, and may be worth trying if it is safe and you've run out of other options.

"Aren't there any studies I can really trust?" Toni pleaded.

The Gold Standard: The Randomized, Controlled, Double-Blind Clinical Trial

Although all studies have shortcomings, the gold standard of scientific evidence is the randomized, controlled, double-blind clinical trial. Randomization means that each child in the study has a 50–50 chance of getting the study treatment or a comparison. The treatment decision is determined by the luck of the draw. That way the group of children who receive the experimental treatment are nearly certain to be similar to the group of children who receive the comparison treatment. This is important because without randomization, certain families would be more likely to believe in and choose one treatment over another. The differences between the families who choose different treatments might very well outweigh the differences in the therapies themselves.

Good studies have a control or comparison group. If you give aspirin to children with fever, the fever will go down. But the fever would go down eventually anyway. A comparison group is needed to see if the fever goes down faster with aspirin than without it. (Yes, aspirin is an effective fever fighter.) The strongest evidence for an effective therapy is that gained from testing children (not adults, animals, or test tubes), randomizing them into active treatment and placebo groups and assessing the results blinded to treatment assignment.

Double-blinding is when neither researcher

nor parent nor child knows whether the child received the study treatment or the comparison treatment until after the study is over. If the child and family don't know what treatment is being given, but the researcher does know, that's *single-blinding*. In a study of the effectiveness of acupuncture, the patient and parent may not know whether the needles are being placed in real points, but the acupuncturist must know whether the needle is going in a real point or not. If the family knew the child was getting the "better" study treatment, their expectation about its benefit would modify the psycho-neuro-immunologic response. This would give the new treatment an unfair advantage or a bias toward appearing to be more effective. Keeping everybody in the dark until the study is over helps minimize the bias that might arise if everyone knew which treatment the child was getting.

In a crossover study comparing two treatments (A and B), all of the patients are divided into two groups. Half receive treatment A and half receive treatment B. Their response to treatment is measured; they usually get a short break from *any* treatment (called a wash-out period because it gives them a chance to wash out all treatment effects). Then they are crossed over to the other treatment. Those who started out on treatment A now go on to treatment B and vice versa. Finally, their response to the new treatment is measured. With this study design, *all* of the subjects try both of the treatments to see which works better for them.

SUMMARY

"Let me see if I've got this straight," Toni said. *"The lowest level of evidence is the case report and the case series. Stories about eventual success with a certain doctor or therapy are really just the same thing. Studies of success in adult patients may not apply to children. Studies in children are good if there is a comparison group to make sure the therapy is better than a placebo. And the strongest evidence is from a randomized, double-blind, controlled trial in children."*

Exactly. If the only evidence for a therapy is based on tradition, a case series, or a case report, I consider it an interesting possibility but unproved. If the evidence is from a comparative trial in adults or children, I'll tell you it's worth trying but not recommended until better studies are done in children. The only therapies I will fully recommend in this book are those that have been tested with a controlled clinical trial in children. I also like to see them used for at least a few years so we know something about the safety and long-term effects of the therapy.

Do people combine faith with evidence? Of course we do. If you generally believe in herbal medicine, you may hear just one neighbor's story about how Echinacea dissipated her daughter's cold before you try it for your own child. On the other hand, if you're skeptical about antibiotics, you may doubt your doctor even when she cites randomized controlled trials. In all cases, you will end up judging my recommendations by your own faith, values, and experiences. We all have our own biases. Be open-minded and remember the levels of evidence when you hear or read about possible therapies for your child.

Ask yourself:

- Have clinical studies in children demonstrated that the therapy is more effective than a placebo treatment?
- How will the therapy affect your family's lifestyle and pocketbook?
- What are the risks and alternatives?
- Who is recommending the therapy, what are their qualifications, and do they have a vested interest in your choice?

"New truths commonly begin as heresies, but all too often end as superstitions."

T. Huxley, 1885

ADDITIONAL READING

Cousins, Norman. *Anatomy of an Illness as Perceived by the Patient.* New York: Bantam Books, 1981.

Dossey, Larry. *Healing Words: The Power of Prayer and the Practice of Medicine.* San Francisco: HarperCollins, 1993.

Siegel, Bernie S. *Love, Medicine and Miracles.* New York: Harper & Row, 1986.

Playing the Research Game. *Nutrition Action Newsletter*, October 7–9, 1994.

3

ACNE

Gerald Taylor came to see me last spring about his acne. He was an indus-
trious seventeen-year-old who was active in the Drama Club at school and
worked part-time at a fast-food restaurant to earn money for college. Gerald
was upset about his skin; the senior prom was coming up in two months,
and he wanted his skin cleared up by then. What had he already tried?
"Oh, the usual," he replied. "I tried some of that benzoyl peroxide stuff, but it
didn't work and it just made my face red. My mom says I should stop eating
french fries, but it's hard because I get them for free where I work. My
friend Marco got this prescription from his doctor for some kind of antibi-
otic, and his face looks real good. I want some of that." Before writing a pre-
scription to clear up Gerald's face, I wanted to clear up some of his ideas
about acne, where it comes from, what causes it, and what he needed to do
to make it better.

The principal players in the acne story are *sebum, hormones, bacteria,* and the *immune system.* Most of the action occurs deep beneath the skin surface in the tiny hair shafts of the face, the chest, and the back. The hair shafts are lined with sebaceous glands which produce a complex oily lubricant called *sebum.* Sebum normally moves smoothly up the hair shaft to the surface. A year or two before other signs of adolescence are visible, increasing levels of *androgen hormones* stimulate the sebaceous glands to make more sebum. Sebum builds up, forming a plug below the skin surface. Dead skin cells mix with sebum in the hair shaft beneath the skin surface, stick together, and worsen plugging. Plugged pores are perfect breeding grounds for the bacteria *Proprionibacterium acnes*. When *P. acnes* proliferate, they break sebum down into irritating *fatty acids* and attract *white blood cells*, starting a cascade of inflammation—redness, swelling, warmth, and pain.

Together the dead cells, sebum, bacteria, and fatty acids form a plug deep within the

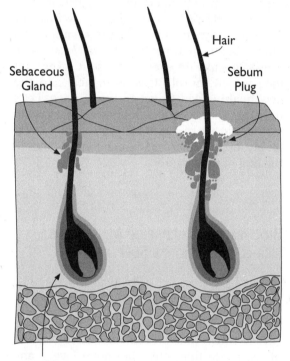

Sebaceous Gland

Hair

Sebum Plug

Hair Bulb

skin. As the plug pushes to the surface, it is visible as a blackhead. Contrary to popular belief, the black color does NOT come from dirt on the skin but from pigment in the dead skin cells. Albinos (people who lack skin pigment) can get acne, but they do not get blackheads. Although blackheads are unsightly, they are eventually extruded without causing redness or irritation.

If a plug blocks its own path to the surface, it makes trouble. The expanding plug eventually bursts the walls of the hair shaft, spilling irritating fatty acids into its surroundings. Immune cells rush to the site, releasing even more irritating chemicals. On the surface, this process initially appears as a whitehead (plugged off hair shaft), eventually becoming a raised, red pimple and then a pustule (a pimple that has come to a head) or, in the worst cases, a scarring nodule or cyst. It takes four to eight weeks for the newly formed plugs to rise to the skin surface as acne. This is why THERE ARE NO OVERNIGHT ACNE CURES; it takes several weeks for changes beneath the surface to become visible at the skin surface.

ACNE AGGRAVATORS

- Higher hormone levels (puberty, males)
- Higher sebum production (from stress) with more fatty acids
- Certain medications (Phenytoin, lithium, isoniazid, iodine)
- Blockage of hair shafts from oily air or oily cosmetics
- Irritation to the skin around the hair shaft

Most American teenagers (over 80%) face acne. About 10% of adults continue to deal with acne into their thirties and forties. Boys tend to have more severe acne because they have more *androgen* hormones. Many women experience acne flares just before menstrual periods when *progesterone* hormones (chemically similar to male hormones) are highest. Athletes who bulk up on *androgen steroids* also tend to get worse acne, among many other more severe side effects. *Stress* from lack of sleep, major exams, or emotional tension also increases sebum production and free fatty acids, increasing acne.[1] Acne-causing medications include the seizure medicine *Dilantin*; a drug for manic depression, *lithium*; an antituberculosis drug, *isoniazid*; and *iodine*. *Oily air* can block pores, contributing to acne. Fast-food restaurants, refineries, garages, and some chemical plants have high oil levels in the air.

I advised Gerald that his job might be contributing to his acne, not so much because of the fries he ate but because of the oily air in the restaurant. If he continued to work there, he would need to wash his face after every shift to help minimize blocked pores.

Common "treatments" can actually worsen acne. Despite the popular idea that sun dries up acne, increased *sweating* from summertime sunbathing on humid days can also block pores, aggravating rather than improving acne. *Over-zealous facial scrubbing*, frequent rubbing, picking, and pinching increase the breakdown of sebum into irritating fatty acids and provoke the immune system. *Friction* from clothing, football pads, hair, headbands, and resting the face on the hand can also aggravate acne. *Oily cosmetic coverups* can block pores, preventing the normal outflow of sebum and dead skin cells. Whenever possible, use water-based rather than oil-based cosmetics. All makeup should be thoroughly removed before bed. Avoid cosmetics containing acne-aggravating ingredients. Read labels carefully.

COSMETIC INGREDIENTS TO AVOID

- Acetylated PEG 15, PEG 75, or plain lanolin
- Butyl stearate
- Cocoa butter or coconut butter
- Glyceryl–3-diisostearate
- Hydrogenated vegetable oil
- Isopropyl anything
- Lauric acid or laureth 4
- Monostearate
- Myristyl myristate
- Oleyl alcohol
- Stearath 10

WHAT CAN YOU DO TO PREVENT OR TREAT ACNE?

You don't have to suffer with acne. There are numerous proved, effective treatments. Many are available without a prescription. If you need professional help, your family doctor, nurse-practitioner, or pediatrician can help with 95 percent of all acne. Refractory cases usually end up at the dermatologist's office. Most treatments take *at least eight weeks to show an effect* because it takes that long for all the old lesions to heal and the new healthy skin to get to the surface. Let's tour the Therapeutic Mountain to learn what works and what doesn't. If you want to skip to my bottom-line recommendations, flip to the end of the chapter.

BIOCHEMICAL THERAPIES: MEDICATIONS, HERBS, NUTRITIONAL SUPPLEMENTS

Medications

Acne medications fall into three categories: those that prevent or destroy sebum plugs, those that affect hormone levels, and those that kill *P. acnes* bacteria. The most effective treatments combine these three strategies.

ACNE MEDICATIONS

PRESCRIPTION AND NONPRESCRIPTION

- Plug Busters: benzoyl peroxide or salicylic acid

PRESCRIPTION MEDICATIONS

- Hormonal treatments
- Antibiotics: lotions or by mouth

Plug Busters

Some of the most effective treatments for busting up sebum plugs are inexpensive and available without a prescription.

Benzoyl peroxide is one of the most effective and widely used nonprescription acne treatments. Numerous brands are available (Acne–10, Benoxyl, Benzashave, Clearasil Maximum Strength Acne Treatment, Cuticura Acne, Fostex 10%, Oxy 5, Oxy 10, and others). You can save money and have the same benefits by buying generic brands. Benzoyl peroxide generates free oxygen radicals deep in the hair follicles, breaking down sebum plugs and killing acne-causing bacteria. Strengths range from 2.5% to 10%. Start with the lower strengths once a day at night until your skin gets used to it. Then advance to twice daily. If there's no improvement after six to eight weeks and your skin tolerates it, advance to the 10% strength at night or to twice daily treatments.

The *side effects of benzoyl peroxide* include irritation, drying, itching, redness, and peeling. Nonprescription benzoyl peroxide is available in either alcohol-based or water-based formulas. Alcohol-based preparations are more irritating than water-based forms. The prescription formulation of benzoyl peroxide comes as a gel rather than a cream; the gel penetrates the skin more deeply and is more effective, but it can also cause more irritation. Benzoyl peroxide is more irritating when applied to wet skin, so wait a few minutes after washing and drying your face to apply it.

About 1 to 2 percent of adolescents who use benzoyl peroxide become *allergic* to it.[2] Because it generates free radicals, benzoyl peroxide could theoretically increase the risk of developing *skin cancer* later in life.[3] However, studies looking at users of benzoyl peroxide have not found any increase in cases of skin cancer.[4] Benzoyl peroxide is a *bleach*; be careful around colored fabrics, especially silk shirts! It can also bleach skin; darkly pigmented teens may prefer nonprescription salicylic acid treatments.

Salicylic acid breaks apart sebum plugs by "ungluing" the dead skin cells. It has been used for over a hundred years to treat acne. Salicylic acid is as effective as benzoyl peroxide for mild acne.[5] It is the active ingredient in many of the over-the-counter acne remedies, such as Stri-Dex, Clearasil Medicated Cleanser, and Therapads Plus. Strengths vary from 0.5% to 2%. Start with the lower concentration; as your skin tolerates it, try higher strengths. As with other topically applied acne medicines, the main side effects are redness and irritation. They are usually mild and don't mean you have to stop treatment; just cut back to a lower strength or once a day use.

Prescription Hormonal Treatments

Birth control pills suppress the body's production of acne-causing hormones. If a young woman is old enough to suffer from moderate acne, she's old enough to use birth control pills. Most birth control pills contain a combination of estrogen and progesterone. Low-progesterone pills are the most effective for reducing acne, especially in women who have signs of hormonal imbalance, such as facial hair.[6] It takes several months for benefits to become apparent, and the course of therapy may last one to two years. Because of their potential side effects, estrogen hormones are *not* recommended for male acne sufferers. Hormones can have serious side effects in women, too, and should not be used without close medical supervision.

Anti-inflammatory *steroids* (not the muscle-building kind) can be injected directly into large cystic acne lesions. This is done only for severe acne.

Antibacterial Agents

Antibiotics kill off *P. acnes* bacteria, thereby decreasing fatty acids and inflammation. They do *not* clear up pimples that are already present. Antibacterial agents can be applied topically (as a soap or liquid) or taken by mouth (orally).

BACTERIA KILLERS

- Soap: chlorhexidine (Hibiclens)—no prescription necessary
- Antibiotics (topical)—require prescription
- Antibiotics (oral)—require prescription

Do NOT use abrasive cleansers and scrubs; they cause too much friction, drawing immune cells into the fray and worsening acne. Most soaps don't penetrate deeply enough or stay on the skin long enough to kill acne-causing bacteria. *Chlorhexidine* (Hibiclens) skin cleanser is widely used in hospitals because it does such a good job of killing skin bacteria. When used twice daily, it has been *proven effective* as an acne fighter in a randomized, placebo-controlled trial. It is as effective as 5% benzoyl peroxide and is less drying and irritating.[7] Washing more than twice daily confers no additional benefits.

The four most widely used *topical antibiotics* are clindamycin (Cleocin), tetracycline, erythromycin, and meclocycline (Meclan). They are all effective, but because people are different, some folks do better with one than another.[8] You might ask your physician for a prescription for the least expensive type for three months. If it is too irritating or doesn't work very well, try another. To stop pimples before they reach the surface, antibiotic medications must be applied to *all* acne-prone places, not just those that have already broken out.

Do NOT apply plug busters and antibiotics at the same time (such as both benzoyl peroxide *and* erythromycin lotion in the morning). Combinations can aggravate side effects, but they do NOT improve acne. By alternating medications—antibiotic lotion in the morning, benzoyl peroxide or salicylic acid in the evening—you can reduce side effects and get better results than with either one alone.[9] Antibiotic lotions are nearly as effective as taking antibiotics by mouth.[10] Very little of the antibiotic lotion is absorbed into the system, so there are fewer side effects than with oral antibiotics. Antibiotic lotions are less irritating than benzoyl peroxide and salicylic acid. Be careful with tetracycline creams; they glow under ultraviolet light. Your face may attract unwanted attention if you apply tetracycline before visiting a nightclub featuring "black" lights!

Oral antibiotics help reduce bacteria over the entire skin surface, reaching beneath the surface to the depths of the hair follicles. Oral antibiotics used to treat acne include tetracycline, erythromycin, and minocycline. Oral antibiotics are more effective than antibiotic lotions in treating severe, widespread acne on the trunk and back, but it takes about four months before the effects are really noticeable. One of the main side effects of tetracycline is vaginal yeast infections. Other side effects include upset stomach, allergies, and increased susceptibility to the sun. Prolonged use increases bacterial resistance and kills normal intestinal bacteria. *Tetracycline should not be taken by children under eight years of age or by pregnant women,* because it turns developing teeth an ugly brown. Erythromycin is usually the least expensive of all the oral acne antibiotics. Minocycline has the fewest side effects but the highest cost ($1.75 to $2.50 per pill).

Isotretinoin (Accutane) is the most powerful prescription antiacne medication available. It reduces sebum production by 90% and helps kill acne-causing bacteria. Along with its power comes the potential for *serious side effects*. It is reserved for patients with severe, deep, widespread acne. Women should not use it unless they abstain from sex or use a reliable form of birth control, because isotretinoin can cause serious birth defects if taken during pregnancy. It can also cause dry eyes, headaches, nosebleeds, and changes in blood lipids. If your acne is bad enough that you are considering this medication, see a dermatologist.

Herbs

Tea tree oil (from the Australian *Melaleuca* alternifolia tree) has proven benefits for acne. An Australian study of 124 acne patients showed that a 5% tea-tree oil *gel* was as effective as 5% benzoyl peroxide.[11] Other herbal preparations have not been evaluated.

Other traditional herbal acne remedies include infusions of catnip, chamomile, comfrey, lavender, thyme, or yarrow root used as facial rinses. Calendula is thought to decrease inflammation, but an oily preparation could just block pores. Folk remedies for acne include poultices of grated carrot, cucumber, or aloe vera, and lemon juice rinses. An Ayurvedic remedy is a paste made with turmeric and sandalwood powder and water. Herbal masks containing equal parts of green clay and corn flour, with one or two drops of the essential oils of chamomile, lavender, juniper, or patchouli have also been recommended. Native American herbal treatments for acne include burdock root, echinacea, Oregon grape, and goldenseal. Until studies document the effectiveness of these herbal remedies, I do NOT recommend them. Too many other effective treatments are available to waste your time and money on unproven remedies.

Nutritional Supplements

VITAMINS AND MINERALS FOR ACNE

PROVEN HELPFUL

- Vitamin A (Retin-A) cream or gel—prescription only

UNCERTAIN BENEFIT

- Vitamin B6
- Zinc
- Vitamin A (oral supplements)—nonprescription
- Selenium
- Chromium

PROVEN HARMFUL

- Vitamin B12
- Iodine

Proven Helpful for Acne

Tretinoin or *topical vitamin A acid (Retin-A)*, the topically applied form of vitamin A, is one of the most effective antiacne preparations available. Tretinoin normalizes skin sloughing, breaks down sebum plugs, and creates an unwelcome environment for *P. acnes*. It works synergistically with plug busters (benzoyl peroxide or salicylic acid) and antibiotic lotions because it makes the skin more receptive to other medications. It should NOT be used at the same time as other medications but should be alternated; for example, tretinoin in the evening and either benzoyl peroxide or an antibiotic lotion in the morning.

Tretinoin comes in several strengths

(0.025%, 0.05%, and 0.1%) and in both a cream and gel; all require a prescription, and all are fairly expensive ($20 to $30 per month). The gel formations and the higher concentrations are more potent and have more side effects (red skin and peeling); side effects can be reduced by starting with lower concentrations. Start by using it at night every other day, gradually increasing to every night as tolerated. Topical vitamin A also makes skin more sun sensitive, so *be sure to use sunblock if you're using tretinoin.* Treatment usually lasts six to eight months. Tretinoin does not cause birth defects or any of the problems associated with overdoses of oral vitamin A supplements.

Retin-A is usually the first medication I prescribe for teenagers who have already tried nonprescription acne remedies. I wrote a prescription for Retin-A for Gerald to use at night after his evening wash with chlorhexidine soap. I suggested that he continue his morning treatment with nonprescription benzoyl peroxide, explaining that he might see some improvements by prom time with persistent use but that he might have some redness and irritation for the first week or so. We took a picture of him in the office to compare to his later appearance because the improvement is sometimes so gradual that you aren't aware of it until you compare before and after pictures.

Uncertain Benefit for Acne

There are case reports (anecdotes) that some women who have acne flare-ups with their menstrual periods benefit from 50 milligrams per day of *vitamin B6, pyridoxine.*[12] However, there are no comparison studies proving its effectiveness. For women who note an association between their acne and their menstrual periods, it may be worth a trial of vitamin B6. To reduce the risk of side effects, start with lower doses such as 10 mil-

ligrams twice daily, increasing as tolerated to 25 milligrams twice daily.

Interestingly, *zinc* levels are lower than normal in many male acne sufferers. Higher zinc levels inhibit sebum production and make sloughed skin less sticky. Studies about zinc's effectiveness are conflicting. A Swedish study showed that 45 milligrams taken three times daily was more helpful than placebo in reducing acne[13]; other studies have not duplicated these results.[14] The body tries to maintain a balance between zinc and copper. If you use zinc as an acne treatment, take a balanced multivitamin as well. If you aren't getting enough zinc in your diet, you may not be getting enough of several other nutrients either. *I'm less in favor of supplements than of a healthy, balanced diet, especially during the teenage years of rapid growth and development.*

Vitamin A supplements were previously recommended to help treat acne based on a series of patients whose acne improved after several months of vitamin A therapy.[15] However, there was no comparison group in this study, and the high doses used (300,000 to 500,000 International Units daily) can result in severe headaches, dry skin, cracked lips, and blurred vision.[16] I do NOT recommend vitamin A supplements in higher doses than are found in nonprescription multivitamins (10,000 International Units daily). *The best plan is to eat a diet rich in vitamin A–containing fruits and vegetables.*

A preliminary study from Sweden indicates that *selenium* supplements (0.2 milligrams taken twice daily) may be helpful in treating acne in areas that have low soil levels of selenium.[17] This study did NOT include a comparison group and has *not* been duplicated in the United States, where soil levels of selenium are higher. If you take a multivitamin that includes selenium, you do *not* need any additional selenium.

Theoretically, supplemental *chromium*

may improve the skin's sugar metabolism, thereby reducing the food supply for acne-causing bacteria. However, there are NO studies indicating that chromium supplements are actually beneficial for acne sufferers.

Proven Harmful for Acne

High doses of *vitamin B12* can promote an acnelike rash.[18]

Excessive *iodine* may worsen acne in some sensitive teenagers. Fast foods often contain extraordinary amounts of iodine. Sushi wrapped in *seaweed* and *kelp* supplements is another potential source of excessive iodine. Regular iodized table salt *is* OK if used sparingly.

LIFESTYLE THERAPIES: NUTRITION, ENVIRONMENT, MIND-BODY

Nutrition

Does a bad diet cause acne? Despite nearly universal fears of fried foods, chocolate, and sweets, there are few scientific studies evaluating their effects on acne. One randomized, controlled study from 1969 showed that eating chocolate did NOT make acne worse.[19] However, the comparison group was eating a very fatty diet. Though frequently cited, this study has NOT been replicated, it did NOT focus on patients who felt that chocolate made their acne worse, and it did NOT control for fat intake.

Studies of acne in different countries suggest that people who eat a diet low in animal fat (especially Mediterranean diets low in red meat, butter, and milk), low in saturated fats, and higher in olive oil have a lower risk of acne.[20] There have not been any scientific studies evaluating the effective-

ness of a low-fat diet (less than 30% of calories from fat) or of switching from saturated animal fats to unsaturated vegetable fats on acne. Nevertheless, the Mediterranean diet has a lot going for it in terms of preventing heart disease and reflecting a healthy lifestyle. I recommend this diet to adolescents interested in life-long nutritional health, whether or not they have acne.

Nor have there been any good studies on the effect on acne of cutting down on refined sugar. Several older studies suggested that poor sugar metabolism made acne worse. A 1937 report from Bellevue Psychiatric Hospital noted that six psychotic teenagers treated with insulin shock therapy (which dramatically drops blood sugar and was standard therapy at that time for schizophrenia) had a marked improvement in their acne.[21] Based on this observation, two British physicians gave insulin injections to nondiabetics in the late 1930s to improve their acne.[22] When oral medications became available to reduce blood sugar in the 1950s, they were given to London patients and reported to be effective.[23] However, these studies did *not* contain comparison groups, and the patients ran the risk of going into shock from low blood sugar. Possible problems with sugar metabolism in the skin form the basis for recommending *yeast supplements* for acne sufferers[24]; yeast contains high amounts of *chromium*, which plays an essential role in helping tissues metabolize sugar. However, there are no studies proving that chromium supplements are effective in treating acne. I do NOT recommend chromium supplements as an acne treatment. Although I think we can all reduce our sugar intake to reduce our risks of obesity and tooth decay, I do *not* believe that a sugar-free diet is a cure for acne.

Clinically, it appears that in a relatively small number of acne sufferers their condition is exacerbated by a particular food, but the effect is inconsistent.[25] For those who are convinced that chocolate, peanut butter, french fries, or some other food makes their acne worse, eliminating the suspected offender is worth a try. Even if your skin is sensitive to a particular food, prepare to endure six to eight weeks of continued symptoms. It takes that long for just about any treatment to start to make a difference.

Environment

Acne is *not* caused by dirt. Washing twice a day is plenty to prevent blocked pores. However, teenagers who work in fast-food restaurants, like Gerald, or in a garage with lots of airborne grease, may find that washing after work helps reduce the oil on their skin.

Some people feel that acne improves during the summertime with increased exposure to the sun. However, there is a condition called tropical acne, in which acne is induced by the high temperatures and humidity in the tropics. With all of the concerns about excessive exposure to sunlight increasing the risks of skin cancer, I do *not* recommend sunbathing as an acne treatment.

Mind-Body

No doubt about it—*stress* makes acne worse. Acne itself is a major stress for most teenagers; it is usually rated among their top health concerns.[26] When British teenagers suffering from severe acne were offered a choice of $1,000 or a cure for their acne, 87% chose the acne cure![27] Failure to get enough rest and relaxation contributes to overall stress levels. Teenagers need a lot of sleep to get through growth spurts and rapid developmental changes.

Adolescents should find a relaxation technique that works for them—listening to music, meditation, self-hypnosis, breathing exercises—and stick with it. *Relaxation techniques are most useful if practiced daily, not just when major stress occurs.* Parents can help by offering emotional support. For severely stressed teens, *hypnotherapy* may be helpful in reducing stress and stopping behaviors that worsen acne such as picking at the pimples.

BIOMECHANICAL THERAPIES: MASSAGE, SURGERY

Massage

Massage oils can block pores, making acne worse. Though massage may be wonderfully relaxing and helpful in stress reduction, there are NO studies evaluating its effectiveness in treating acne.

Surgery

Some dermatologists use a long-handled thin extractor to remove blackheads. The extractor has a round end that fits around blackheads. By pressing down on the round loop, the plug is forced up and out. Extraction is a less irritating technique than pinching or pushing. It does *not* prevent pimples but can help reduce the number of cosmetically disturbing blackheads.

A variety of plastic surgery treatments are available to treat scarring from acne. With cryosurgery, acne scars are sprayed with a freezing cold liquid; the frozen surface layers eventually peel away, leaving smoother skin. *Chemical peels* work the same way. Dermabrasion, in which the skin is scraped with a wire brush, is reserved for more severe scarring. For deep scars, the individual areas are cut out, then grafted or stitched. Collagen or silicon can be injected under the skin to push up broad, flat, scarred areas. These procedures should only be undertaken by a plastic surgeon after the acne is no longer active.

BIOENERGETIC THERAPIES: ACUPUNCTURE, HOMEOPATHY

Acupuncture

Two case series report that acupuncture is a helpful treatment for acne.[28, 29] Before you get your hopes up, you should know that there was *no* comparison group in either study, so it is impossible to tell how many patients would have improved without acupuncture. There was also no mention of concurrent treatments that may have played a role. It took an average of sixteen treatments for improvements to appear. If you are paying out of your own pocket, acupuncture becomes a very expensive therapy with very uncertain benefits.

Homeopathy

Homeopathic remedies for acne include Antimonium crudum, Carbo animalis, Hepar sulfur, Kali bromatum, and Sulfur. But save your money. There are *no* scientific studies documenting their effectiveness for treating acne. I do NOT recommend them.

WHAT I RECOMMEND FOR ACNE

PREVENTING ACNE

1. *Lifestyle—nutrition.* Eat a healthy diet, rich in fruits, vegetables, and grains and low in red meat, whole milk, and butter. If you don't eat a balanced diet, consider taking a multivitamin containing zinc, B6, and antioxidants.

2. *Lifestyle—environment.* Avoid prolonged exposure to oily environments such as fast-food restaurants and car repair shops. Avoid sunbathing, especially on hot, humid days. Avoid abrasive soaps or scrubs. Do *not* pick at your pimples. Minimize friction to your face and other acne-prone areas.

3. *Lifestyle—mind-body.* Get enough rest and practice some form of relaxation daily to reduce stress levels. Remind yourself that your worth is not determined by your skin's appearance.

4. *Biochemical—medications.* Avoid cosmetics or use only water-based kinds. Avoid the following ingredients: acetylated lanolin; PEG 15, PEG 75, or plain lanolin; butyl stearate; cocoa butter or coconut butter; glyceryl-3-diisostearate; hydrogenated vegetable oil; isopropyl anything; lauric acid or laureth 4; monostearate; myristyl myristate; oleyl alcohol; oils of avocado, mink, or sesame; propylene glycol; red dyes; stearath 10.

See Your Health Care Professional If

- Home remedies have not resulted in any improvement in two months. You may benefit from

  - *vitamin A cream, retinoic acid.* Retinoic acid can make skin sun sensitive, so avoid sun exposure and use a good sunscreen—at least SPF 15.

  - *antibiotic lotions* such as tetracycline, clindamycin, erythromycin, or meclocycline. Do not use at the same time as other skin creams. If you're using another treatment such as benzoyl peroxide, use one in the morning and the other in the evening.

  - for *women, birth control pills.* Ask your health care professional.

  - *oral antibiotics,* for severe acne that has not responded adequately to the other therapies. Talk with your doctor.

- You have severe, cystic acne. You may consult a dermatologist for a thorough evaluation and consideration of even stronger medication (such as isotretinoin [Accutane]).

- You have severe acne scars. See a dermatologist about surgical therapies.

TREATING ACNE

Remember: it will take eight to twelve weeks to see the effect of almost any therapy. Treatment must be persistent, and you must be patient!

Biochemical—medications. Wash acne-prone areas twice daily with chlorhexidine or a mild antibacterial soap. Try nonprescription medications such as

- tea-tree oil gel
- salicylic acid
- benzoyl peroxide

4

ALLERGIES

Every spring Yvonne gets itchy, watery eyes, a runny nose, and sneezes.

Every time Cory eats strawberries, his tongue swells and he breaks out in hives.

Aaron has chronic diarrhea, eczema, and asthma. He also has dark circles under his eyes and is not growing as well as his brothers.

Every time Anne wears inexpensive earrings, her earlobes swell and become painful.

These are all examples of allergies. Allergies affect more than 30 million Americans, account for 2 million days lost from school, and cost approximately $1 billion annually in doctor visits and medications. According to recent surveys, food allergies affect about 2 to 5 percent of children,[1] skin allergies affect 3 to 10 percent, and nasal allergies such as hay fever affect as many as 30%.[2,3] Allergies are responsible for symptoms ranging from fussiness to fatal shock. Allergies are the top health problem leading parents to take their children to nonmedical health care providers.[4]

Allergies are confusing to most parents and many physicians because the body reacts to what it perceives as allergies in different ways; many allergic symptoms mimic other illnesses. Many symptoms have been blamed on allergies that are NOT true allergies. Despite their complaints to the contrary, most kids are *not* allergic to homework, algebra, or Latin! The vast majority of people who can't tolerate milk aren't allergic to it, but they lack the enzyme needed to digest milk sugar. Kids who have an upset stomach after eating a chili dog slathered with onions may have poor judgment, but probably aren't allergic to chili or onions. Belching and passing gas after eating raw vegetables or beans are not due to allergies either. Chinese restaurant syndrome is a direct chemical effect of the flavor enhancer MSG, monosodium glutamate, not an allergy to bean sprouts. Red eyes after swimming are due to irritation, not allergies.

COMMON ALLERGY SYMPTOMS

Skin: hives, eczema, swelling, itching

Nervous system: headache,[5] fatigue, confusion, difficulty concentrating, decreased attention span,[6] depression, insomnia and other sleep problems[7]

Eyes: red, itchy, watery eyes; dark circles under the eyes; swollen eyelids

Nose: watery, itchy, sneezing, congestion; horizontal wrinkle across tip of the nose

Mouth: itchy roof of the mouth, swollen tongue, lips; sore, scratchy throat

Respiratory system: asthma, wheezing, coughing, feeling of tightness in the chest

Heart: rapid heart rate, irregular heartbeats

Muscles and joints: muscle pain, joint pain, arthritis

Intestines: colic, diarrhea, nausea, vomiting, constipation, abdominal pain, itchy anus, bloody diarrhea[8]

Urinary system: sense of urgency or frequent need to urinate

Allergies are symptoms of an *oversensitive immune system*. They occur when the immune system decides that something that has come in contact with the body is dangerous and needs to be fought. There are four main types of allergic immune reactions, sensibly called Type 1, Type 2, Type 3, and Type 4.

Type 1 reactions are immediate; they are usually due to reactions of the immune molecule immunoglobulin E (IgE). IgE triggers the mast cells in the immune system to release histamine—the chemical that causes swelling, itching, and watering. Type 1 reactions cause watery eyes, sneezing, hives, itching, swelling, and in the most extreme cases, shock. Fortunately, severe Type 1 reactions are very treatable with medication.

Just as we were about to close the clinic one warm summer evening, Bill Aylers rushed in the door carrying his pregnant wife, Judy. She was weak to the point of collapse, wheezing and dotted with hives. Bill told me that he and Judy had been visiting relatives in the country. As they got in the car, Judy was stung by a bee. She felt weak and started wheezing almost immediately. As he frantically drove down the road, he saw our clinic lights on and pulled in. Within minutes after a shot of Adrenalin (epinephrine) and a dose of Benadryl (diphenhydramine), Judy roused, the hives faded, and the wheezing improved. Bill's quick action and our clinic's readiness for this kind of emergency saved his wife's (and unborn baby's) life.

This kind of immediate, life-threatening, Type 1 allergic reaction is called *anaphylaxis*. It can be caused by insect stings, certain medications, or even common foods, such as eggs, nuts, strawberries, or shellfish. Parents whose children have had an anaphylactic reaction to common foods such as eggs or wheat must be vigilant about the ingredients in prepared or processed foods such as breads, cakes, snacks, and candy because they may contain the fatal allergen.[9]

Most of the time, the IgE molecule causes Type 1 immediate reactions that are less serious but are still uncomfortable. The reactions most people get to ragweed pollen or cats happen within an hour or two of exposure—watery, itchy eyes, sneezing, wheezing, coughing, and hives. This less serious variety of Type I reaction is far more common than anaphylaxis. It is the main reason for the booming industry in antihistamines.

Type 2 allergic reactions are much less common. They are the reactions that destroy red blood cells if the wrong type of blood is given during a transfusion.

Type 3 allergic reactions are rare. They occur when antibodies bind to foreign substances (antigens), forming big clusters that deposit in various tissues such as the kidneys and the joints. Wherever they settle, the antibody-antigen clusters cause problems such as the allergic arthritis that sometimes follows infectious diarrhea. It usually takes several days after the initial antigen-antibody clusters form to develop symptoms.

The *Type 4 allergic reaction* is typified by the common response to poison ivy and to nickel jewelry (contact dermatitis). They usually take twelve to twenty-four hours to become visible. Type 4 reactions cause intense itching and a blistering rash but are rarely life-threatening.

Some allergies don't depend on the dose of allergen—one bee sting or one bite of eggs may be enough to trigger a severe reaction. Other allergies do depend on the dose. A child who is allergic to cow's milk may tolerate half a cup of milk on his cereal in the morning but have severe bloody diarrhea if he drinks a whole quart of milk. Some allergies (such as that to animal dander) are perennial (all year round), and some only occur during certain seasons (such as ragweed season in the fall or tree pollen allergies in the spring). Some allergies are developed during adulthood or are lifelong (such as hay fever), and some allergies are outgrown (most cow's milk allergies).

COMMON ALLERGY TRIGGERS

OUTDOORS

- Plants—such as poison ivy and poison oak
- Chemicals—such as insecticides, pesticides, fertilizers, fumigants
- Pollens—such as ragweed

INDOORS

- Animal dander, saliva, or urine
- Dust and dust mites
- Insect venom—such as bee stings
- Foods—such as nuts, milk, soybeans, shellfish, eggs, wheat, oranges, strawberries, chocolate, tomatoes, corn
- Herbs—such as feverfew, chamomile, yarrow, tansy[10]
- Irritants—such as wool, fabric finishes, dry cleaning solvents
- Chemicals—such as perfumes, soaps, detergents, cosmetics, cleaning products, disinfectants, solvents, turpentine, paint, formaldehyde
- Food colorings, additives, preservatives, hormones, antibiotics
- Medications—such as aspirin, antibiotics, morphine, X-ray contrast material

In addition to not feeling well, children who suffer from allergies frequently suffer from other problems. For example, they tend to grow poorly. So much of their energy is consumed with the allergy, there just isn't enough left over to grow. Chronic nasal allergies lead to nasal obstruction, mouth-breathing, and can eventually lead to deformities of the face, necessitating later orthodontic treatment. Children with hay fever–type allergies may have more frequent ear infections, sinus infections, and delayed language development.

When children eat foods to which they are allergic, the normal intestinal barrier is breached, promoting sensitivity to even more foods.[11] Fortunately, many children outgrow food allergies over one to three years.[12, 13] Those whose symptoms come on immediately or within a few hours are more likely to outgrow their allergies than those whose symptoms occur several hours or days after eating the allergenic food.[14]

Could It Be Something Else?

Yes. It is often difficult to diagnose allergies in babies because allergic symptoms can easily be attributed to other problems: colds, diarrhea, eczema, and sleeping problems. Sometimes it's hard to tell the difference between a cold and an allergy—both cause runny or stuffy noses and sneezing. Children who have diarrhea and gas after drinking milk due to lactase deficiency have similar symptoms to children suffering from true milk allergies. If you are not sure whether your child's symptoms are due to allergies or something else, take him to be evaluated by a professional who is experienced in treating allergies.

Diagnosing Allergies

The basis of all allergy diagnosis is the relationship of the child's symptoms to his exposure to allergens. Physical examination is also useful. Health professionals rely on a variety of tests as well as symptoms and the physical exam to diagnose allergies.[15] *Skin prick or skin scratch tests* are the most widely available and widely used allergy tests. In a skin test, the child's skin is scratched and a liquid containing the suspected allergen is dropped on the scratched or pricked area. The test is positive if the skin gets red and has hives at the scratch site. Unfortunately, the prick or scratch tests are sometimes falsely positive. This means that your child could have a positive test and not really have an allergy. Skin tests are most useful for diagnosing Type 1 allergies such as hay fever.

For diagnosing food allergies, the most common test is a *double-blind, placebo-controlled food challenge*. In this test, all potentially allergic foods are withheld for several days; then the child is given a capsule containing either a suspected allergen or an inert substance (placebo). Neither the child, the parents, nor the physician knows whether the capsule contains the allergen or the placebo. After taking the capsule, the child is carefully watched for any type of reaction. A more extreme evaluation requires hospitalization in a special low-allergy unit and going on a fast or severely restricted diet, gradually reintroducing substances and assessing the child's reactions as each thing is added—a food, a pollen, dust, etc. This kind of evaluation is expensive, time-consuming, and stressful for the family and child, so it is not often done. In severe cases, it may be the best alternative.

The *RAST (radioallergosorbent test)* is one of the most commonly used tests for allergies because it is convenient (it only requires a blood test), but it can also be inaccurate. The *FICA (food immune complex assay)* is another blood test, but it is expensive and not widely available. *Cytotoxic blood tests* for allergies are very controversial. In this test, the child's white blood cells are mixed with the suspected allergen; if the white cells react, the child is thought to be allergic to that substance. The problem is that white cells isolated in a test tube don't necessarily react the same way they do in a human body. The test is also very dependent on the skill of the person looking at the white blood cell reaction; there is a lot of variability in interpreting the results.

The recently popular intradermal provocation/neutralization skin tests are not accurate or reliable[16]; do not rely on practitioners who base their allergy treatments on these techniques. Though practitioners who use them come up with rationales that sound convincing, there is no scientific basis for recent fads such as urine autoinjection, kinesiology testing, or electroacupuncture as diagnostic techniques for allergies.

The best test for allergies is *careful observation* over a long period of time. Keep a diary of your child's symptoms and exposures. You may be able to figure it out yourself with some careful detective work. If your child's symptoms are severe or incapacitating, get professional guidance.

WHAT'S THE BEST WAY TO PREVENT AND TREAT ALLERGIES?

The best preventive strategy is to avoid the allergen (Lifestyle-environment). When children are inundated with allergens, their immune systems get revved up and it takes very little of another allergen to trigger a big reaction. On the other hand, if your child is allergic to three things—cats, dust, and pollen, for example—and you markedly reduce her exposure to two of those things (say cats and dust), she will be much less likely to react to the third (pollen). If you can eliminate most of your child's allergy triggers by changing things you can control (dust and

pets), you may also reduce her sensitivity to other triggers over which you have less control (pollen). Let's tour the Therapeutic Mountain to find out what treatments have proven effectiveness. If you want to skip to the bottom line, flip to the end of the chapter.

BIOCHEMICAL THERAPIES: MEDICATIONS, HERBS, NUTRITIONAL SUPPLEMENTS

Medications

The overwhelming variety of allergy medications can be very confusing. There are several classes of effective medications that work different ways.

ALLERGY MEDICATIONS

- Antihistamines
- Mast cell stabilizers
- Steroids
- Desensitization therapy
- Epinephrine
- Decongestants
- Saline
- Others

Antihistamines are the mainstay of medical allergy treatments. They work by blocking the action of histamine released from mast cells. There are many types, varieties, and brands of antihistamines. It's impossible to tell which antihistamine is most effective for your child without trying different kinds. Most people start with the least expensive nonprescription remedy. If these don't help or have unacceptable side effects, see your physician about other (more expensive) prescription medications. More expensive antihistamines are NOT necessarily more effective.

ANTIHISTAMINES

Over-the-counter (nonprescription):
triprolidine (Actidil), diphenhydramine (Benadryl), chlorpheni-
ramine maleate (Chlortrimeton),
brompheniramine (Dimetane),
clemastine fumarate (Tavist)

Prescription: hydroxyzine (Atarax),
cyproheptadine (Periactin),
promethazine (Phenergan)

*Prescription (nonsedating) for children
twelve years and older:* loratadine
(Claritin), astemizole (Hismanal),
terfenadine (Seldane)

Many antihistamines are available without a prescription. Nearly all of them require
doses every four to six hours and have side
effects such as a dry mouth, difficulty concentrating, and drowsiness; a few children
also have problems with urination and constipation. A few children become irritable and
hyperactive from antihistamines. Antihistamines do a good job with runny noses, but
they don't help much with congestion. That's
why many allergy preparations contain a
decongestant as well as an antihistamine.
Decongestants have additional side effects:
increased blood pressure, increased heart
rate, and decreased appetite.

Because most people don't want to spend
the entire hay fever season sleeping, they
often ask physicians for prescription antihistamines that are less sedating, such as
Claritin, Hismanal, or Seldane.[17] These medications only require dosing every twelve to
twenty-four hours. They are, however,
extremely expensive compared to nonprescription antihistamines and are only
approved for use in children twelve years and
older. They should *not* be taken at the same
time your child is on erythromycin-type
antibiotics or antifungal medications such as
ketoconazole because of the risk of liver toxicity. A few adults have had seriously irregular
heart rhythms while taking terfenadine
(Seldane) and astemizole (Hismanal).

When using an antihistamine, give it to
your child *before* symptoms occur rather
than after he is miserable. Antihistamines
work by blocking the reaction to allergens. If
your child's symptoms are triggered by visits
to his cat-loving friend, giving him an antihistamine thirty to sixty minutes before he gets
to the friend's house is more effective than
delaying treatment till after he's coughing and
sneezing.

You can also increase your child's tolerance to the sedating effect of antihistamines
by starting him on doses before he goes to
bed, so he can get used to it when it doesn't
matter if he's sleepy. Then add low daytime
doses and gradually increase the dose as his
body gets used to it.

Although antihistamines do help relieve
allergic symptoms, they do not address the
underlying sensitivity that causes allergies.
Go ahead and use them if your child has mild
or occasional symptoms and to help your
child feel more comfortable while you take
other measures to address the underlying
problem.

Mast cell stabilizers are medications that
help *prevent* allergic symptoms by calming
down the mast cells that release histamine.
These medications all require a prescription.
They are also best given *before* symptoms
start. Unlike antihistamines, they have very
few side effects, and I recommend them for
children who have predictable allergies, such
as hay fever, or year-round allergies, such as
dust mite allergies. Cromolyn is effective in
preventing symptoms of food allergy as well
as allergic asthma.[18]

MAST CELL STABILIZERS
(ALL REQUIRE PRESCRIPTION)

- Loxamide (Alomide eyedrops)
- Cromolyn (Nasalcrom) nasal spray
- Nedocromil (Tilade) inhaler and
  eye drops

Mast cell stabilizers have fewer side effects than other medications because they target the affected area. For example, Alomide eye drops are just put in the eye, Nasalcrom is sprayed in the nose, and Tilade is inhaled into the lungs or dropped in the eyes. They prevent histamine release from the mast cells in those areas but do not affect other tissues such as the brain or heart. They have specific rather than general effects. They are safe to use in combination with other more general treatments such as antihistamines or steroids.

Steroid medications are available in several forms to treat different kinds of allergic reactions. Steroid medications are very similar to the body's own anti-inflammatory messengers. They help reduce swelling, pain, and irritation.

STEROID PREPARATIONS FOR ALLERGIES

Creams or ointments—such as Cortaid
  (prescription and nonprescription)

Nasal sprays—such as Vancenase,
  Beconase, and Nasalide (prescription only)

Metered dose inhalers for allergic
  asthma—such as Aerobid,
  Azmacort, Beclovent, Decadron,
  Vanceril (prescription only)

Oral steroids for systemic symptoms—
  such as cortisone, Decadron,
  Medrol, Pedi-pred, Prelone,
  Prednisone (prescription only)

The mildest kind of *steroid creams* (0.5% and 1% hydrocortisone, Cortaid) are available without a prescription. They are helpful for allergic rashes such as poison ivy. Steroids also come as *nasal sprays* to treat runny nose and congestion due to allergies. The stronger sprays are effective even with once a day dosing[19]; all steroid nasal sprays require a prescription and are best used as a preventive therapy before symptoms start.[20] It usually takes several days for improvements to be noticeable. Steroids are also available in *inhaled form* (metered dose inhalers or MDIs) to treat allergic asthma. For children with more severe, system-wide symptoms, *steroid pills or liquid* may be needed to get symptoms under control. When taken by mouth, steroids can have powerful side effects, which include suppressing the immune system, raising blood sugar, and increasing blood pressure; they should be used for as little time as possible. When steroids are applied directly to the affected area (such as creams to rashes and sprays to the nose), they have very few side effects and are safe even for young children.

Allergy shots (desensitization therapy) are a series of injections of minute amounts of whatever is causing the allergy. They stimulate the immune system to produce the "good" kind of immune globulin, IgG, which blocks the allergy-causing immune globulin, IgE. Allergy shots are most effective for allergies to bee stings,[21] pollen, dust mites, and animals[22]; they are less effective for mold and food allergies.[23] Desensitization therapy usually lasts three to five years. It can be dangerous if the dose is advanced too quickly, resulting in a severe allergic reaction. That's why allergy shots should only be given in the office of a physician who is trained in treating severe allergic reactions and who has emergency equipment on hand.[24]

If your child ever has a major allergic

reaction (anaphylaxis) to a food, bee sting, or anything else, please have him wear a *Medic-Alert bracelet* and ask your physician for a prescription for two *epinephrine* kits. Keep one at home and one with the child wherever he may come in contact with the allergen. I keep one at home and one in my backpack. These kits (such as *Epipen*) can be life-saving if your child has an anaphylactic reaction. You don't have to know how to give a shot. The medication comes preloaded; all you have to do is push the syringe against the child's thigh and the needle will automatically inject the right dose at the right depth.

If your child's main symptom is a stuffy nose, you may be tempted to use a nonprescription *nasal decongestant spray*. Don't. Although these products do reduce congestion, they do so at a price. Because the blood vessels swell when allergies strike, shrinking them with decongestants helps open up the nasal passages and results in symptomatic relief. However, the blood vessels quickly become dependent on the decongestants, requiring higher and more frequent doses to achieve the same effect. It only takes a few days to become dependent on (or addicted to) decongestant nasal sprays. If your child suddenly quits taking them, he could have rebound swelling and worse congestion than ever.

For those children who have become dependent on their nasal spray, don't make them quit cold turkey. The rebound swelling will just make them miserable and tempted to return to the spray for relief. Instead, spray only one nostril for three days. The unsprayed nostril will initially swell up and feel stuffy, but your child can still breathe through the sprayed side. When the unsprayed side returns to normal in two to three days, stop spraying the other side. It will be congested for a day or two, but your child can breathe through the now normal side. Within a week, both sides will have returned to normal and your child will have

overcome the dependence on nasal sprays nearly painlessly!

If you want to help keep nasal secretions loose, give your child simple *saline nose drops* (1/4 teaspoon of salt in 8 ounces of water—or buy premixed saline drops, NaSal). One or two drops on each side can be given as often as you like to help with congestion. In fact, some parents find that frequent saline nose washes help rinse out the allergy-causing pollen.

You may be hearing about two new medical treatments for children with allergies. *Atrovent (ipratropium bromide)* has been used for several years to treat adults with nasal allergies and asthma. There is preliminary evidence that it may be useful for children, too.[25] *Thymomodulin* is an extract of calves' thymus glands which may modulate the immune response. Several European studies have demonstrated its effectiveness in treating children with food and nasal allergies,[26,27] but it has not yet been approved by the U.S. Food and Drug Administration.

Herbs

HERBAL REMEDIES

Scientifically Proven Useful: ephedra

Scientifically Unproven but Widely Used: angelica, skullcap, coleus root, eyebright, goldenrod tea, goldenseal, licorice root, wild yam, magnolia, nettle leaf tea, plantain, green clay, and calendula

Ephedra tea (Ma huang) has long been used by the Chinese as a treatment for allergies, asthma, hay fever, and the common cold. It is the original source of *ephedrine,* which is an ingredient in many cold and allergy medications. Ephedra is a decongestant, and it has some anti-inflammatory effects.[28] It is contraindicated for long-term use because with frequent, repeated use, higher and higher doses are required to achieve the same results. Ephedra also has side effects such as high blood pressure and rapid heart rate, so it should not be used by children who have weak hearts or who already have high blood pressure.

In addition to having a beautiful ornamental flower, the *angelica (dong quai)* plant root has been used by Chinese herbalists since ancient times to treat allergies, eczema, and hay fever.[29, 30] Angelica extracts have several effects on the immune system. *Chinese skullcap tea* helps decrease inflammation and inhibits the immune system's allergic response. One of the chemical constituents of *coleus* root has demonstrated antihistamine properties in animal studies.[31] However, there are NO studies that demonstrate the effectiveness of angelica root, Chinese skullcap, or coleus root in treating children with allergies.

Eyebright tinctures have long been used to treat the burning watery eyes and runny nose associated with hay fever–type allergies. *Euphrasia* is also one of the most commonly recommended homeopathic allergy remedies (see the Homeopathy section below). The anti-inflammatory properties of *goldenseal* have made it a favorite herbal remedy. Scientific studies have *not* evaluated the effectiveness of any of these three herbs in treating childhood allergies.

Goldenrod tea or tincture are controversial allergy remedies because goldenrod actually *causes* allergies when it is inhaled. Some physicians believe that drinking goldenrod tea may cause a severe allergic reaction; others who believe in the healing principle of "like cures like" believe that goldenrod tea or tinctures make the perfect preventive medication and antidote to inhaled allergens. Although both sides of the argument can be

quite vocal, there are *no* studies showing either marked benefits or severe risks of goldenrod tea in treating childhood allergies.

Licorice root and *wild yam* have antiallergy and anti-inflammatory effects, perhaps due to their similarities to the body's own anti-inflammatory steroid chemical, cortisol.[32, 33, 34] Because licorice root mimics an innate hormone which affects the kidneys, large doses or chronic use can result in fluid retention, high blood pressure, headache, and significant potassium loss.

Magnolia flower buds reduce histamine release in test tube studies but have *not* yet been evaluated in children.[35] *Nettle tea* also has a good reputation for preventing and soothing allergic reactions. Although brushing up against a nettle plant usually causes stinging and hives, it is also a commonly recommended homeopathic remedy for allergies. Again, there is *no* scientific evidence that it is useful.

For those suffering from allergic skin rashes, *plantain* poultices are said to be soothing. Others recommend an application of a paste made of *green clay* and water to the affected area. Many people find *calendula* creams and ointments soothing for allergic skin irritation. However, there are NO scientific studies documenting the effectiveness of any of these remedies.

Nutritional Supplements

NUTRITIONAL SUPPLEMENTS FOR ALLERGIES

- Vitamin C
- Essential fatty acids—evening primrose oil
- Other vitamins and minerals
- Red peppers (capsaicin)

Large doses of *vitamin C* (2 grams per day) have been shown to decrease symptoms in adults with allergic asthma and hay fever but have not been studied in children.[36] If you'd like to try vitamin C, start with smaller doses (50 to 100 milligrams). Vitamin C is excreted very rapidly, so doses must be given several times daily to maintain blood levels. Increase the dose gradually. If your child develops diarrhea (an early symptom of vitamin C overdose), reduce the dose. Frequently recommended supplements include *vitamins A, B6, E, beta-carotene, selenium,* and *zinc.* Although these vitamins and minerals are essential for normal immune function, there is little research to support their use in treating children with allergies, and I do *not* recommend them as allergy remedies.

Supplemental *essential fatty acids (EFA)* are sometimes recommended for children with allergies and eczema. Some allergic families have a blockage in fatty acid metabolism which destabilizes the immune system. By giving large doses of EFA, the blockage can be bypassed and the immune system more stabilized. EFA are found in linseed, safflower, and sunflower oils, nuts, mackerel, and sunflower seeds. *Evening primrose oil, blackcurrant oil,* and *borage oil* are very high in EFA. Evening primrose oil (EPO) is available in many health food stores as 500-milligram capsules. In scientific studies of EPO, doses of two capsules (1,000 milligrams) three times daily were helpful in treating children suffering from eczema (see Eczema chapter).

Capsaicin, the spicy, pungent molecule in *red peppers*, decreases airway sensitivity to irritants such as tobacco smoke. Spicy foods such as peppers, horseradish, and hot mustard have long been part of folk remedies for allergies. In animal studies, capsaicin decreases a variety of airway allergic responses.[37] There are no studies yet evaluating the effects of hot peppers in allergic children, but you might try keeping track of your child's symptoms following a spicy meal.

One theory holds that food allergies are due to the passage of small molecules of undigested food across a leaky gut wall into the bloodstream. Those who hold to this theory believe that *digestive enzymes* such as *papaya enzyme tablets* and *bromelain* may be helpful in preventing allergies. Others believe that allergic reactions are *causes,* not consequences, of leaky intestines.[38] Although papaya is one of my favorite foods, it has *not* been scientifically evaluated for its effectiveness in treating childhood allergies.

Bee pollen supplements are another favorite folk remedy for allergies which have *not* been scientifically studied in children.

LIFESTYLE THERAPIES: NUTRITION, EXERCISE, ENVIRONMENT, MIND-BODY

Nutrition

Children who are fed a variety of solids before four months of age are more susceptible to developing allergic skin rashes.[39] Do *not* feed your child anything besides mother's milk or formula in the first few months of life.

Omitting an allergenic food from the diet may be your only practical alternative if your child has a serious food allergy. Some clinicians recommend that a severely suffering patient go on a total fast for four to five days to clean all potential allergens out of the system before reintroducing possible offenders one every few days. I do *not* recommend fasts for children under six years old; nor should they be undertaken in older children without the supervision of a dietitian or nutritionist. Eliminating major dietary staples such as milk or wheat runs the risk of producing serious nutritional deficiencies.[40] Most children who are fed milk-free diets get too little calcium unless they receive supplements.

Be aware of potential cross-reactions between inhaled allergens and foods. For example, many who suffer from ragweed allergies are also allergic to melons (cantaloupe, honeydew, or watermelon). Those who are allergic to pollen from birch trees may react to apples, carrots, cherries, pears, peaches, or potatoes. Keep a diary of your child's exposures to foods and pollens and the allergic symptoms to help sort out these associations.

I do not recommend that most children eat much red meat because of its high fat and cholesterol content, the widespread use of hormones and antibiotics in the meat industry, and the tremendous drain on the ecosystem involved in producing meat. However, there is *no* scientific evidence that red meats provoke more allergies than other kinds of meat or soy protein. Lamb is one of the least allergenic foods available. Try to buy meats labeled as organic or free of hormones and antibiotics or use wild game to reduce your child's exposure to these chemicals.

Sugar has been blamed for a variety of childhood problems, from acne to tooth decay to hyperactivity to allergies. Sugar comes in a variety of forms, including table sugar (sucrose), milk sugar (lactose), and fruit sugar (fructose). There are *no* studies proving that children who avoid sugar have fewer allergy symptoms. However, kids don't need candy or soft drinks to grow well. I recommend that most parents keep a lid on their child's sugar consumption, but you don't need to take extra precautions if your child has allergies.

Despite widespread recommendations to avoid "mucus-producing foods" such as dairy products, there have not been any scientific studies showing that dairy products produce more mucus than any other kind of food. If your child does not have other symptoms of milk allergy, you do not need to avoid dairy products. Milk allergy typically causes symptoms such as diarrhea and upset stomach, anemia, chronic lung problems, and eczema.[41] One dairy product, yogurt, may be a helpful preventive therapy for allergy-prone children. Yogurt containing live cultures increases gamma interferon, one of the body's own infection- and allergy-fighting chemicals. Start feeding your child yogurt daily several months *before* allergy season to start building up gamma interferon levels.

Exercise

Vigorous exercise can make allergy symptoms worse. Not only does outdoor exercise expose children to pollens and air pollution, but some children actually get hives just from getting overheated. Two recent studies showed that some children have worse food allergy symptoms if they exercise immediately after eating.[42, 43] They had no symptoms if they ate wheat (to which they were all allergic) and didn't exercise but had a severe reaction if they ate wheat and then exercised. One adult had repeated life-threatening allergic reactions when exercising after eating hazelnuts.[44] No one knows exactly why this happens, but consider having a rest period between eating and exercising.

Environment

The primary treatment for allergies is environmental: avoid the allergen! The majority of people who are allergic to one thing are sensitive to others too. If you reduce children's exposure to some allergens, it may reduce their reaction to others.

If your child is allergic to pollens, take a

few minutes to check the daily pollen count. Radio and television stations usually have this information, or call your local weather service. Pollen counts are generally highest in the morning, so you may want to limit your child's outdoor activities until the afternoon and keep the windows closed in the morning.

Between 5 and 10 percent of Americans are allergic to cats or dogs. About twice as many children are allergic to cats as are allergic to dogs. Children can also be allergic to guinea pigs, mice, hamsters, and rats. Even if the animal is removed from the home and you start an aggressive cleaning campaign, it can take four to six months for animal allergen levels to clear.

TIPS FOR REDUCING ALLERGENS IN THE HOME

1. Thoroughly dust (using a damp cloth or mop) and vacuum the house every week. Change the vacuum's dust bag frequently. Keep your child out of the vacuumed room for an hour after you've finished to allow the dust to settle.

2. Avoid using chemical cleaners that leave a lingering smell. Cleaning with bleach helps eliminate molds from damp areas.

3. Remove all dust-catchers from your child's room. This means carpeting, stuffed animals, ruffled bedclothes, and draperies. Avoid wool blankets, down, and feather or foam pillows in your child's room. Dacron is much less allergenic. Wash all of your child's bedding in hot water weekly to destroy dust mites. To avoid additional pollen, do not dry the bedding outdoors. Dry cleaning does not reduce allergens as much as cleaning in very hot water.[45]

4. Encase your child's mattress and pillow (favorite homes of the dust mite) in allergy-proof nylon or vinyl casings.

5. Install a high-efficiency particulate arresting (HEPA) air filter in your child's room. Keep the windows closed between 5 and 10 a.m. when pollen counts are highest. Install an electrostatic air filter on your furnace or air conditioner.[46, 47]

6. Add air-cleaning house plants (such as philodendrons and spider plants) to your child's room. They help remove indoor air pollutants.

7. Do not allow furred or feathered pets in your child's room. Preferably, pets should be kept outside. If your pets are as much a loved and integral part of your family as mine are, you can keep them in the house if you bathe them weekly.

8. Keep the humidity in your house below 50% to discourage molds and dust mites.[48]

9. Kill dust mites by spraying an acaricide-dust mite killer (such as Acarosan)[49] or tannic acid (Allersearch-Ads) on all your carpeting, upholstery, and draperies at least twice yearly; thoroughly vacuum a day later to clean up the residue of dead dust mites. You can obtain Acarosan by calling 1(800)882–4110, 1(800)621–5545, or 1(800)422–3878.

10. DO NOT SMOKE AND DO NOT ALLOW OTHERS TO SMOKE IN YOUR HOME.

To treat reactions to bee, wasp, and hornet stings, immediately apply ice. Ice numbs the pain and reduces swelling. Remove the stinger by scraping it off; pulling it can release more venom into the skin. Children whose reaction consists of hives and swelling at the sting site are *not* at increased risk of a life-threatening reaction in the future.[50]

OTHER HOME REMEDIES FOR POISON IVY AND OTHER ALLERGIC RASHES

1. Rub them with ice. Ice helps numb the area, reducing itch.

2. Make a paste of baking soda and water and rub it in. Baking soda seems to be most helpful for blistering rashes, not plain old hives.

3. Some of my patients have tried applying Milk of Magnesia (MOM)—usually used for upset stomachs—when they were desperate and there was nothing else in the house. They reported that it was useful. I've recently learned that some of my colleagues actually recommend MOM as a soothing lotion for itchy rashes. It's readily available and free of side effects, but I don't think anyone has actually studied its effectiveness in treating allergies.

4. Other parents report that zinc-oxide (the active ingredient in the strongest sun blocks and diaper rash preparations) is also an effective anti-itch treatment.

Heat and cold also affect allergic symptoms. Some people break out in hives wherever an ice cube is rubbed on their skin. The runny nose caused by going in and out of the cold is called skier's nose. On the other hand, allergy sufferers can achieve four to six hours of relief from inhaling hot steam.[51]

Running the air conditioner may help reduce pollen inside your home. I know many parents hate air-conditioning, but it can make allergy sufferers much more comfortable because it filters allergens out of the air. For maximal benefits, keep the windows and doors closed (even when the temperature isn't high) and keep the pollen out! If you don't need the cold air, just run the fan to circulate air through the filter. Clean the filter at least twice yearly with a bleach or vinegar solution or use disposable filters.

Tepid baths may be soothing for a child suffering from irritating skin allergies. Try putting a cup of plain, dry oatmeal in an old stocking and tossing it in the bathwater. Oatmeal is very soothing to irritated skin, no matter whether the underlying problem is allergies, eczema, or chicken pox.

Bathing and shampooing at night will help wash out all the pollens and other allergens that have clung to your child's skin over the day. Rinsing off in the evening ensures that your child doesn't have to deal with allergens when he's asleep.

Mind-Body

Several startling experiments have proved that the mind and mood affect allergic reactions.[52] In one experiment, hypnotized subjects were told that a leaf was poison ivy. After the leaf touched their skin, all of the subjects broke out in a typical poison ivy rash, even though the leaf was from a maple tree! In another experiment, subjects who were tested with varying strengths of allergen reacted differently depending on what mood they were in when the test was placed; they had much smaller reactions when they felt happy or lively than when they felt down or listless.[53]

Anecdotes from psychiatry also lend credence to the power of the mind in mediating allergic reactions. Some patients suffering from multiple personality disorders display an interesting allergic phenomenon: one of their personalities can be severely allergic to a food, such as oranges, while another personality has no reaction to that food at all. So if the person eats an orange in personality A, she may break out in hives, but if she eats oranges while she is personality B, she can eat as many oranges as she wants without any reaction.

Stories such as these tell us that the connection between the mind and the immune system is far more complex than our current understanding of it. Clearly, hypnotized subjects and patients with multiple personalities have only one body and one immune system, but their allergic reactions vary depending on their mental state. We don't need to fully understand the mechanism of this interaction to use it. Hypnosis and even conscious suggestion can markedly reduce symptoms of food and inhaled allergies in children.[54]

If your child suffers from chronic annoying allergies, consider taking him to a hypnotherapist. Hypnotherapy can help uncover the source of the problem (if it is emotional), provide powerful suggestions to prevent reactions, and give you and your child useful images to help deal with reactions when they do occur. Images of cold are particularly useful. The image need not be elaborate. As you apply whatever treatment you use for your child's allergy, remind him that this is a healing treatment and that it will make him better.

Anne was able to cool off the itchy reaction to her earrings by imagining herself skiing down a snowy mountain on a clear, cold day with her cap off.

It has been said that allergic reactions are a manifestation of unexpressed emotions, particularly anger. Although it is difficult to imagine that a six-month-old's anger results in an allergy to cow's milk, it is easy to imagine how the stress of pent-up emotions in the family can trigger a variety of physical symptoms. Infants and children are particularly sensitive to the emotions of other family members. Emotional stress affects the immune system (the key factor in allergies) in profound and as yet unexplained ways. Whether or not your child's allergy symptoms are directly due to family emotional issues, it makes sense to put such issues on the table and resolve them. Professional counseling may help.

BIOMECHANICAL THERAPIES: SPINAL MANIPULATION

Osteopathic manipulation was the most commonly recommended treatment by the American psychic Edgar Cayce during his trance readings for children suffering from allergies. Cayce recommended relaxing adjustments of the upper neck and back areas and stimulating adjustments for the lower back. Although these recommendations are fascinating and the patients reported remarkable improvements, osteopathic treatment for allergies has *not* undergone scientific evaluation.

BIOENERGETIC THERAPIES: ACUPUNCTURE, HOMEOPATHY

Acupuncture

Acupuncture has been a mainstay of allergy treatment in China for hundreds of years. Acupuncture treatment fifteen minutes prior to exposure to an itch-inducing allergen can markedly reduce itch. Acupuncture is best when used as *preventive* therapy, given *before* symptoms occur. It is less effective after symptoms have already appeared.[55] Recently, acupuncture treatment was compared to antihistamine treatment in forty-five adults with nasal allergies. Antihistamines were taken three times daily for seven weeks, and acupuncture treatment was given for fifteen minutes every other day. Both treatments resulted in significant improvement.[56] In another study acupuncture treatment was compared with desensitization injections in 143 adults. The desensitization group was treated for a year; the acupuncture group was treated every one to three days for a total of five to ten treatments (less than a month). Significantly more patients treated with acupuncture improved than patients who were treated with desensitization therapy. This was true whether their primary symptoms were asthma, nasal allergies, or hives.[57] These results are impressive. If you are tired of the side effects of chronic allergy medication and are considering taking your child to an allergist for desensitization shots, you may want to try acupuncture first. Please seek an acupuncturist who has extensive experience in dealing with children and their fears of needles.

Homeopathy

Homeopathy is more closely related to conventional allergy desensitization treatments than it is to any other medical therapy. Based on the principle of "like cures like," the primary homeopathic remedy for hay fever is Ambrosia (ragweed). Like all homeopathic remedies, it is given in extremely minute doses. Allium cepa (spring onion) is a common homeopathic remedy for burning, watery eyes. Apis homeopathic remedy is an extract of crushed bees—rather like a crude form of the allergists' injections for bee sting allergies. Euphrasia (eyebright) is used for the allergic symptoms in which the eyes are primarily affected (redness, watering, burning, feeling rough or gritty). Euphrasia is also used in larger doses by herbalists to treat allergic symptoms. Urtica urens (stinging nettle) is the homeopathic remedy for treating hives.

Other homeopathic remedies for hay fever–like allergies (usually to inhaled allergens such as pollen) include Arsenicum, Kali bic, Natrum mur, Nux vomica (poison nut), Pulsatilla (windflower), Sabadilla (cevadilla seed), Sulfur, and Wyethia (poison weed). Many of these remedies are very poisonous undiluted. Homeopathic remedies are *extremely* dilute, and there is no danger of poisoning.

Homeopathic remedies for skin allergies (contact dermatitis) include Bryonia (wild hops—said to be good for food allergies as well), Rhus, and Sulfur.

Homeopathic remedies are widely used in Europe to treat allergies. In a 1990 survey of nearly 300 Dutch general practitioners, almost half reported that they believed homeopathic remedies are effective in treating hay fever.[58] Several European studies have demonstrated that homeopathic remedies are superior to sugar water placebos in treating hay fever.[59, 60] A review of the world's scientific studies on homeopathic remedies concluded that the trials on treating hay fever showed an overall positive result.[61] If you choose homeopathic remedies, please take your child to a homeopathic physician who has extensive experience in treating children with allergic disease. Do *not* rely on homeopathy alone for severe, life-threatening allergic reactions.

WHAT I RECOMMEND FOR ALLERGIES

PREVENTING ALLERGIES

1. *Lifestyle—environment.* Cleanup. No matter whether your child's allergies are from pollen, poison ivy, or potatoes, the best prevention is to reduce your child's exposure to the allergen. Also reduce exposure to pollution and irritants. Do NOT smoke and do not allow others to smoke around your child.

2. *Lifestyle—nutrition.* Do NOT feed your child solids before she is at least four months old. When you do introduce solids, try one new food a week; not several new foods within a day. If your child has allergies at predictable times of year (spring or fall pollen season), try giving him 1/2 to 1 cup of yogurt daily for two months preceding allergy season.

TREATING ALLERGIES

1. *Biochemical—medications. For severe, life-threatening allergic reactions such as ana-phylaxis from a bee sting, seek emergency care immediately.* If your child has a severe reaction, ask for a prescription for an epinephrine kit. Get your child a Medic-Alert bracelet.

For symptomatic relief of minor symptoms, try nonprescription antihista-mines. Follow package directions on doses and be aware of potential side effects.

For minor relief of itchy allergic rashes, try a mild steroid cream such as Cortaid to treat rashes that do appear.

For moderately severe respiratory allergies (affecting the eyes, nose, sinuses, and lungs), consider prescription medications such as cromolyn (Intal), nedocromil (Tilade), or steroid nasal sprays.

For respiratory allergies to pollens and pets, consider desensitization therapy (*after* cleaning up the environment to prevent symptoms and *after* trying nonpre-scription antihistamines and prescription mast cell blockers.

2. *Biochemical—nutritional supplements.* For respiratory allergies, try vitamin C supplements; start slowly and gradually increase to 250 to 500 milligrams three times daily. Back off if diarrhea develops. For children whose food allergies appear as skin rashes, consider evening primrose oil supplements, one gram three times daily.

3. *Lifestyle—nutrition.* If you suspect that your child has moderate or severe food allergies, seek the help of a health professional, nutritionist, or dietitian in devel-oping an elimination or few foods diet.

4. *Lifestyle—environment.* Wash thoroughly immediately after contact with poison ivy or other skin sensitizers. Use ice compresses to reduce swelling and itching. Try tepid baths with or without oatmeal to relieve itching.

5. *Lifestyle—mind-body.* For any type of allergy, consider taking your child for hypnotherapy or biofeedback therapy with a therapist trained in treating children.

6. *Bioenergetic—homeopathy.* For hay fever symptoms, consider seeing a homeopathic physician who is experienced in treating children.

7. *Bioenergetic—acupuncture.* If your child is comfortable with the idea of needle therapy, consult an acupuncturist who is trained in treating children.

RESOURCES

Food Allergy Network
4744 Holly Avenue
Fairfax, VA 22030–5647
1(703)691–3179
1(800)929–4040

Enviracaire HEPA Air Filters
Honeywell Environmental
   Air Control
747 Bowman Avenue
Hagerstown, MD 21740
1(800)332–1110

5

ASTHMA

Yolanda Jefferson awoke suddenly in the middle of the night, hearing her youngest son, Devante, cough again. Neither of them was getting any sleep. Yolanda was exhausted from the lack of sleep, caring for three children and two cats, getting the kids to day care while she worked, making meals, and trying to keep the house clean. Devante seemed to cough more than other kids when he caught a cold. His cough was worse at night; sometimes he coughed even when he didn't have a cold. Yolanda was beginning to wonder if he had asthma. Her mother, who lived with them, continued to smoke though she had asthma, and Devante's two older brothers had asthma, too. Yolanda couldn't believe Devante was starting to get sick already; he was only eighteen months old. She wanted to know what she could do to ease his symptoms.

If your child suffers from asthma, you are not alone. Asthma is the most common chronic illness of childhood, affecting 4 to 5 percent of American children—that's about 3.2 million kids![1] Asthma has become even more common and more severe in recent years. Between 1980 and 1990 the number of Americans suffering from asthma climbed from 6.8 million to over 10 million and the asthma deaths jumped a whopping 40%.[2]

Asthma starts earlier in boys than in girls (three years old vs. eight years old on average). Asthma is epidemic in American inner cities—14% of children living in the Bronx have asthma.[3] Asthma is more common among children living with a single parent, those living in crowded conditions and in poverty, and those living with a smoker. Although asthma is more common in Puerto Rican and African-American children, the fastest increase in cases has been among middle-class Caucasian children.[4, 5, 6] Premature babies born with lung problems often suffer from asthma, too. Asthma, along with allergies and eczema, tends to run in families. Symptoms improve for many children when they reach adolescence. On the other hand, some children first experience asthma as teenagers.

Children with asthma can do just as well in school, sports, and social situations as their peers without asthma. In the 1984 Olympics, 67 of 597 U.S. athletes had exercise-induced asthma. They brought home fifteen gold, twenty-one silver, and five bronze medals.[7]

ASTHMA SYMPTOMS

- Dry cough (especially at night)
- Wheezing (high-pitched whistling sounds) during exhalation
- A feeling of tightness in the chest
- Having difficulty breathing

Sometimes children will have only one of these symptoms—usually the cough. Many children have symptoms just once or twice and never have them again. Coughing and wheezing can be caused by other health problems, too.

OTHER CAUSES OF COUGH AND WHEEZING

- Viral infections
- Aspirating food or other objects into lungs
- Genetic lung diseases

Viral infections, such as colds and bronchitis, aspiration (when food or a small object is inhaled into the airways), and genetic diseases such as cystic fibrosis are all marked by coughing and wheezing. X rays, blood tests, and lung function tests may be necessary to make the correct diagnosis. A child is called asthmatic only if his symptoms occur at least three times, several family members have asthma, or there is some other reason to suspect that symptoms will recur.

It sounded as if Devante had the classic symptoms of asthma. His diagnosis was confirmed by his physical examination and response to treatment. Yolanda wanted to know what was happening in his lungs to cause Devante's symptoms. She also wanted to know what might trigger his asthma, so she could prevent flare-ups.

Three changes in the small airways (*bronchioles*) cause asthma symptoms.

LUNG CHANGES IN ASTHMA

- Inflammation and swelling of the walls of the bronchioles
- Increased mucus production, blocking the bronchioles
- Bronchospasm, constriction of the muscles surrounding the bronchioles

When the airways become inflamed during an infection or allergy, the walls of the bronchioles become swollen and irritated, blocking air flow to the tiny air sacs (*alveoli*) at the end of the bronchioles. The irritation also triggers coughing. Normally mucus helps clear the airways, but too much mucus clogs air passages. Irritation also stimulates the muscles around the bronchioles to tighten or constrict, further reducing airflow. These changes lead to cough, wheezing (the sound the air makes as it tries to flow through narrowed tubes), and feelings of tightness.

Very few children have asthma symptoms all the time; most just have symptoms triggered occasionally. Sometimes the effect of a trigger is immediate—the child starts wheezing as soon as he walks outside on a pollen-filled spring day. Sometimes triggers have delayed effects; a child is exposed to a cat in the afternoon and does not have symptoms until he goes to bed. Keeping a diary of your child's asthma symptoms can help you figure out what triggers the flare-ups.

COMMON ASTHMA TRIGGERS

- Airway irritants: cigarettes, air pollution, wood smoke
- Allergies, including food sensitivity
- Exercise
- Cold air
- Infections: colds, sinus infections, bronchitis
- Medications (aspirin)
- Stress

Cigarette smoke is the #1 preventable trigger of asthma. Even if your child doesn't smoke, being around smokers will almost certainly make your child's asthma worse. Maternal smoking during pregnancy affects a child's lung development and increases his risk of having asthma later. *Do* NOT *smoke and do not allow other people to smoke around your child!*

Air pollution also aggravates asthma. Today's energy-efficient houses tend to trap indoor air pollutants such as mold, dust mites, and animal danders in the house, aggravating asthma symptoms. Children who live near busy roads, factories, power stations, and other sources of air pollution often suffer from bad asthma. City emergency rooms log more asthma visits when pollution levels are higher. Children who live in the country suffer from their own sources of pollution: wood smoke from stoves and fireplaces, dust, animal dander, and agricultural chemicals. Worsening air pollution may be indirectly responsible for the increasing frequency and severity of asthma among American children and children living in other industrialized countries.[8]

Ragweed and pollen provoke seasonal *allergies* in some children and asthma in others. Other asthma-inducing allergens are molds, grasses, goose down, feathers, dust, dust mites, fleas, and cat and dog dander. *Food allergies* (such as to peanuts, egg white, cold drinks, soda, and citrus juice) can also trigger asthma symptoms in some sensitive children.[9] Cow's milk is a well-known but rare trigger for asthma symptoms.[10] Children who are truly allergic to milk almost always have other symptoms besides cough and wheezing, such as hives, diarrhea, or eczema. *Food additives*, such as yellow dyes, sodium benzoate, and sulfites, also trigger asthma in some children.[11, 12] If you think your child might be allergic to foods or food additives, please have him tested by an allergist before you make radical changes in his diet. Many children outgrow their food allergies, though no one knows why (see Chapter 4, Allergies).

Exercise, especially in cold, dry air, triggers symptoms in nearly 90% of asthmatics.[13] Frequent, vigorous exercise in cold, dry air may actually induce chronic asthma.[14] More than half of Swedish elite cross-country skiers, for example, have asthma. Many healthy speed skaters also wheeze after a race.[15] Fortunately, exercise-induced asthma can be effectively prevented and treated. *There is no reason for your child to avoid exercise just because he has been diagnosed with asthma.*

Colds and sinus *infections* are among the most common triggers for asthma. Cold viruses trigger wheezing in 80 to 85 percent of asthmatic children.[16] They can even provoke wheezing and coughing in people who don't have asthma.[17] Sinus infections in children can be subtle and difficult to diagnose. If your child has frequent bouts of asthma, is troubled by nighttime coughing, or has had a cold that lasts more than ten days in a row, talk with your health care provider about the possibility of a sinus infection. Treating the infection can dramatically improve asthma symptoms.

The most common *medication* causing asthma flare-ups is aspirin.[18] Steer clear of aspirin, ibuprofen, and naproxen-containing compounds. Acetaminophen products (e.g., Tylenol) do *not* trigger asthma attacks. Prescription medications known as beta-blockers (such as propanolol), used to prevent migraine headaches, can also trigger asthma symptoms.

Emotional *stress* can cause a tight chest and labored breathing in almost anyone. It's not surprising that children with asthma are more prone to having symptoms at stressful times such as the first day of school, following a death in the family, or during a divorce. Previously it was believed that dysfunctional parents contributed to childhood asthma, and children were sent away to boarding schools to get away from their "toxic" families. A recent study demonstrated that, on the contrary, children's illnesses contribute to parental stress and dysfunction. The more serious the child's illness, the more disruptive for the family.[19]

Asthma can be deadly. If your child has any of the following symptoms, take him for professional care.

SEEK IMMEDIATE PROFESSIONAL CARE IF YOUR CHILD IS

- Having a hard time breathing
- Breathing much more rapidly than usual
- Making a grunting noise when he breathes out
- Getting tired or agitated with his shortness of breath
- Getting blue in the lips or fingertips
- Sucking in the spaces between his ribs with each breath.

MAKE AN APPOINTMENT IF

- Symptoms interfere with sleep or other activities
- The child has a high fever
- The child has a poor appetite

DIAGNOSING AND MONITORING ASTHMA

Observations of coughing, wheezing, and breathing patterns have long been the mainstays of monitoring asthma symptoms.

MONITORING ASTHMA SYMPTOMS

- Daily diary: symptoms, triggers, treatments
- Peak flow meter
- Visits to health care professional four times yearly

Today you can measure your child's lung function at home using a peak flow meter.

You can purchase a peak flow meter for less than $30. Your insurance may cover the cost. A peak flow meter measures how forcefully your child can exhale. Breathing is blocked with asthma, so a low reading on the peak flow meter is an early warning sign that symptoms could soon deteriorate. Children as young as six years old can learn to use a peak flow meter reliably. Children with frequent symptoms should measure their peak flow at least twice daily (morning and evening) and record it in an asthma diary along with symptoms and triggers. Such information will be very helpful to your child, you, and your health care provider in mapping out the best treatment plan for your child.[20] See your doctor four times yearly to monitor your child's growth and response to therapy and to receive support and information about new treatment strategies.

PREVENTING AND TREATING ASTHMA

There are no cures for asthma, but many treatments can help control its symptoms. Optimal treatment is based on careful observation and relies on a combination of biochemical, lifestyle, and other therapies. Let's tour the Therapeutic Mountain to find out what works; if you want to skip to my bottom-line recommendations, flip to the end of the chapter.

BIOCHEMICAL THERAPIES: MEDICATIONS, HERBS, NUTRITIONAL SUPPLEMENTS

Medications

Although modern medication has a lot of shortcomings when it comes to treating colds, it is lifesaving for acute asthma attacks.

MEDICATIONS
(ALL ARE PRESCRIPTION ONLY)

- Preventive: cromolyn or nedocromil, influenza vaccine
- Steroid (sprays and oral forms): maintenance and treatment
- Beta-agonists (albuterol): prevent exercise-provoked symptoms; treat symptoms
- Other: theophylline, ipratropium, adrenalin, terbutaline

Inhaled cromolyn (Intal) and nedocromil (Tilade) help *prevent* asthma symptoms. When sensitive lungs are irritated (by tobacco smoke or cold viruses, for example), they release small amounts of histamine. Histamine causes inflammation and thus asthma symptoms. Cromolyn and nedocromil reduce histamine release and asthma symptoms. They only work when taken *before* the lungs get irritated; they are useless in treating acute attacks. They are my first choice for preventing symptoms in children who have symptoms three or more days a week.[21]

For maximal effectiveness, cromolyn and nedocromil must be taken several times daily for at least two to four weeks before improvements are detectable. Although few side effects have been reported from either medication, nedocromil has only been approved for use in children twelve years of age and older.

Asthma medications can be delivered directly to the lungs by either a nebulizer (a device that turns the medication into a fine mist) or a metered dose inhaler (MDI or "puffer"). Cromolyn is available as either an MDI or a nebulizer solution; nedocromil only comes as an MDI. Home nebulizers are the best way of delivering asthma medication to infants and young children. Some families find it helpful to have a special "nebulizer time" story, game, or puzzle so that treatment is more enjoyable. If your child is very resistant to the nebulizer, try giving him treatments when he's asleep.

Metered dose inhalers are the most widespread and convenient way for older children to take asthma medication. A metal canister containing the medication is inserted in a plastic dispenser. By depressing a button on the canister, a premeasured amount of medication is released into the air. The child inhales the medication, delivering it right where it's needed in the lungs. Metered dose inhalers are as effective as nebulizers if they are used correctly.[22, 23, 24, 25] Children as young as two years old can learn to use MDIs *if they use a spacer.*[26]

HOW TO USE AN MDI

- Shake canister while taking deep breath in and out
- Hold can 1 inch from mouth
- Depress button at the beginning of the next breath in (inhalation)
- Breathe the medication mist in deeply
- Hold breath to count of 10; exhale
- Wait one minute; repeat

Although these directions sound simple, it takes a fair amount of coordination to get the timing right for dispensing the medication just at the beginning of inhaling. If the child has finished breathing in by the time the medicine is dispensed, the medicine evaporates into the surrounding air rather than reaching the lungs where it is needed. That is why spacers were invented.

A *spacer* is a device that holds the medicine in a confined space after its release from an MDI. The medication remains suspended in the space, waiting for the child to take the next breath. Before commercial spacers became available, we used empty toilet paper rolls as spacers. The child put the medication dispenser in one end and his mouth around the other end of the tube. The medication was dispensed, the tube held the aerosolized drug, and the child inhaled the medication during the next breath. Nowadays, more elaborate, aesthetic, and durable spacers are made commercially. Some fold up so they can be carried in a purse or backpack; some make sounds to let the child know when the medication has been inhaled properly. I always write a prescription for a spacer at the same time I write the initial prescription for metered dose medications.

Even very young children can use a metered dose inhaler by using a spacer and a simple trick: after having the child put his mouth around the mouthpiece of the spacer, gently pinch his nostrils together so he has to breathe through his mouth; then dispense the medicine. This forces the child to breathe the medicine in through his mouth and gets it right to his lungs. Some spacers come with face masks that cover the nose and mouth, so even infants can receive MDI medication with the proper spacer and technique.

Children with asthma can have especially severe symptoms with *influenza.* New strains of influenza appear every winter. If your child has asthma, please see your health care provider to get the *influenza vaccine every fall.* Because I am exposed to so many sick children, I get the vaccine myself every year to reduce my chances of getting influenza and passing it on to others.

More physicians are prescribing *inhaled steroids* (such as Aerobid, Azmacort, Beclovent, Decadron, and Vanceril) nowadays to both prevent and treat moderate or severe asthma.[27] Steroids effectively decrease airway inflammation and swelling. If they are given immediately for an acute attack, steroids can often prevent hospitalization.[28] Given when peak flow meter readings start to fall, steroids can prevent asthma flare-ups[29] and are among the most cost-effective treatments for children with chronic asthma symptoms.[30]

These are *not* the kind of steroids that athletes use to bulk up. When steroids are given by MDI, they go directly to the lungs; very little is absorbed into the bloodstream, resulting in very few side effects. A recent analysis of over 800 children showed that inhaled steroids do *not* impair growth.[31] Inhaled steroids can cause throat irritation, hoarseness, and yeast infections in the mouth. These side effects can be reduced by using a spacer (so more of the medicine goes to the lungs and less stays in the mouth) and gargling with plain water after taking it to rinse it out of the mouth.

Children with severe asthma may need to take *steroids by mouth*. Because of the potential side effects of oral steroids (e.g., decreased growth, unstable blood sugar levels, impaired immunity), they should be taken for as short a time as possible. Generally, three to five days of oral steroid treatment are sufficient for most children with a severe asthma attack and may help prevent a hospitalization.[32] For children who are coughing too hard to take medicine by mouth, a steroid injection is as effective as three days of oral therapy.[33]

Beta-agonists (such as albuterol) are the most commonly prescribed asthma medications. They relax airway muscles, allowing the air passages to expand. Beta-agonists effectively prevent exercise-induced asthma; inhaled twenty to thirty minutes prior to vigorous exercise, they reduce breathing problems. You may have seen Olympic athletes using them before practices and competition. Beta-agonists are also useful for the quick relief of flare-ups caused by an allergy or a cold. They start to work in about twenty minutes; benefits last for four to six hours. A new, longer-acting (twelve-hour) beta-agonist medication, *salmeterol,* is more effective than

albuterol, but so far it has only been approved for use by teenagers and adults.[34] Beta-agonist medications are best given by MDIs or nebulizers. For infants and toddlers, beta-agonists can also be given by mouth, but this is not as effective as inhaled treatments, because not as much medicine goes directly to the lungs, and there are more side effects.

The main side effects from beta-agonists are like the side effects from drinking too many cups of coffee: racing heart, high blood pressure, high blood sugar, reduced appetite, or feeling a little "hyper." With overuse, the lungs get used to beta-agonists, requiring higher and higher doses to achieve the same benefit. If your child requires more than three doses in a day or more than three times a week, see your doctor about additional or alternative treatments.

Previously, *theophylline* and its cousin, *aminophylline,* were the therapeutic mainstays for children with asthma. Theophylline is chemically related to caffeine; it helps relax the muscles around the bronchioles, allows the airways to expand, and decreases inflammation.[35] Blood levels need to be monitored closely to minimize side effects.[36] Theophylline fell out of favor because of its many reported side effects: hyperactivity, decreased attention span, decreased appetite, and increased risk of seizures. Theophylline's bad reputation may not be entirely deserved.[37, 38, 39] On the other hand, for children who are already taking other asthma medications such as albuterol, theophylline is probably not helpful, not necessary, and simply adds expense, complication, and aggravation.[40, 41]

Inhaled *ipratropium bromide* (Atrovent) has proven useful for children suffering from severe attacks who needed emergency room treatment, but it is not yet a widespread pediatric asthma treatment.[42] One of my patients with severe asthma uses it daily to prevent the need for hospital care.

One of the quickest treatments for children with an acute attack of severe asthma is a shot of epinephrine (Adrenalin). Adrenalin works well, but it wears off quickly. In the 1970s clinicians started using *terbutaline* injections instead of adrenalin because it is longer lasting. Because adrenalin and terbutaline require injections, they were replaced in the 1980s in most places by inhaled medications, such as albuterol. For children with severe asthma who are hospitalized in intensive care units, terbutaline is still sometimes given by vein to help open up the airways.

Herbs

Herbs have been used to treat asthma by traditional healers around the world. However, there are few scientific studies evaluating their effectiveness compared with other treatments. They do *not* appear to be as effective as medications.

TRADITIONAL CHINESE HERBAL REMEDIES FOR ASTHMA

- Ephedra (*Ma Huang*)
- Chinese skullcap
- Angelica (*Dong Quai*)
- Licorice root

Perhaps the most well-known herbal asthma remedy is *ephedra*, the original source of the old asthma medication ephedrine and the modern decongestant pseudoephedrine. The Chinese have used ephedra for nearly 5,000 years for short-term relief of asthma symptoms. It is chemically related to epinephrine and it has similar side effects: high blood pressure, rapid heartbeat, decreased appetite, and feeling overstimulated, eventually resulting in severe fatigue. Other mainstays of Chinese herbal therapy are *Chinese skullcap*, which has anti-inflammatory properties similar to cromolyn,

angelica (Dong Quai), which relaxes bronchospasm and reduces reactivity to allergens, and *licorice root,* which has anti-inflammatory properties similar to steroids.

Other healing traditions rely on other herbs: Indians use mullein leaf to treat cough, bronchitis, and asthma; Native Americans used black haw bark to treat asthma and other problems. Other traditional remedies for asthma include: coltsfoot, yerba santa, wild cherry bark, ginger root, peppermint, red clover, coleus root,[43] comfrey, lobelia, marsh mallow root, nettle, parsley, and thyme. Adding a strong solution of thyme tea to bath water is believed to help all kinds of coughing illnesses. Thyme is also added to home steam inhalation treatments to soothe irritated airways.

Like medications, herbs can have powerful benefits and side effects. Unfortunately, herbal remedies are sometimes contaminated; strengths and dosing are not standardized. Until there is better research on their safety and effectiveness, I do *not* recommend herbal remedies for asthmatic children.

Nutritional Supplements

NUTRITIONAL SUPPLEMENTS FOR ASTHMA

- Vitamin B6 (pyridoxine)
- Vitamin B12
- Vitamin C
- Magnesium
- Fish oils

Supplemental *pyridoxine* has proven helpful in reducing the number of asthma attacks, the severity of symptoms, and the need for medications in a double-blind study of asthmatic children.[44] Pyridoxine doses of 50 to 200 milligrams per day for at least one month were required before benefits were seen. A similar trial did *not* demonstrate pyridoxine's effectiveness for adults with severe asthma who were already receiving powerful asthma medications.[45] Do not try more than 100 milligrams daily without consulting your doctor; higher doses can lead to side effects such as numbness or tingling in the hands and feet.

One adult study suggests that adverse reactions to sulfites can be prevented by taking 1.5 milligrams of *vitamin B12* before ingesting sulfites.[46] There have not been any controlled comparison studies, and it is difficult to anticipate such exposures in time to pretreat. I do *not* recommend it.

In ancient days, the relationship between scurvy (severe vitamin C deficiency) and asthma was well known. However, the benefit of megadoses of *vitamin C* in reducing asthma remains controversial. Vitamin C reduces reactivity to histamine, the lung chemical that causes bronchospasm.[47] Adults whose diets are naturally high in vitamin C have the fewest breathing problems such as asthma[48]; at least 300 to 500 milligrams of vitamin C daily are necessary to have a noticeable effect. That's about five times the Recommended Daily Allowance, or four to six tall glasses of orange juice. Vitamin C given prior to exercise does *not* reduce symptoms. Six months of daily vitamin C (1 gram per day) did *not* improve asthma symptoms in one study.[49] On the other hand, a double-blind comparison study of 1 gram of vitamin C taken daily significantly improved symptoms in adult Nigerian asthmatics.[50] Giving your child 500 to 1,000 milligrams (1/2 to 1 gram) per day is probably safe, though its effectiveness remains controversial.

Lower dietary *magnesium* intake is associated with more wheezing.[51] Higher dietary magnesium is associated with fewer breathing problems. Magnesium (300 milligrams to 2 grams depending on the child's weight)

given by vein during a severe asthma attack helps reduce symptoms in both adults and children.[52, 53, 54, 55] There are no studies evaluating the effectiveness of oral magnesium supplements in preventing childhood asthma episodes. Oral magnesium therapy remains experimental.

Oils from *fatty fish* such as mackerel, salmon, sardines, and tuna may reduce the body's production of inflammatory chemicals.[56] However, the impact of these changes on asthma symptoms is unclear.[57] Adults who eat more fish tend to have better lung function than those who avoid fish.[58] In one study, adults who took supplemental fish oils for nine months had fewer asthma symptoms than others who took placebo pills. Another study showed that fish oil supplements were no more helpful than olive oil placebos.[59] No similar studies have been done on asthmatic children. I do *not* recommend that you spend your money on fish oil supplements for your wheezing child, but a moderate intake of fish is part of a healthy diet.

LIFESTYLE THERAPIES: NUTRITION, EXERCISE, ENVIRONMENT, MIND-BODY

Nutrition

NUTRITIONAL THERAPIES FOR ASTHMA

Do:

- Breast-feed
- Give plenty of water
- Try onions and spicy foods
- Try coffee

Don't:

- Ingest sulfites, preservatives, yellow dyes
- Ingest excessive tryptophan

Start your child's life right by *breast-feeding.* Breast-feeding reduces wheezing in the first month of life,[60] and the benefits persist throughout the first six *years* of life.[61] Make sure that your child gets plenty of *water.* Water helps keep secretions thin and loose, preventing mucus in the lungs from getting dry, sticky, and difficult to clear.

It appears that certain active compounds in *onions and spicy foods* such as red peppers can reduce the release of histamine, the chemical responsible for much of asthma's symptoms.[62, 63] There are no scientific studies to assess onion's effectiveness in treating asthma in humans, but one study in guinea pigs suggested that eating onion extracts might reduce subsequent reactions to allergens.[64] I have no idea how many onions a child would need to eat to affect asthma symptoms. Some parents believe that hot spices such as horseradish, mustard, and chili peppers are also helpful in preventing asthma symptoms. Since onion and hot spices are common cooking ingredients, you may want to experiment yourself: note onion and spice intake and asthma symptoms in your child's asthma journal to see how much better (or worse) he is on the days he eats (or doesn't eat) these foods.

Coffee for asthma? In the 1800s it was the treatment of choice. Caffeine is chemically related to the asthma medication theophylline. Large Italian and American studies show that adults who drink 2 to 3 cups of coffee daily have about 25% less asthma than those who abstain.[65] There is no benefit to drinking more than 3 cups daily. There are *no* recent studies evaluating the effects of caffeine on childhood asthma. Don't try to substitute caffeine-containing colas; colas can actually trigger asthma symptoms in some children.[66] Coffee is relatively inexpensive and widely available. If you want to try it for your child, remember that less coffee would be needed for smaller chil-

dren than for adults and that coffee can have significant side effects.

Sulfite preservatives, benzoic acid, MSG, and *yellow dyes* may trigger your child's asthma.[67, 68] Sulfites (chemically related to the sulfur dioxide in smog) are commonly sprayed on fresh fruits and vegetables (beware of restaurant salad bars!), added to certain snacks, orange drinks, beer, and wine. It may be that the real culprit for coughs associated with foods is either allergies to additives or sensitivity to the temperature or acidity of the food being eaten.[69] If you are not sure if your child is sensitive to preservatives or dyes, read labels for all prepared food, wash all fresh fruits and vegetables thoroughly before serving them, and consider serving only organically grown produce.

Common foods may trigger asthma in some people. A Swedish study of asthmatic adults showed an improvement on a diet low in *tryptophan,* an amino acid found in milk, cheese, turkey, and bananas.[70] Asthmatic adults improved when they were placed on a very strict diet (no meat, fish, fowl, dairy, eggs, chocolate, coffee, apples, or citrus) for a year.[71] In a Danish study, the symptoms of hospitalized adult asthmatics improved when they were placed on a hypoallergenic, elemental diet.[72] It is not clear which of the eliminated foods was the culprit. It is possible that the discipline required to follow this strict diet stimulated the psycho-neuro-immunologic system to improve symptoms. These studies have *not* been duplicated in children. If you decide to radically rearrange your child's diet, seek the guidance of a professional nutritionist to avoid deficiencies of essential nutrients.

Many parents believe that *milk* increases mucus and worsens asthma symptoms. This idea was tested in a randomized, controlled trial in asthmatic adults. Milk did not cause coughing, wheezing, or impaired lung function.[73] Milk does *not* make asthma worse.

Exercise

Yoga, particularly yogic breathing (prana-yama), helps reduce the frequency of asthma attacks in young adults.[74, 75, 76] The proven breathing exercises emphasize slow, regular breaths in which the ratio of inhalation (breathing in) to exhalation (breathing out) is 1:2. For example, have your child breathe in for a count of five and breathe out to a count of ten. The benefits can be enhanced by breathing hot, moist air. It is not known whether yoga is helpful because of general relaxation or because of specific effects in the lungs. Nevertheless, it is straightforward, inexpensive, and free of side effects. Try it!

Another good breathing exercise for asthmatic children is called *pursed lips breathing*. In this technique, children purse their lips and blow out as if blowing a kiss. Adults with severe lung disease who practiced this technique were able to increase their blood oxygen levels during pursed lips breathing alone without any other therapy.[77]

Swimming is a great exercise for youngsters with asthma because the humidity in pools is very high; on the other hand, some kids are sensitive to the high chlorine levels.[78] There's no way to tell beforehand, so give it a cautious try.

PREVENTION STRATEGIES FOR EXERCISE-INDUCED ASTHMA

- A fifteen- to thirty-minute warm-up period before vigorous exercise[79]
- Breathing in through the nose—not the mouth—to warm and filter outside air before it hits the lungs
- Covering the nose and mouth with a loose-fitting scarf or bandanna when exercising outdoors on especially cold days

Environment

Avoiding environmental triggers is the best way to prevent your child from having asthma flare-ups.

REDUCING AIRBORNE ASTHMA TRIGGERS

- *No smoking* anywhere near the child
- HEPA air filters; furnace and air-conditioner filters
- Houseplants: philodendrons, spider plants
- Windows closed 5 a.m. to 10 a.m. when pollen counts are high
- Reduce air pollution: ride a bike or take a bus

Avoiding cigarette smoke reduces the risk of many heart and lung diseases, including childhood asthma. Free-standing HEPA electronic air filters efficiently remove airborne asthma triggers inside the home.[80] Recent research has shown that potting soil and common house plants (such as spider plants, philodendron, bamboo palm, and English ivy) absorb some indoor air pollutants.[81] Change or replace your furnace filter and air-conditioning filter regularly. Consider installing an electrostatic air filter on your furnace; some filters can effectively remove over 90% of airborne irritants and allergens. Check *Consumer Reports* for the best buys. Keep your child indoors when air quality is bad. Pollen counts are usually highest between 5 and 10 a.m., so keep the windows closed during early morning hours. To reduce outdoor air pollution, think of carpooling, using buses or bicycles, and working for tougher antipollution laws as ways of helping your child stay healthy throughout life.

Many children who suffer from chronic asthma are sensitive to *dust* and microscopic *dust mites*.[82] By reducing the levels of household dust and dust mites, you can help your child reduce asthma and allergy symptoms.[83, 84] Eliminate dust-catchers such as old carpeting, feather pillows, dust ruffles around the bed, wool blankets, and down comforters in the child's bedroom. Consider switching from foam or feather pillows to Dacron, which is much less allergenic. Dust mites love to live in mattresses and pillows. Keep them away from your child by encasing the mattress and pillow in a plastic or vinyl fitted sheet.[85] Wash your child's sheets, pillow cases, and blankets weekly in hot water to kill dust mites. Engage in a weekly cleanup campaign to fight dust and mold in the child's room; damp mopping helps remove dust without stirring it up.[86] Consider spraying carpets and upholstery with a dust mite killer.[87] Spray carpet and upholstery with a 3% tannic acid solution or benzylbenzoate (chemicals that kill the dust mite) every two to three months.[88] Clean thoroughly after spraying to remove all of the dead dust mite particles.

Furry pets should not sleep in your child's bedroom. Furry pets should be confined either to the outdoors or to a noncarpeted room that is easily cleaned and in which the child does not spend a lot of time. If your child is visiting a home with furry pets, pretreat the child with asthma medication prior to the visit.

Mold, a common asthma trigger, is a problem in humid climates and in households that cook a lot of pasta or rice because of all the water vapor in the air. Try to keep household humidity less than 50% with a dehumidifier, and frequently clean any visible mold or mildew with a 10% bleach solution.

Negative *ion generators* have *no* proven benefits for asthmatic adults or children.[89] I do *not* recommend them. While *mist* and steam from vaporizers are often soothing for children with colds, sinus infections, and bronchitis, they are not very helpful for children with asthma.

Mind-Body

Stress is a major trigger for asthma symptoms. Asthma symptoms are very susceptible to the power of suggestion. In numerous comparison studies of asthma medications, 20 to 30 percent of patients improve with placebo treatment alone.[90]

Hypnosis or therapeutic imagery has proven useful in improving lung function and symptoms in asthmatic children.[91, 92, 93] Relaxation and breathing exercises are a worthwhile addition to a comprehensive asthma management program for children because hypnosis and relaxation exercises are so straightforward and safe.[94] A trained therapist should be able to get you started on a home program of your own.[95] In the meantime, it is important for parents to remain calm and confident when their child has an asthma attack. Plan your strategy in advance. When parents stay calm and relaxed, children have an easier time relaxing, addressing the problem, and reducing symptoms.

Like self-hypnosis, *autogenic training* has proven effective in reducing chronic asthma symptoms.[96] (See Appendix B for more information on how to do autogenic training.) Daily practice is essential for maximal effectiveness of mind-body therapies.

Biofeedback can also be a useful therapy for asthmatics. In a fifteen-month follow-up of seventeen adult asthmatics who were trained with biofeedback devices to improve their breathing, there were fewer and less severe asthma attacks, requiring less medication and resulting in fewer visits to the emergency room for over a year following training.[97] Other studies have reported success in children as well[98, 99]; if your child has persistent, recurrent symptoms, biofeedback may be worth trying.

Seek *support* from other families who have asthmatic children. Sharing stories and strategies helps decrease isolation and make stress more manageable.

BIOMECHANICAL THERAPIES: PHYSICAL THERAPY, SPINAL MANIPULATION

Physical Therapy

Physical therapy treatments (pounding on the chest to help clear mucus) have been proved *not* to benefit asthmatic children.[100] I do *not* recommend it for asthma.

Spinal Manipulation

Spinal manipulation is used by chiropractors, naturopaths, and osteopaths in treating adults with asthma. There have NOT been any comparison trials documenting the effectiveness of spinal manipulation in preventing asthma, and I do *not* recommend it.

BIOENERGETIC THERAPIES: ACUPUNCTURE, THERAPEUTIC TOUCH, PRAYER, HOMEOPATHY

Acupuncture

Acupuncture can reduce asthma symptoms if given during an acute attack, but it must be done by someone highly trained, the child must be willing to be treated with nee-dles, and even then it is not as effective as medical therapies such as albuterol. Asthmatic children treated with acupuncture twenty minutes before *exercise* have milder symptoms,[101, 102] but acupuncture has had mixed results in treating chronic asthma symptoms.[103, 104] Even in China, acupuncture is not usually used as the only remedy for people with asthma, but it is used in combination with herbs or Western medications.

Therapeutic Touch

There have not been any studies of the effectiveness of Therapeutic Touch in treating asthma symptoms. However, in my own practice I have watched children's oxygen levels climb and breathing relax during Therapeutic Touch treatment. I incorporate Therapeutic Touch into my therapy for children during acute asthma attacks.

Prayer

Prayer helped reduce symptoms in one study of asthmatic adults.[105] I recommend prayer if it is consistent with your family's values and beliefs.

Homeopathy

Homeopathy shows some promise in treating allergic asthma in adults.[106] Common asthma remedies include Arsenica, Antimonia, Chamomilla, Ipecac, Lobelia, Nux vomica, and Pulsatilla. However, there are *no* published studies of homeopathy in preventing or treating asthmatic children. Homeopaths themselves advise parents not to treat symptoms of acute asthma with homeopathic remedies alone.

WHAT I RECOMMEND FOR ASTHMA

PREVENTING ASTHMA

1. *Lifestyle—nutrition.* Start your child off right by breast-feeding. Give plenty of fluids, especially when your child has a cold.

2. *Lifestyle—environment.* Do *not* smoke and do not allow others to smoke around your child. Avoid allergy triggers. Work for clean air in your community.

See Your Health Care Professional If Your Child Is

- Having a hard time breathing
- Breathing much more rapidly than usual
- Making a grunting noise when breathing out
- Getting tired or agitated with his shortness of breath
- Getting blue in the lips or fingertips
- Sucking in the spaces between his ribs with each breath
- Having symptoms that interfere with sleep or other activities or has a high fever or poor appetite
- Or if you have *any* concerns about your child's breathing or he is not improving with home therapies

---

TREATING ASTHMA

Help children monitor their symptoms using a peak flow meter and keep a record of symptoms, triggers, treatments, and peak flow meter readings. If they have symptoms, treat them promptly.

1. *Biochemical—medications.* Work with your physician or other health care professional to develop the best plan for using medications to prevent and treat asthma. In general, cromolyn and nedocromil help prevent symptoms, and beta-agonists and steroids are useful once symptoms have begun. Have your child immunized against influenza every fall. Do *not* rely on nonprescription medications.

2. *Lifestyle—environment.* Avoid triggers such as allergens, dust and mold, and foods that trigger your child's asthma. Don't let furry pets sleep in your child's room. Work for cleaner air in your home and in your environment. Thoroughly clean your child's room weekly. Consider using an electronic air filter and adding house plants such as philodendron to your child's room.

3. *Lifestyle—exercise.* Don't limit your child's exercise. Asthma symptoms can be controlled even during vigorous exercise. Have your child try yoga (especially yogic breathing), pursed lips breathing exercises, or swimming. Have your child warm up before exercise; breathe through the nose, not the mouth; and cover nose and mouth with a scarf when exercising in very cold weather.

4. *Lifestyle—mind-body.* Consider training in self-hypnosis or autogenic training. Communicate with other adults who care for your child about your child's asthma. Get support. Teachers, day care workers, baby-sitters, and relatives need to know what symptoms to look for, what your care plan is, and how to reach your child's health care professional in case of an emergency. Remind yourself and your child to have fun! Asthma can be serious, but with an appropriate treatment plan, your child should be able to have a happy, normal childhood.

5. *Lifestyle—nutrition.* Consider supplemental onions and spicy foods. Give your child foods rich in vitamin C and magnesium, and include fish in his diet. Avoid sulfite preservatives.

6. *Biochemical—nutritional supplements.* Consider supplemental pyridoxine, and vitamin C.

7. *Bioenergetic—prayer.* If it is consistent with your family's beliefs.

RESOURCES

American Lung Association
1740 Broadway
New York, NY 10019–4374
1(800)LUNG USA or
1(212)315–8700

Asthma and Allergy
    Foundation of America
1717 Massachusetts Avenue
Washington, DC 20036
1(800)727–8462

National Allergy and Asthma
    Network
1(800)878–4403

National Asthma Education
    Program
National Heart Lung and
    Blood Institute
1(301)251–1222

Sources for Peak Flow Meters

Armstrong Industries, Inc.
PO Box 7
Northbrook, IL 60062
1(800)323–4220

Healthscan Products, Inc.
908 Pompton Avenue
Cedar Grove, NJ 07009
1(800)962–1266

Sources for Peak Flow Meters (cont.)

Mini Wright's Peak Flow
Clement Clarke
1(800)848–8923

Source for Asthma Diaries

Asthma Peak Flow Diary
Pedipress, Inc.
125 Red Gate Lane
Amherst, MA 01002

Books

Astor, Stephen. *Empty Your Bucket: Practical Steps to Overcome Allergy and Asthma.* Mountain View, Calif.: Two A's Industries, 1992.

Plaut, Thomas F. *Children with Asthma: A Manual for Parents.* 2nd ed. Amherst, Mass.: Pedipress, 1988.

Rogers, A. *Luke Has Asthma Too.* Burlington, Vt.:Waterfront Books, 1987.

Parcel G., Tiernan K., Nader P., Weiner L. *Teaching Myself about Asthma.* Columbia, S.C.: Health Education Associates, 1984.

6

BED-WETTING
(ENURESIS)

Maggie Murphy brought her seven-year-old son, Matthew, in to see me several months ago for his annual checkup. When I asked what concerns they had about Matt's health, they looked at each other sheepishly. "Well," Maggie began, "Matt wants to join the Scouts this year, but they have overnight camping trips, and he can't always make it through the night without an accident." Matt looked down at the floor. I looked directly at him. "There's no need to be embarrassed about this, Matt. Lots of boys your age have the same problem. Let me ask you a few more questions, and then we'll do some tests on your urine, and I can give you a few ideas for things to try at home." Matt looked cautious but hopeful. "OK, but am I going to have to take drugs or have a blood test?" "No. You definitely don't need a blood test today, and most boys learn to manage this problem just fine without any medication."

Bed-wetting (or enuresis, as it's known in medical circles) is the most common bladder problem affecting children. Everyone starts life without control over their bladder. We don't expect babies or toddlers to stay dry by themselves. Bladder control is usually learned after bowel control. Most children are dry during the daytime many weeks or even months before they are dry at night (usually by three to four years old). Many children don't develop full control of their bladders until about school age, and some take even longer.

Bed-wetting was noted as a medical problem in papyrus writings dating back to 1550 B.C. Between 5 and 15 percent of seven-year-old boys occasionally wet the bed.[1] There are two kinds of enuresis: *primary* (never has been dry at night) and *secondary* (was dry at night at one point and is now wetting again). Primary enuresis is the most common kind of bed-wetting. It is more common in boys and tends to run in families.

Matt had never been completely dry at night, though he had been fine during the daytime for two years. He didn't wet every night, but there was a problem at least three nights a week. His mother told me that Matt's father had had the same problem when he was a boy and hadn't outgrown it until he was ten. Both parents wanted Matt to be spared the embarrassment of having an accident while he was out camping or spending the night with friends. It sounded to me as if Matt had a classic case of primary enuresis, but I wanted to check his urine, just to make sure he didn't have a secondary reason for bed-wetting.

Secondary enuresis can be a sign of an underlying medical problem (such as a bladder infection, constipation, or diabetes) or a sudden emotional stress (such as moving or having a new baby at home), causing the child's behavior to regress. Unfortunately, another cause of bed-wetting in girls who have been dry in the past is sexual abuse or molestation. If your child has been dry at night for a while and suddenly starts wetting again, have him checked by your health care professional.

Constipation is a common cause of secondary enuresis.[2] When the colon is stretched full, it rubs up against the bladder, irritating it, putting pressure on it, and making the child feel as if he has to urinate even though his bladder isn't full. If your child is constipated and wets the bed, treat the constipation first (see Chapter 12). Once the constipation has been resolved, the bed-wetting may no longer be a problem.[3]

Children suffering from enuresis also frequently suffer from *allergies* such as hay fever, hives, and eczema. This has led many people to believe that enuresis is just another manifestation of allergy, especially food allergy.[4] Rather than causing a skin rash or wheezing, these allergic reactions are thought to irritate the bladder, sending it into spasms. Commonly blamed food allergens are cow's milk, chocolate, eggs, wheat, and citrus fruit. *Caffeine* is a known bladder irritant. Like coffee and tea, *chocolate* contains caffeine and should be avoided by children suffering from enuresis.

Many parents think that bed-wetting is a sleep problem.[5] It's not. Extensive studies have shown that children who wet the bed are *not* necessarily more sound sleepers. Children who wet the bed sleep normally. Bed-wetting doesn't just occur during deep sleep or dreaming sleep; it occurs when the child's bladder is full.

Enuresis is also *not* necessarily a sign of psychological or emotional problems. It is *not* a sign of bad parenting or a sign that the child is bad, willful, or lazy. On the contrary, enuresis can *cause* humiliation and lower self-esteem.[6] Punishing a child who suffers from enuresis just adds to the burden of guilt and makes it less likely that the child will be able to summon up the inner resources to overcome the problem. Successfully resolving the problem boosts a child's self-esteem and improves performance in school and social situations as well.[7]

Matt's urine test showed no sign of infection or diabetes. Neither he nor his mother could identify any recent stresses, except the stress of bed-wetting. His parents were divided about how to handle it. Maggie just wanted to use a plastic mattress cover, change the sheets when they needed it, and wait until Matt outgrew it. His father thought Matt should lose TV privileges for his wet nights and not be allowed to go on overnight trips until he learned better. It sounded as if both parents needed to learn more about enuresis.

At school age, about 10% of children still wet the bed regularly; this means that one out of every ten children (or three children in a class of thirty) in first grade has a problem with nighttime wetting. By fifteen years of age, 2% of children still suffer from occasional bed-wetting. Remember, unless there is an anatomic problem or underlying illness, everybody eventually outgrows enuresis.

CAUSES OF ENURESIS

- Genetic—runs in families
- Small bladder
- Slow hormonal maturation

Like many problems, enuresis tends to *run in families*. A child whose father was a bed-wetter has a 40 to 50 percent chance of being one too. If both parents suffered from enuresis, the child has a 70 to 80 percent chance of being a bed-wetter! For unknown reasons, enuresis is more common in boys than girls. Enuresis is *not* caused by poverty or ignorance,[8] but it is more common in crowded living conditions and families in which one or both parents smoke.[9]

Children with enuresis tend to have *smaller bladders* than other children.[10] Children with small bladders have to make frequent trips to the bathroom. You can check your child's bladder capacity by having him hold his urine as long as he can after he feels he has to go (in the daytime), and then have him void into a container. A normal child should be able to hold (and void) his age in years plus two in ounces.[11] For example, a seven-year-old should be able to void

7 + 2 = 9 ounces.

The adult bladder capacity is reached between ten and fourteen years of age.

NORMAL BLADDER CAPACITY	
AGE IN YEARS	*VOLUME IN OUNCES*
6	8
8	10
10	12
12	14

The brain monitors the balance of salt and water throughout the body. It sends hormonal messages to the kidneys about how much salt and water to save and how much to release. The brain's hormonal messenger, antidiuretic hormone (ADH), tells the kidneys how much urine to make. *Lower* ADH levels tell the kidneys to make *more* urine and to make the urine more dilute (watery). *Higher* ADH levels tell the kidneys to make *less* urine and to make the urine more concentrated.

As a child grows and develops, the brain gradually makes more ADH during the nighttime and less ADH during the day. More ADH at night means less urine is produced, so the bladder doesn't fill as quickly. This is what saves us from having to urinate every three to four hours at night. Low daytime ADH levels tell the kidney to make more urine when it is easy to empty a full bladder.

Children suffering from enuresis secrete the same amount of ADH around the clock. They don't develop the difference in daytime vs. nighttime ADH secretion at the same age as other children.[12] This means their kidneys produce urine as fast at night as during the day, filling their (relatively small) bladders every few hours.[13] Some enuretic children have such low levels of nighttime ADH they produce enough urine to fill four normal bladders at night.[14] A full bladder needs to be emptied. If the child doesn't wake up when the bladder is full, it empties while he's asleep, and the bed is wet. Most children *do* eventually develop the day-night differences in ADH secretion that allow them to go through the night without urinating. In the meantime, they need to be trained to wake up when their bladder is full, so they can empty it in the toilet rather than in the bed.

How to Treat Enuresis

No matter how you decide to help your child with enuresis, *make at least one visit to your health care professional* to make sure your child doesn't have a bladder infection, early diabetes, or some other reason for excessive urination. These kinds of disease account for less than 5% of enuresis, but they are the kinds of things you wouldn't want to overlook. Let's tour the Therapeutic Mountain to find out what works for treating enuresis. If you want to skip to my bottom-line recommendations, flip to the end of the chapter.

Biochemical Therapies: Medication, Herbs

Medications and herbs are *not* the first choices for treating enuresis. The primary treatments for enuresis are changes in lifestyle: diet, exercise, environment, and behavior (mind-body). Nevertheless, if changes in lifestyle alone do *not* cure the problem, biochemical therapy may be helpful for some children.

Medication

No *nonprescription* medications are useful in treating enuresis.

PRESCRIPTION MEDICATIONS FOR ENURESIS

- Imipramine (Tofranil)
- DDAVP pills or nasal spray (Minirin)
- Oxybutynin (Ditropan)

Several types of powerful medication have been used to treat enuresis. For several years, the most commonly prescribed medication was *imipramine (Tofranil).*[15] Imipramine is in the antidepressant family of drugs, but it works in enuresis by increasing bladder capacity and decreasing spontaneous bladder contractions. It is taken just before bedtime. It is effective for many children while they are taking it, but many children relapse after they stop the medication. *Overdoses of imipramine can be fatal.* Many physicians have stopped prescribing imipramine because of the obvious hazards of having a potentially fatal drug around a child who has low self-esteem or depression because of his enuresis.

The new favorite medication for enuresis is *DDAVP.* DDAVP is a synthetic form of antidiuretic hormone, which tells kidneys to make less urine. DDAVP is one of only a few drugs that is as effective when given as a nasal spray as it is when taken by mouth.[16] DDAVP is very effective in children over nine years old.[17] It reduces the average number of wet nights per week from an average of four or five to an average of two or three compared with placebo pills.[18]

Unfortunately, bed-wetting frequently reoccurs when the medication is stopped because DDAVP doesn't really change hormonal maturation.[19] DDAVP is also pretty expensive ($50 to $100 per month). About 4% of children have significant side effects with DDAVP.[20] Their kidneys overconcentrate the urine, resulting in water-salt imbalances throughout the body, and even seizures in some children.[21] This risk can be minimized if the child does not drink anything after dinner. Nevertheless, DDAVP is safer than imipramine; it has become the medication of choice (when medications are needed) for treating children who wet the bed.[22] Over the long term, however, DDAVP is less effective than *Lifestyle* approaches. I do *not* recommend it unless other treatments have failed or the child needs it occasionally to avoid embarrassment on an important overnight trip.[23] Even then, DDAVP is far from 100% effective.

A third drug, *oxybutynin (Ditropan)*, decreases bladder contractions, but in a controlled trial it was *not* found to be helpful in treating children with enuresis.[24]

Herbs

There are no scientific studies evaluating the effectiveness of any herbal remedy in treating childhood enuresis. Children who suffer from enuresis should *avoid* hops, valerian, skullcap, and passion flower. These herbs promote deep sleep, potentially impairing the ability to awaken when the bladder is full.

Teas made of chamomile, corn silk, comfrey root, couch grass, horsetail, juniper, oatstraw, Saint-John's-wort, uva ursi (bear berry leaves), and yarrow have been recommended to decrease bladder irritation and improve bladder tone. Horsetail and juniper are actually weak diuretics (increase urination); they may dehydrate the child during the day, so there is less water in the system to cause problems at night. Despite this rationale, it just doesn't make sense to me to treat a child who is suffering from excessive wetting with an herb or medication that increases urination. Juniper irritates the kidneys and can cause problems if taken when the kidneys are already afflicted with an infection. Uva ursi is a diuretic that also calms bladder spasms and decreases bladder inflammation; it is a common ingredient in kidney and bladder teas sold in Europe. Until studies are performed comparing herbal remedies to other effective treatments, I do *not* recommend them for bed-wetting.

LIFESTYLE THERAPIES: NUTRITION, EXERCISE, ENVIRONMENT, MIND-BODY

Nutrition

Do not let your child drink any fluids for at least one or two hours before going to bed. This helps reduce the strain on a small bladder's capacity to make it through the night without being emptied.

Some have suggested that enuresis can be caused by *intolerance or allergy* to *cow's milk* or other foods (chocolate, eggs, grain, citrus fruit). This belief has led to trials of hypoallergenic diets as treatments for bedwetting. Although some investigators have reported success with elimination diets,[25, 26] their studies did *not* include control groups, and there was probably a strong placebo effect at work. A later study that compared dietary restriction to imipramine (medication) showed that the medication was far more effective.[27] I do *not* recommend that you embark on an elimination diet for your child unless

- he has other allergy symptoms (eczema, hay fever, wheezing, diarrhea),
- other treatments for the enuresis have failed, *and*
- you seek professional guidance from a nutritionist to make sure your child maintains a balanced diet.

Exercise

If your child has a small bladder, try *bladder-stretching exercises* during the day. Bladder-stretching exercises have proven effectiveness in treating enuresis.[28]

BLADDER-STRETCHING EXERCISE 1

1. Agree in advance on some small reward (stickers or vouchers that can be redeemed for a larger reward such as a trip to a ball game) for successfully delaying voiding.
2. Ask your child to notice when he has to urinate, and ask him to hold his urine.
3. Set a portable timer for five minutes, and have him try to wait until the timer goes off before he voids.
4. Gradually increase the time on the timer to ten minutes during the second week of practice, then fifteen minutes the third week.

This exercise gets the child in the habit of overcoming the initial bladder spasms.

BLADDER-STRETCHING EXERCISE 2

1. Have your child drink 8 to 12 ounces of water.
2. Have him note his initial urge to urinate.
3. Have him count as high as he can while he holds his urine until it becomes uncomfortable.
4. Measure and record the amount voided and the number reached during counting.
5. Give rewards for being able to hold the urine longer and counting higher before voiding. Make it a game to see how high the child can count before he has to void.

A third exercise helps kids gain a sense of control over the urination process.

BLADDER-STRETCHING EXERCISE 3

WHILE THE CHILD IS VOIDING, HAVE HIM PRACTICE

1. Stopping (interrupting the stream),
2. Holding it a second, and
3. Restarting the stream.

Practice at least once a day until the child gains a sense of mastery in being able to start and stop at will.

Bladder-stretching exercises work best if you are calm about both success and failure. Progress is gradual, as it is with all types of exercise. Relapses are common when a child is overexcited, overtired, afraid, or anxious. Don't emphasize your child's misses; instead, reward successes. Remeasure his bladder capacity once a week to see how well the bladder is stretching. Celebrate successes!

Environment

If your child is still potty training and has a hard time making it to the bathroom in the middle of the night, put the potty chair in his bedroom so he doesn't have as far to go.

Mind-Body

Bed-wetting is *not* a sign of parental or child failure. It is simply a sign of a small bladder and a possible delay in developing hormonal rhythms for antidiuretic hormone. While the bladder is stretching and the hormones are coming into balance, a number of mind-body remedies have proven effectiveness.

MIND-BODY THERAPIES FOR ENURESIS

- Behavior
- Punishment is *not* helpful
- Responsibility
- Tracking on a calendar
- Rewards
- Alarms
- Hypnotherapy
- Biofeedback

Some parents believe that **punishment** will stop enuresis. This is misguided. It is *not* helpful to yell at, humiliate, allow siblings to tease, or physically punish the child. These punishments just make the child feel more ashamed and lower the child's sense of self-esteem. It is helpful to be calm and to give the child **responsibility** for cleaning up his clothing and bedding (changing clothes and putting the wet things in the washing machine or laundry basket). It is helpful to **track** dry nights on a calendar. It is also helpful to give praise, stickers, and other **rewards** for dry nights.

One of the most effective treatments for enuresis is the *bed-wetting alarm*. Bed-wetting alarms have a cure rate of 70 to 90 percent, which is higher and longer lasting than any medication. Alarms also raise a child's self-esteem because they actually train him to wake up rather than simply create a dependency on a drug.[29] They are especially useful to train children with small bladders to awaken when the bladder is full.[30, 31] Most alarms are lightweight and are easily attached to the child's pajama bottoms. The devices are sensitive to just a few drops of urine. When urine is sensed, the alarm rings, awakening the child and alerting him to finish voiding in the bathroom.

Several different brands of alarms are available. Many cost less than $50—about the price of one visit to the doctor. Some doctors and clinics have programs in which the alarm can be rented for even less. Some insurance policies will cover an enuresis alarm if the health professional writes a prescription for it as a medical device.

Make sure you tell your child that this is *his* alarm and that he is responsible for hooking it up, testing it out, and responding to it. Success with this treatment is directly tied to the child's motivation and the family's support.[32] Do help your child by making sure he wakes up the first few times the alarm goes off; encourage him to get to the bathroom, change pajamas, reattach the alarm, and put a towel over the wet spot on the bed or change the sheets. It usually takes a couple of months to achieve consistent dryness. Continue using the alarm for a few weeks after dryness has been achieved, just to be sure the child has learned to wake up on his own. Alarms are especially effective in combination with bladder-stretching exercises (described in the Exercise section).[33] Nearly 100% effectiveness can be achieved by combining alarms with rewards for following the instructions.

ALARM INSTRUCTIONS

1. Turn off the alarm.

2. Get out of bed.

3. Go to the bathroom to finish voiding.

4. Reset the alarm.

5. Go back to bed.

If you want to try something even simpler and less expensive, set an *alarm clock* for three hours after he goes to sleep. When the alarm goes off, wake the child up and have him empty his bladder in the toilet. Do this several nights in a row. Do *not* set the alarm for more than two awakenings at night or you could interfere with his sleep so much that he has trouble functioning during the day. Gradually reduce the time to two hours, then one hour, then have the child wake himself. One study showed a 92% success rate within one month of using the alarm clock treatment.[34] Another study showed that alarm clock wakening did *not* add anything to the usual treatment of bladder stretching and rewarding dry nights.[35] A third study showed that alarm clock wakening in combination with bladder-stretching exercises was more effective than medication.[36] Give it a try!

Hypnotherapy is another technique that has helped thousands of children. It is my treatment of choice during an initial visit for enuresis.[37] Actually, I combine hypnosis with

(1) keeping a calendar, (2) rewarding dry nights, (3) bladder–stretching exercises, and (4) having the child change his own pajamas and sheets. If these treatments do not start working within six weeks, I recommend the alarm clock approach, awakening the child every three hours so he can void in the toilet. Hypnosis or *imagining therapy* has proven as effective as medication, and the results are more long-lasting.[38] You do *not* need to be a professional therapist to use these techniques yourself at home.

The technique I use involves using the child's imagination to visualize the connections between his brain, his bladder, and the muscles that allow the urine to flow out or keep it in. Help the child visualize these parts by drawing a picture.

Staying Dry

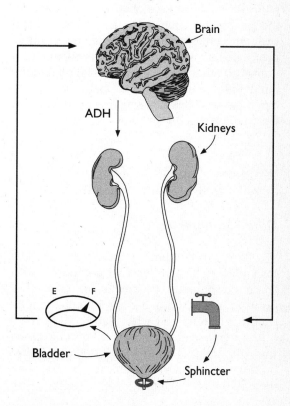

He can imagine or pretend what it feels like to have a full bladder, see the nerves telling the brain the bladder is full, and imagine the brain deciding whether to tell the nerves and muscles to keep the urine in or let it flow out. If the brain decides to let the urine flow out, it can wake up the rest of the body so the child can urinate in the bathroom rather than in bed. The brain can tell the nerves and muscles to keep the urine in until he gets out of bed and goes to the bathroom. Remind your child that the bladder, nerves, brain, and muscles are already doing this job very well during the day. Assure your child that you are confident that they can do this job at night, too. You can help your child practice imagining this picture during the day and right before he goes to sleep. Reward your child for success in making it to the bathroom before he urinates.

Biofeedback therapy can effectively treat enuresis in those rare children who have an incoordination between the bladder and sphincter contractions.[39] Biofeedback requires professional guidance. I do *not* recommend it unless all other treatments have failed *and* the child has a rare functional-anatomical problem that will almost certainly need surgical treatment if this doesn't work.

BIOMECHANICAL THERAPIES: SPINAL MANIPULATION, SURGERY

Spinal Manipulation

One study found a small, statistically insignificant benefit for real compared with sham chiropractic treatment for enuresis.[40] Another showed no benefit of chiropractic treatment compared with just keeping track of the number of dry nights.[41] The chiropractors who did this study concluded that chiropractic was *not* a useful therapy in the treatment of enuresis. I agree.

Surgery

Surgery is unnecessary for treating ordinary enuresis. If your child dribbles urine throughout the day or has frequent bladder infections, have him evaluated for an anatomical problem of his bladder or kidneys. Surgery can often correct these problems.

BIOENERGETIC THERAPIES: ACUPUNCTURE, HOMEOPATHY

Acupuncture

Several studies report good success using acupuncture (traditional, electrostimulation, and scalp acupuncture) to treat enuresis.[42, 43, 44] However, because of the pain from the needles, scalp acupuncture, in particular, is *not* acceptable to many children, even in China.[45] Most treatments require repeated needle treatments over several weeks. However, two series of Chinese cases indicate that a single treatment is sufficient to cure enuresis in over 80% of children.[46, 47] An Italian study showed that acupuncture decreases bladder spasms.[48] A study comparing acupuncture to DDAVP indicated that the combination of both treatments was most effective and that acupuncture alone was comparable to DDAVP.[49] If acupuncture needles are acceptable for you and your child, it may be worth a try if other treatments (rewards for dry nights, bladder-stretching exercise, alarms, and imagery techniques or hypnosis) have failed.

Homeopathy

Homeopathic remedies traditionally used to treat bed-wetting include Belladonna, Causticum, Equisetum, Kreosotum, Phosphorus, Pulsatilla, Sepia, and Sulfur. There are *no* studies evaluating the effectiveness of homeopathic remedies in treating children with enuresis. I do *not* recommend them.

WHAT I RECOMMEND FOR TREATING ENURESIS

See your health care professional for an evaluation to make sure the child doesn't have a bladder infection, diabetes, or some other treatable condition.

Also consult a professional if

- home treatments don't seem to help after two to three months,
- your child has burning or pain with urination,
- your child starts wetting during the day,
- your child's stream of urine seems abnormal to you,
- you have any other questions or concerns.

---

1. *Lifestyle—mind-body (behavior).* Keep a calendar marked with dry nights and wet nights. Give your child positive rewards (such as stickers or vouchers) for dry nights. Do *not* punish your child for wet nights.

Put your child in charge of changing pajamas, changing the wet sheets, and putting the wet bedding in the laundry basket. It should be clear that he is *responsible* but *not* guilty or being punished.

Have your child imagine the nerves going from his bladder to his brain, telling his brain that the bladder is full and needs to be emptied. Have him visualize the nerves from the brain to the bladder muscle, telling it to hold the urine a little longer. The brain then sounds the alarm so he can wake up and go to the bathroom before his brain tells his bladder it's OK to go. Help him practice this imagination exercise twice a day, especially before he goes to sleep.

Set an alarm and awaken your child three hours after he goes to bed so he can get up and void again. If this is not successful within six weeks, try an enuresis alarm.

2. *Lifestyle—nutrition.* Do not give your child anything to drink in the two hours before bed. Have him avoid caffeine and chocolate. If he has other symptoms, consider having him evaluated for food allergies.

3. *Lifestyle—exercise.* Have your child try one or more bladder-stretching exercises described in this chapter. Remeasure bladder capacity every week.

4. *Biochemical—medication.* If the child is still wet at night, see your health care professional about the possibility of medication, especially if your child needs short-term help (e.g., going to camp or slumber parties).

5. *Bioenergetic—acupuncture.* Alternatively, consider acupuncture therapy if lifestyle remedies haven't worked.

RESOURCES

Sources of Enuresis Alarms

Nite Train'r Alarm

> Koregon Enterprises
> 9735 SW Sunshine Court
> Beaverton, OR 97005
> 1(800)544–4240

Nytone Alarm

> Nytone Medical Products
> 2424 S. 900 West
> Salt Lake City, UT 84119
> 1(801)973–4090

Wet Stop Alarm

> Palco Laboratories
> 8030 Soquel Avenue
> Santa Cruz, CA 95062
> 1(408)476–3151 or
>   1(800)346–4488

Books

Allison, Mack. *Dry All Night: The Picture Book Technique That Stops Bed-wetting.* Boston: Little, Brown, 1990.

Other Information

> Center to Assist Regulation
>   of Enuresis
> Division of Urology
> The Children's Memorial
>   Hospital
> 2300 Children's Plaza
> Chicago, IL 60614
> 1(312)880–4000

7

BURNS

Brian West brought his two-year-old daughter, Cora, into clinic to be treated for a scald burn first thing one morning before dropping her off at day care. Heavy hearted, he told me he'd had a cup of coffee and a bran muffin sitting on the sink, so he could eat breakfast while getting ready for work. Before he knew it, Cora had come in and pulled his cup off the sink, splashing hot coffee on her left shoulder, arm, and chest. The coffee had been sitting out for a few minutes, so he didn't think it was very hot, but Cora had cried immediately. He'd put cold water on the burn, which was pink and had a few small blisters. He'd also given her some Tylenol. Brian's wife was out of town on a business trip, and he wasn't sure what else to do. He'd called his mother, who said to put butter on it. Brian wanted to know if there was anything else he could put on the burn to prevent complications. Because Cora was screaming, he also wanted something stronger to help with her pain.

Each year over 23,000 American children are hospitalized and nearly 1,500 die from burn injuries.[1] Burns can be caused by heat, caustic chemicals, electricity, or radiation. The most common burns in children are sunburns and scald burns. The most deadly burns are due to fires and electricity.

It may take a day or two after a burn before you can really tell how deep it is. Have you ever spent the day at the beach and returned home thinking you had escaped a sunburn only to awaken the next day to red, painful skin? Many burns appear to be less serious initially than they are. It sometimes

DEGREE OF BURN	HOW DEEP	APPEARANCE
First degree burn	Superficial	Pink, no blisters; dry; painful
Second degree	Partial thickness	Pink or red with blisters; moist; very painful
Third degree	Full thickness	Red, white, or charred; not painful in center

takes forty-eight hours after the burn before even a physician can accurately determine how deep it is.

Sunburn typifies the *first-degree burn*. The skin is pink or red, dry, and painful. Even a soft sheet or breeze can cause agony, but the pain resolves in a day or two. Regardless of how you treat it, it heals in three or four days without scarring; within a week the burned skin becomes itchy and peels. Severe sunburn can damage deeper layers of skin; *second-degree burns* are signaled by the development of blisters within twelve hours after sun exposure. Sunburns increase the later risk of skin cancer and premature aging of the skin.

Scald burns are the most common *second-degree* or *partial thickness* burns, accounting for more pediatric hospitalizations than any other type of burn. The peak age for scald burns is between six months and two years of age—another reason toddlers need constant, close supervision. Scalds typically occur when a toddler pulls a container of boiling water or a cup of coffee off the counter, splashing it onto her face and upper body. Also, dipping braids into boiling water to "set" them can unintentionally scald the scalp, face, or back.[2]

Even tap water can cause burns if the hot water heater thermostat is set too high. Tap water at 130°F takes less than thirty seconds to cause a second-degree burn. Prior to 1978, 80% of homes had hot water heaters set at these dangerous levels![3] In 1983 Washington State began to require that new hot water heaters be preset at the factory to 120°F. As a result of this simple law, the number of hospital admissions for tap water scald burns was cut in half within five years.[4]

Scalds can also cause deep burns. Between 1979 and 1986, there were 459 deaths due to scald burns; 20% of these deaths were in children under five years old.[5] Flame burns, electrical burns, and contact with hot stoves, hot wood stoves, irons, or space heaters are the most common causes of deep *third-degree* or *full thickness* burns. Flame burns from fires are often accompanied by smoke inhalation, which can be even deadlier than the burn itself. *These burns should be evaluated by a health care professional immediately.*

Many small, mild burns such as sunburns can be handled at home. Deeper or more extensive burns should be evaluated by a professional. Your child may need more fluids than she can take at home by mouth and may need stronger pain medications, antibiotic creams, physical therapy, or even surgery to minimize disfiguring scars.

TAKE YOUR CHILD TO YOUR HEALTH CARE PROFESSIONAL IF

- Any burn (other than a mild sunburn) covers more than 5% of her skin
- Your child is less than two years old with any kind of burn
- The burn contains blisters that cover more than a palm-size area of skin (1 percent of total skin surface)
- A blistering burn occurs on the hands, feet, face, or genitals
- Any burn encircles the child's arm or leg
- It is an electrical burn
- You suspect possible smoke inhalation, regardless of the size of the burn
- The burn is deep or contains white, charred areas or nonpainful areas
- The burn looks infected
- Your child is in severe pain or refuses to eat or drink
- You are concerned about the appearance of the burn
- Your child has swallowed a caustic chemical (such as lye or Drano). You can't tell if the chemical has caused burns in the esophagus or stomach without special tests.

Cora's burn looked like a typical scald burn with a mixture of first- and second-degree burns. It covered about 5% of her total skin area. It was bright pink, and a few spots had blistered and peeled already, leaving raw, tender skin exposed.

WHAT IS THE BEST WAY TO PREVENT BURNS?

The best way to prevent burns is to use common sense, create a safe home environment, and supervise your child closely.

PREVENTING SUNBURN

- Minimize sun exposure between 10 a.m. and 2 p.m.
- Beware of reflective surfaces such as water or snow.
- Don't count on clouds—up to 80% of burning rays can get through.
- Wear protective clothing, such as a hat with a broad brim.
- Use sunscreen with an SPF of 15 or higher.

Keep your child out of the sun between 10 a.m. and 2 p.m. Be especially cautious around water or snow because they can reflect burning rays back and intensify the trouble. Don't count on clouds to reduce sun exposure; they let about 80% of burning rays through to the skin. When your child is outdoors, protect her face with a brimmed hat. Use sunscreen generously. The higher the SPF (sun protection factor), the more protection your child has against the sun's burning ultraviolet rays. Choose a sunscreen rated at SPF 15 or higher. Zinc oxide (the white cream worn by lifeguards) is the most effective sunscreen. Newer sunscreens containing avobenzone and titanium oxide also protect against the ultraviolet rays which are thought to cause skin cancer.

You can also take steps to reduce burn hazards in your home.

REDUCING BURN HAZARDS IN THE HOME

- Lower hot water heater temperature to 120°F.
- Have smoke detectors and fire extinguishers on every floor.
- Cover electrical cords and outlets.
- Be careful with space heaters, radiators, wood stoves, and fireplaces.
- Practice stove and microwave safety.
- Ban baby walkers.
- Keep vaporizers and steam machines out of children's reach.
- Keep matches and lighters out of children's reach.
- Prohibit use of gasoline and fireworks.

Make sure your *hot water heater* is set no higher than 120ºF. Your dishwasher and washing machine can still do an excellent job at these temperatures. Many dishwashers now include heat boosters to increase the water temperature in the unit without overheating the rest of the water in the house. By turning down your hot water heater, you'll not only reduce the chances of a scald burn, you'll save money on your gas or electric bill, too.[6]

Install a *smoke detector and fire extinguisher* on every floor of your home. A smoke detector is the single most inexpensive investment you can make to protect your family from fire injuries. Most states require landlords to have working smoke detectors in every apartment. Change the batteries regu-

larly; I change mine every fall, the same day I turn the clocks back. I also keep two fire extinguishers on the main floor of my home—one in the kitchen and one in the living room next to the fireplace. I've never had to use them, but I review the directions and check the expiration dates every fall when I turn the clocks back and replace the batteries in smoke detectors.

Toddlers chew everything they can get their hands on. The word *no* just doesn't make sense to an exploring fifteen-month-old. She isn't being bad, she's simply trying to figure out the world. You can't expect toddlers to behave safely; you have to protect them from hazards in the environment. Keep appliances close to outlets, so the cords don't trail across the room. Install *outlet covers,* so your curious toddler isn't tempted to explore electrical outlets with fingers, paper clips, or hair clips. Outlet covers are available at many toy stores and hardware stores.

Space heaters get very hot. Clothes or draperies near the space heater can easily catch fire. All too often space heaters are left on when adults fall asleep. Turn off your space heaters when you go to bed. Keep all clothing and fabric well away from them whenever they are on. *Radiators* have caused burns in infants who rolled off of beds onto the radiator and toddlers who tried to pull themselves to a stand by holding onto the radiator. Put a barrier between toddlers and wood stoves or fireplaces.

Keep the handles of pots and pans turned away from the edge of the *stove top* to prevent curious toddlers from pulling hot pans onto themselves. Whenever possible, use the back burners of the stove to put more distance between your child and the burner. Before giving your child anything from the *microwave,* test the temperature first yourself. Despite widespread advice against it, many parents heat their child's formula in the microwave.[7] If you heat liquids in the microwave, shake the container thoroughly to distribute the heat throughout the contents, and test the temperature on yourself before giving it to your child.

Infant walkers are a menace, and they do *not* help children learn to walk any faster. Walkers were the culprits behind many of the scalded children I saw in the Harborview Hospital Burn Unit. The children "walked" over to the stove or table, and quicker than the parent could stop them, pulled pots of boiling water, coffee, or spaghetti down onto themselves, resulting in severe burns. If you already have a walker, remove its wheels. Better yet, when friends and relatives want to get you something for the baby, ask for a high chair, a baby gate, a car seat, or an infant swing instead.

Vaporizers are a boon for many children struggling with coughs and colds, but steam vaporizers and steam machines can burn curious toddlers.[8] If you have a hot air or steam vaporizer or steam machine, make sure it is safely out of reach of children.

Matches and lighters should always be kept out of children's reach. I have seen several tragic house fires in which families lost everything they owned and children were scarred for life because a youngster got hold of his parent's cigarette lighter. Children can unintentionally ignite their clothes while playing with matches or lighters, resulting in severe burns to the face and chest. This is another good reason for parents to stop smoking.

Gasoline and kids just don't mix. Some of the worst burns I saw in the Burn Unit were in boys between eight and fifteen years old who were burning leaves and threw gasoline (or lighter fluid) on the fire to get it going. Gasoline spilled on their pants, caught fire, and resulted in severe, disfiguring burns. Don't let a child use gasoline or lighter fluid until she is at least old enough to pay to put it in the family car.

Fireworks also cause disproportionate damage among school-age boys. I have seen fingers, hands, feet, and other body parts blown off or burned from fireworks. Do *not* let your children use fireworks without your direct supervision.

Brian took advantage of his day at home to do a careful inventory of burn and fire safety in his house. He drew up a checklist to show his wife and decided they would review it every year on the anniversary of Cora's burn as a way to remind themselves of the importance of prevention. They also decided to make a fire escape plan and practice that every year as well.

No matter how safety-conscious their parents are, some children still get burned. What treatments work for burned children?

TREATMENTS FOR BURNS

Children who have suffered different kinds of burns (mild vs. deep) require different kinds of therapy. Children who suffer severe burns go through several predictable stages, and they need different therapies at different times. For the first day or two, they are likely to be in shock, sleepy and withdrawn from the world. The burned area and other areas may become swollen, and the child requires much more fluid than usual. After a day or two, as the child begins to mobilize reserves to begin healing, the heart rate and blood pressure rise and the child may run a fever. As a burn heals, it gets very itchy. Finally, deep burns tend to leave ugly scars without appropriate therapy. Let's tour the Therapeutic Mountain to review the effectiveness of different kinds of therapies for burns. If you want to skip to my bottom-line recommendations, flip to the end of the chapter.

BIOCHEMICAL THERAPIES: MEDICATIONS, HERBS, NUTRITIONAL SUPPLEMENTS

Medications

BURN TREATMENT MEDICATIONS

- Pain medications (prescription and nonprescription)
- Tetanus immunization
- Antibiotic ointments
- Other salves

Effective *nonprescription analgesic medications* include aspirin, acetaminophen (Tylenol), ibuprofen (Advil), and naproxen (Aleve). These medications are safe, but they need to be repeated every few hours to help the child remain comfortable while the burn is healing.

If the burn is deep or extensive, your child may need stronger *prescription pain medications*. The most commonly prescribed pain medication is codeine or a combination of codeine and acetaminophen (Tylenol III). If your child is hospitalized, other pain medications such as morphine may be used. Burns are very painful. Your child will heal much faster if the pain is effectively managed so she can sleep, eat, and drink. No matter how much pain medication your child requires during the early phases of treatment, she will not become a drug addict. In all the years I worked at the Harborview Burn Center, I never saw a child whose pain was effectively managed become a drug addict. People do crave drugs if they are not given enough medication frequently enough. Far more damage is done by withholding pain medications or undertreating pain than by giving the large doses necessary to make her as comfortable as possible.

Burns are highly prone to *tetanus* infection. If your child is burned and has not fin-ished her initial series of immunizations (usually given at two, four, and six months of age), she needs a tetanus shot and a dose of tetanus immune globulin to prevent tetanus. If she has had all of her required immunizations but it has been more than five years since her last tetanus shot, she needs a booster. Nobody likes getting shots, but the risk of tetanus is far worse.

Burn wounds are extremely susceptible to other infections, too. *Antibiotic ointments* help reduce the risk of infection. The most commonly used antibiotic cream is a prescription sulfa drug, silver sulfadiazine (Silvadene). If your child is allergic to sulfa drugs, let your physician know. Other effective antibiotics are available.[9] Antibiotic ointments are applied once or twice daily following thorough wound cleaning. The process of removing dressings, washing the burn, and replacing the antibiotic ointment can be very painful. Hospitals and burn centers routinely give pain medications before changing dressings. Oral antibiotics are not helpful and are not necessary unless your child has another infection such as pneumonia.

The most interesting burn salve I have run across is Preparation H. Believe it or not, many people put the famous hemorrhoid medication on minor burns to "soothe inflamed tissues." Even more amazing, someone actually studied the active ingredient, live yeast cell derivative (LYCD), and found that skin grafts did heal faster with it than with a placebo ointment![10] The ointment stings a bit, but nothing that the patients weren't willing to tolerate. These results are intriguing, and I'd like to see more studies in children; you might give Preparation H a try on *minor* burns.

Cora was up to date on all her immunizations. We gave her some Tylenol III in the office and carefully cleaned her burns. The nurse applied Silvadene antibiotic ointment and cov-

ered the whole thing with a large dressing. Brian decided to take the day off from work to stay home with Cora, renting some cartoon videos to distract her from the pain. I gave them a prescription for Tylenol III to help keep her comfortable and asked him to return the next day for another assessment and dressing change.

Herbs

A number of herbal remedies have been traditionally used to treat minor burns.

HERBAL REMEDIES FOR BURNS

- Aloe vera
- Gotu kola
- Calendula and arnica
- Oil of geranium
- *Avoid* raw herbs, tea tree oil, garlic

Aloe vera gel first gained popularity during the 1930s with reports of its success as a treatment for radiation burns.[11] It is now a common ingredient in many nonprescription burn remedies. Be sure to read the ingredients to ensure that the product you use contains 70% or more aloe. The gel from fresh leaves is applied directly to the burn. Aloe grows well on windowsills with minimal care, and many cooks and restaurants keep it on hand for minor kitchen burns. In animal studies, aloe vera is as effective as antibiotic cream in keeping burns free of bacteria.[12] Although there are no studies specifically evaluating its effectiveness in treating burned children, I use aloe vera myself and recommend it to my patients as a remedy for minor burns such as sunburns.

Gotu kola (Centella asiatica) is a native herb of Eastern Asia and the Pacific Islands used for numerous skin problems and wounds including burns,[13] skin grafts,[14] and scars.[15] Gotu kola extracts stimulate wound healing by promoting collagen (connective tissue) formation.[16] Excessive collagen, however, can cause disfiguring scars. Gotu kola extracts can also cause irritation and allergic reactions in some people.[17] Gotu kola remains an experimental treatment in the United States; I do *not* recommend it until additional studies of its safety and effectiveness have been completed.

Calendula, another popular skin soother, is available in several brands of skin cream sold in health food stores. Calendula seems to have anti-inflammatory properties, and I use it on minor skin irritations. There are *no* studies evaluating its effectiveness in treating burns. *Arnica* is an ingredient in many herbal salves, creams, ointments, and oils. Applying arnica to broken or irritated skin can lead to a rash. I do *not* recommend arnica applications for burns.

Geranium oil is a traditional remedy for cuts, bruises, and burns. Oil of geranium has shown some antibacterial, antiviral, and antifungal properties in the test tube and in experimental mice.[18, 19] There are *no* studies evaluating its effectiveness in treating burned children. Because of the risk of causing irritation, I do *not* recommend that you apply any aromatherapy or essential oil directly to burned skin.

Folk remedies for burns include marsh mallow root, plantain, comfrey, and mullein leaves, and slippery elm bark powder. Many of these herbs are added to herbal ointments as skin salve for minor skin irritations or made into poultices. Despite their popularity, they have not been evaluated in scientific studies in the treatment of burns. Because of their potential for contamination with bacteria and fungal toxins,[20] I do *not* recommend raw herbal products as burn treatments.

Other home remedies include cider vinegar, lemon juice, and baking soda. For minor burns (without blisters), you can use whatever has worked for you. Do *not* use home remedies on second- or third-degree burns.

Tea tree oil is an increasingly popular remedy, which contains phenol, a potent bacteria killer. However, tea tree oil can be very irritating and cause allergic reactions, especially when used undiluted or straight.[21] It can be absorbed through the skin, causing severe side effects such as depression, weakness, incoordination, and tremors.[22] Because of its potential for causing skin irritation, I do *not* recommend it as a treatment for burns.

Garlic can also lead to irritation and burns when applied directly to a child's tender skin.[23] Do *not* use garlic poultices on burns.

Nutritional Supplements

Vitamin and mineral supplements are often given to children hospitalized with serious burns. The most commonly supplemented vitamins and minerals are vitamin C, B vitamins, and zinc.[24] Mineral supplements (copper, selenium, and zinc) have resulted in significantly shorter hospital stays in adult burn patients with extensive burns.[25] Iron supplements are avoided because extra iron seems to feed the bacteria that thrive in burn wounds.

POSSIBLE NUTRITIONAL SUPPLEMENTS FOR BURNS

- Vitamin A (orally)
- Vitamin C (orally)
- Vitamin E (orally or as a salve)
- Zinc and copper (orally)
- Honey (salve)
- *No* iron (orally), milk, butter, shortening, or lard (salves)

Vitamin A is essential for wound healing. Supplemental vitamin A (approximately 10,000 International Units [IU] daily) seems to decrease the risk of diarrhea that frequently complicates burns.[26] There are no studies evaluating the effectiveness of higher doses of vitamin A. Vitamin A overdoses can cause serious side effects. I do *not* recommend vitamin A supplements higher than the doses typically contained in multivitamins (10,000 IU daily) for burned children.

Vitamin C is also necessary for healing. Many seriously ill and injured children can tolerate large doses of vitamin C. High doses of vitamin C given immediately after a burn help decrease swelling in animal studies.[27] You can try anywhere from 60 milligrams to 250 milligrams given three to four times daily for a burned child. If your child develops diarrhea (an early side effect of vitamin C overdose), reduce the dose.

Vitamin E has been recommended both as a nutritional supplement and as a salve for minor burns. In a study of seventeen patients with extensive burns, vitamin E supplements led to higher counts of immune T-cells, possibly improving resistance to infection.[28] On the other hand, a recent study showed that vitamin E *salve* did not help burns; it also had more side effects than the placebo cream.[29] Vitamin E *may* be useful, but until more studies are done in humans, vitamin E supplements and salves must be regarded as experimental, not proven therapy.

Children with major burns lose a lot of minerals, particularly *zinc and copper*.[30] Zinc is important for immune function and healing. Zinc and copper normally exist in balance, so their replacement needs to be balanced as well. The amount of replacement minerals needed depends on the size of the child and the severity of the burn. For most small burns, foods rich in zinc or a multivitamin/multimineral is sufficient.

Honey was cited in an Egyptian papyrus from 2000 B.C. as a treatment for burns; it continues to be used today in many parts of the world as a burn salve. A recent study from India showed that on minor burns, honey did a better job than the standard antibiotic cream, Silvadene, in reducing infection, speeding healing, and minimizing pain and scarring.[31] A later study confirmed that honey dressings were more effective than standard dressings in terms of infection and healing rates.[32]

Like all natural products, honey varies in its purity and potency. New Zealand scientists have investigated the antibacterial properties of different kinds of honey against different kinds of bacteria.[33] Manuka honey (from the pollen of Leptospermum scoparium) is the most potent honey against *Staphylococcus* bacteria.[34] Despite its killer effects on *Staphylococcus* and fungi, manuka honey has *no* impact on another deadly, burn-infecting bacterium, *Pseudomonas*.[35] Other kinds of honey, including much of what is available in the grocery store, have *no* effect on the usual burn-infecting bacteria and fungi.[36]

Some honey is contaminated with bacterial spores that can cause botulism. People who are allergic to certain flowers or trees can have an allergic reaction to honey made from the pollen of those plants.[37] Honey derived from Turkish rhododendrons (Rhododendron ponticum) has been known for centuries as "mad honey" because of its intoxicant effects; it was cited by several Greek historians as playing a key role in military history because of its devastating effects on the armies who ate it.[38] Any honey used for medicinal purposes should come from a known source and be tested for purity and potency before being applied to wounds.

Do *not* put *milk, butter,* or *lard* on a burn. Though they may initially feel soothing, they provide a great environment for bacteria to grow and multiply.

LIFESTYLE THERAPIES: NUTRITION, EXERCISE, ENVIRONMENT, MIND-BODY

Nutrition

One of the biggest challenges in caring for severely burned children is getting them to eat. Severe burns are a major stress, resulting in metabolic rates (and calorie needs) 50 to 100 percent higher than normal.[39] Children feel miserable, are often nauseated, and just aren't hungry. However, several studies show that hospitalized burned children heal much faster and have fewer infections if they are fed from the day they are admitted to the hospital, even if they aren't hungry. High-protein diets help maintain immune function and blood levels of essential amino acids in severely burned children.[40] On the other hand, excessive protein intake puts an extra strain on the kidneys. If your child is severely burned, consult a professional nutritionist.

Extra fluids are very important, especially in the first few days after a burn. Our bodies are mostly water, and our skin helps prevent all of our body fluids from evaporating. Burns destroy this barrier between body fluids and the environment. Children whose burns cover more than 10% of their skin often lose so much fluid they need intravenous fluid to replace their losses.

Brian stopped at the grocery store on the way home to pick up extra orange juice and some of Cora's favorite foods (ice cream and peanut butter) to encourage her to eat. He also purchased a chewable children's vitamin to make sure Cora got the vitamins and minerals she needed to help heal her burns.

Exercise

Initially, children suffering from burns need to rest, so their body's energy can go into healing the burn. For the first few days, it may help to keep the burned area *elevated.* Just as in a sprained ankle, the injured area is likely to swell. Swelling is not only uncomfortable, but it may impede blood flow and slow the healing process. Elevating an injured extremity means keeping it above the level of the heart.

After the initial healing phase, it is important for children with healing burns to keep *moving their joints,* even though it may be very painful. Burns that extend across joints can cause scars that eventually contract and limit movement. Physical therapists can help a child keep motivated and keep moving, preventing long-term disabilities. Exercise programs improve self-esteem and speed returns to work and school.[41] Slow stretching such as yoga or tai chi can be very helpful in maintaining limber joints.

Environment

When a child is burned, the first and most effective therapies are environmental. *Remove the child from the source of the heat.* Usually in scald burns, the hot water or coffee has already run off or evaporated, but if the hot liquid or grease is still on the child's clothes, remove the clothes. If your child's clothes have caught on fire, smother the flames.

Second, *put cool water on the burned area.* Don't use ice. Ice may cause even more damage to already injured skin.[42] Your child doesn't need to get frostbite on top of the burn. Cool water helps numb the pain. If your child's burn covers more than 10% of her skin, do not run cold water over her; she will get chilled and be even more uncomfort-

able. *Large burns need immediate professional treatment.*

Third, *cover the burn with a clean, dry dressing.* You can use bandages or a clean handkerchief, sheet, or towel. Covering the burn reduces pain and lessens the risk of infection.

Pressure dressings similar to Ace wraps are used to prevent scars from becoming heaped up and disfiguring. For maximal effectiveness, they should be measured, applied, and monitored by a physical therapist.[43]

Pigskin for burns? It's not just for football any more. Pigskin makes an excellent dressing for minor burns. It is used at major burn centers for some second-degree (blistering) burns. Pigskin immediately reduces pain and the risk of infection and speeds up healing. On the other hand, it is expensive and is not widely available in most doctors' offices. It does not work well if the burn has already been treated with any kind of ointment or salve. If you are planning to take your child to a burn center for evaluation and treatment, just wash the burn with cool water, cover it with a clean bandage, handkerchief, or sheet, and bring the child right away. For anything other than a very minor burn, a health care professional should be consulted regarding appropriate burn dressings and dressing changes.

Mind-Body

Hypnosis has been used in both adults and children to help manage the pain of burns and the pain of dressing changes.[44, 45] At the Northwest's regional trauma center, the staff psychologist who provides hypnotherapy is a key member of the burn team. Hypnotherapy can help decrease pain and improve sleep and appetite.[46] In addition to reducing pain, hypnosis also reduces the anxiety associated with dressing changes. Effective hypnotherapy can markedly reduce the need for pain medications in seriously burned children.

Distraction with cartoons, stories, and songs can also help burned children deal with the pain of their injuries and dressing changes.[47] Most hospitals have cassette tape players on pediatric wards, so parents can leave recordings of their child's favorite stories and songs to play when the parent can't be there. The Nintendo machine and VCR are favorites among the children on the burn ward. You can also use these simple distraction techniques at home to help your child manage the pain of a burn or other injuries.

At the opposite end of the spectrum from distraction is having the child *fully engaged* in treatment. Some children scream and fight dressing changes despite maximal pain medication and attempts at distraction. Often these children feel wildly out of control. When they are offered the opportunity to help change their dressings, they do much better.[48] Giving children a sense of predictability and control decreases their anxiety and pain, making the whole experience much easier for everyone. Parents know best whether their child will do better with distraction from or increased participation in burn treatments.

BIOMECHANICAL THERAPIES: MASSAGE, SURGERY

Massage

There are *no* studies evaluating the effectiveness of massage in treating burned children. Exposing the burn to air or touching it can be excruciating. I do *not* recommend massage on burns themselves while they are healing. Some children find massage to other areas comforting. Massage is very helpful *after* the burn has healed; it decreases itching, tightness, and pain, improves circulation, and promotes comfort and flexibility.

Surgery

If a burn blisters, leave it alone unless the blister is larger than a quarter or has already broken. A small, intact blister helps protect the burn from further injury. Once the blister breaks and the fluid drains out, removing the dead skin on the top of the blister minimizes the chances of infection.

If your child's burn is very deep, *skin grafts* may be necessary to minimize scarring and maximize function. It takes a few days for the burn to declare itself; that is, to be able to tell how severe the burn really is. Young children can sometimes heal burns that adults can't heal on their own. Most burn surgeons wait at least ten days before doing any skin graft surgery. The child remains in the hospital before surgery to receive fluid therapy, dressings, pain medications, and other necessary treatments. Hospitalization is also required after the surgery to make sure that the skin graft "takes" and the child continues to receive optimal therapy.

BIOENERGETIC THERAPIES: ACUPUNCTURE, THERAPEUTIC TOUCH, HOMEOPATHY

Acupuncture

Acupuncture is becoming more and more widely used to treat pain. One comparison study in hospitalized adult burn patients indicated that acupuncture significantly improved their pain.[49]

Therapeutic Touch

In an excellent double-blind study, Therapeutic Touch (TT) proved to be an effective treatment for skin wounds in adult volunteers. In this study, forty-four healthy men volunteered to undergo a standardized skin wound (made with a skin biopsy instrument). Half the subjects received TT and half did not. The treatment sessions lasted five minutes daily. By means of an elaborate setup of study rooms, subjects did not know whether or not they received TT. A physician who also did not know which men had been treated measured their wounds at the beginning of the experiment and eight and sixteen days later. The wound sizes in the treated and untreated groups were identical initially (about 59 square millimeters). But eight days later, the wounds in the treated group had healed significantly faster than the untreated group (down to 4 millimeters in the TT-treated group versus 19 millimeters in the comparison group). Sixteen days after the initial injury, thirteen of the twenty-three men in the TT group were completely healed, whereas none of twenty-one men in the comparison group had completely healed.[50] These results are highly significant statistically, although they remain unexplained scientifically. Despite the lack of scientific rationale, these results have convinced me to recommend Therapeutic Touch for my patients with burns and other minor injuries. (See Appendix A for more books about TT; see Appendix B for basic information on how to perform TT.)

I did Therapeutic Touch with Cora in the office and showed Brian what I was doing. He decided to practice it at home with Cora while she was relaxed and watching cartoons.

Homeopathy

Commonly used remedies for minor burns include Arnica, Calendula, Causticum, Hypericum, and Urtica urens. Only one scientific study evaluated homeopathy's effectiveness for treating burns, and it found that the remedy was no more effective than a placebo.[51] I do *not* recommend homeopathic remedies for burn therapy.

WHAT I RECOMMEND FOR BURNS

PREVENTING BURNS

1. *Lifestyle—environment.* Take sensible precautions regarding sun exposure: avoid the hours between 10 a.m. and 2 p.m.; don't count on clouds; wear a hat; use sunscreen.

Make a burn safety inventory for your house:

    a. Hot water heater temperature 120°F
    b. Smoke detectors and fire extinguishers on every floor
    c. Electrical cords and outlets covered
    d. Space heater, radiator, and steam vaporizer safety
    e. Stove top and microwave safety
    f. No wheeled walkers
    g. Matches and lighters out of reach

h. Gasoline, fireworks out of reach
i. Escape plan

Take Your Child to a Health Care Professional If

- Any burn covers more than 5% of her skin
- Any burn is electrical
- Your child is less than two years old with any burn
- The burn contains blisters
- Any blistering burn occurs on the hands, feet, face, or genitals
- Any burn encircles your child's arm or leg
- There is any chance of smoke inhalation
- The burn contains white, charred areas or nonpainful areas
- Your child is in severe pain
- Your child refuses to eat or drink
- You are concerned about the appearance of the burn
- Your child has swallowed a caustic chemical

TREATING BURNS

1. *Lifestyle—environmental.* Get the child away from the heat; smother flames; remove clothing that has had hot food or liquid spilled on it. Run cool water over the burn.

2. *Biochemical—medications.* Give your child an analgesic medication such as acetaminophen. (Use an antibiotic cream or ointment on the burn.)

3. *Biochemical–herbs.* For minor burns, use nonprescription skin salve containing at least 70% aloe vera.

4. *Biochemical—nutritional supplements.* Consider giving a multivitamin supplement. Consider additional vitamin C–60 to 250 milligrams three to four times daily.

5. *Lifestyle—nutrition.* Encourage your child to drink plenty of fluids and eat a balanced, high-protein diet.

6. *Lifestyle—mind-body.* Distraction may help make dressing changes more bearable; consider stories, songs, and videos. Other children do better if they can participate in their dressing changes.

7. *Lifestyle—exercise.* As the burn heals, keep your child moving to decrease scarring and limited joint movement.

8. *Bioenergetic—Therapeutic Touch.* Learn how to use Therapeutic Touch to help your child relax and heal faster from burns and other injuries.

8

CHICKEN POX

Julie Frazier called me on a March Monday because her three-year-old, Tom, had come down with the chicken pox. Her six-year-old, Jeff, had broken out the previous week. Tom had been well until the weekend, when he started to develop cold symptoms and a fever. This morning Tom developed a few little pimples on a reddish base, known as "dewdrops on a rose petal," which are characteristic of chicken pox. Julie bought some nonprescription diphenhydramine (Benadryl) to treat Jeff's itching and help him sleep, but it just made him more irritable. She wanted to know what else she could try because she did not want two irritable, itching little boys running around the house. She also wanted to know how long this whole thing would last, when the boys could return to school and day care, and if there was any chance that their cousins could have caught it from them over the weekend.

Chicken pox is an itchy rash caused by the varicella virus. It is very contagious. No matter how healthy, if they are not immunized, almost all kids will catch it. More than 3 million Americans, most of whom are between two and eight years old, are affected with chicken pox every year, usually in the springtime. If your child is basically healthy, chicken pox is more annoying than serious. However, chicken pox can be serious for adults and for children who have weakened immune systems. It kills between fifty and a hundred people every year.

The varicella virus remains dormant in

the body even after the acute illness is over. It can recur in adulthood as the painful disease shingles or zoster. Children can actually catch the varicella virus from an adult who has an active case of shingles.

A child is *most contagious* in the day or two *before* he breaks out in the rash. After exposure to chicken pox, a newly infected child develops symptoms in two to three weeks. Usually the rash is preceded by one or two days of cold symptoms and a low-grade fever. Unless you know that chicken pox is going around and your child has been exposed, it's hard to tell if he just has a cold or is having the first chicken pox symptoms. Children are contagious until the last blister has scabbed over, so they should stay out of school or day care until all the blisters have dried up.

The rash itself usually starts on the chest or abdomen as fluid-filled blisters on small patches of red skin. In a day or so the fluid turns cloudy, the blisters break, and they later dry and scab over. The pox are extremely itchy. There may be only one or two on the first day, but they rapidly spread over three to four days to involve the entire body. All of the pox dry up and scab over within ten days.

Jeff's and Tom's visiting cousins were likely to have been infected over the weekend because Tom was very contagious just before he broke out in the rash. Both Jeff and Tom could return to school and day care as soon as all the pox had dried and scabbed over.

Children with chicken pox also occasionally suffer from headaches, swollen lymph glands under the neck, fever, tiredness, and irritability. Mood management is an important part of therapy. Seek professional help for chicken pox if your child has any complications, has a weakened immune system, or is an adolescent.

TAKE YOUR CHILD TO THE DOCTOR IF

- You suspect he is developing a complication such as
  — chicken pox on the eyeball itself
  — bacterial superinfection of the chicken pox spots
  — pneumonia, encephalitis, or Reye's syndrome
- Your child has a weakened immune system from
  — taking steroid medications (such as for asthma[1] or arthritis)
  — leukemia or AIDS
  — an organ transplant
- Your child is an adolescent

If your child develops blisters or pain on the eyeballs, take him to an eye doctor quickly to prevent damage to the eye. In 1 to 4 percent of children, the chicken pox blisters become infected with strep or staph bacteria, leading to problems as minor as a little extra redness and pain to as major as a life-threatening infection.[2] The 1994 outbreak of flesh-eating bacteria (strep) struck several children with chicken pox. Rarely, children with chicken pox develop serious complications such as pneumonia and encephalitis.[3] Children with weakened or suppressed immune systems are at particularly high risk of developing serious complications and even dying from chicken pox–related infections.[4] Reye's syndrome is a rare (3 cases per 100,000 children with chicken pox) but serious complication that affects the brain and liver of children with chicken pox and certain other viral diseases, especially if they have been treated with aspirin.

Effective *preventive therapies* for chicken pox are now widely available. These include a chicken pox vaccine, acyclovir medication, and immune globulin.

The chicken pox or varicella vaccine has finally been approved by the U.S. Food and Drug Administration. It is recommended by the American Academy of Family Practitioners and the American Academy of Pediatrics. The vaccine is about 90% effective. Even immunized children who do get chicken pox tend to have much milder cases than unimmunized children. Children from twelve months to twelve years old receive one injection. Teenagers require two doses, given one to two months apart. The vaccine should *not* be given during pregnancy or to those taking aspirin every day. Children who have already had chicken pox do *not* need the vaccine. Since most teenagers have had chicken pox already (even if they didn't have symptoms at the time), they do *not* need the vaccine *unless* they've had a blood test showing that they lack antibodies to chicken pox.[5]

Since chicken pox is usually so benign, the main reasons to immunize are (1) to prevent illness in children who have serious chronic diseases and (2) to prevent parents from losing work when their children are sick. Chicken pox can be devastating and even fatal for children whose immune systems are suppressed by leukemia, AIDS, steroid medications, or organ transplants. All of these children should be immunized. Families save an average of $66 per child vaccinated, mostly due to time *not* lost from work.[6] From a societal perspective, vaccination saves $5 for every dollar spent on chicken pox vaccine.[7]

Acyclovir and immune globulin injections can help prevent chicken pox if given shortly after a susceptible child is exposed to the illness. Acyclovir is very effective in reducing the severity of chicken pox if it is given after a child has been exposed to the illness and before the disease has broken out.[8] For maximal effectiveness, immune globulin must be given within four days of exposure to the illness.[9] These medications are usually reserved for children with weakened immune systems, premature babies, and infants less than one month old because these children suffer the most serious complications of chicken pox.

It was too late for preventive therapy for Tom and Jeff; they already had chicken pox. No one in their family had a weakened immune system, so there was no need for preventive therapy for anyone else. It was time to focus on therapies to help make the illness more bearable for Tom, Jeff, and their mother.

WHAT IS THE BEST WAY TO TREAT CHICKEN POX?

Although there are no *cures* for chicken pox, there are a number of therapies that can help you manage your child's symptoms. Let's take a trip around the Therapeutic Mountain and find out what works.

BIOCHEMICAL THERAPIES: MEDICATIONS, HERBS, NUTRITIONAL SUPPLEMENTS

Medications

Several medications help shorten the course of chicken pox, reduce complications and make the symptoms more bearable.

MEDICATIONS FOR CHICKEN POX

- Acyclovir (prescription only)
- Antibiotics (if the pox become infected)
- Antihistamines (nonprescription brands are available)
- *Avoid* antihistamine lotions (Caladryl), aspirin, acetaminophen, and steroid creams

Acyclovir effectively treats the illness and

prevents complications, *but only if it is started within the first twenty-four hours of the rash.*[10] There is no point in waiting until your child has been sick for three days and you are all miserable before starting acyclovir, because it just doesn't work if it is started late. Acyclovir must be taken four times daily for maximal benefits.

Antibiotics are used only if the chicken pox blisters become infected (look redder and become painful as well as itchy). If only one or two blisters are infected, you can use a nonprescription antibiotic ointment, but if the situation doesn't improve in a day or two or if several spots look infected, see your health care professional. Serious bacterial infections can spread rapidly. Call your doctor if you have any questions about an infection starting in the chicken pox blisters.

Anti-itch (*antihistamine*) medicines are somewhat effective and also help children sleep. The most widely used antihistamine, diphenhydramine (Benadryl), is available without a prescription. Antihistamines have 3-D side effects: *d*ry mouth, *d*izziness, and *d*rowsiness. On the other hand, they make some children, like Jeff, more irritable. It is impossible to predict in advance how your child will react.

You can try Calamine lotion to help dry up the pox and decrease itching, but do *not* use *Caladryl*, the combination of Calamine and Benadryl. Some children absorb a great deal of the Benadryl through their skin, causing an overdose.

DO *not* give *aspirin* to a child with chicken pox. Aspirin has been associated with Reye's syndrome, a very serious complication of chicken pox that affects the brain, liver, and other organs. *Acetaminophen* (Tylenol, Panadol, and other brands) is *not* a helpful treatment for children suffering from chicken pox. Although acetaminophen helps kids feel better temporarily, it may actually delay healing from chicken pox.[11] Do *not* put *steroid cream* on chicken pox. Though it is tempting to treat an itch with a nonprescription steroid cream, the steroid suppresses the immune system and may worsen the rash or predispose toward a bacterial infection.

Herbs

There are no herbal cures for chicken pox. Some herbal poultices are time-honored itch remedies, but there are no scientific studies showing that any of them are more effective than placebo creams or ointments. If you are intent on trying an herbal poultice, the following are traditional remedies. (See Appendix B for "how to" information on making poultices.)

TRADITIONAL HERBAL POULTICES FOR ITCHING

- Plantain leaves (can be applied directly)
- Burdock root, peppermint leaves, yarrow sage leaves
- Calendula
- Sedative teas

Plantain leaf poultices are traditional remedies for itchy rashes such as chicken pox and poison ivy.[12] Plantain is a common weed growing by roadsides and in abandoned lots. You can apply the leaves directly to the chicken pox. Plantain is very safe.

Peppermint tea can be added to bath water to help soothe itchy skin. Peppermint has a pleasant smell, and your child will probably enjoy playing in this bath for at least fifteen minutes. Some herbalists combine peppermint leaves with other skin softeners such as burdock root and sage and yarrow leaves.

Calendula (pot marigold) has become such a popular skin remedy that many health food stores carry calendula-containing creams and ointments. *Witch hazel* is a traditional liniment used for skin problems. It evaporates quickly, cooling hot, itchy skin.

Sedative herbal teas that might calm your itchy, irritable youngster include chamomile, catnip, skullcap, hops, passion flower, and valerian. Combinations of chamomile and mint are commercially available in grocery stores and health food stores. You may have to try an herbalist to obtain some of the others.

Julie decided to try her boys on a combination of chamomile and mint tea (available in her grocery store) as an alternative to diphenhydramine (Benadryl). She also found calendula cream to rub into their drying, itchy scabs. She reported that the tea helped them relax at bedtime, and the cream seemed to soothe their dry skin.

Nutritional Supplements

There is no evidence that supplementary vitamins or minerals speed healing from chicken pox.

Apple cider vinegar is a widely used home remedy for skin problems. Many parents dab it on sunburns and other minor skin problems. I have some misgivings about using it for chicken pox because of the potential for stinging and burning. If you want to try it, go slowly at first to see how well your child tolerates it before applying it to the whole body. Baking soda can be mixed with a bit of water until it becomes a paste, then dabbed onto the weeping chicken pox to dry them.

LIFESTYLE THERAPIES: NUTRITION, EXERCISE, ENVIRONMENT, MIND-BODY

Nutrition

Appetites are usually decreased during the first few days of chicken pox. You needn't force your child to eat. Keep offering fresh foods, broths, and plenty of liquids. Cool treats such as popsicles, ice pops, and frozen juices are favorites among kids with hot, itchy rashes. Within a few days, your child's appetite will return to normal.

Exercise

As with other infections, it is helpful to have your child *rest* so that the body's energies can be directed toward healing. Getting overheated from vigorous exercise may make your child even itchier! Most children with chicken pox have normal energy levels within a few days and would just as soon play. That's OK; just don't overdo it.

Environment

Several environmental therapies can help ease the discomfort of chicken pox.

ENVIRONMENTAL THERAPIES

- Tepid baths
  — *with* oatmeal, barley, cornstarch, arrowroot, or baking soda
  — with*out* bubble bath
- Cool temperatures
- Short fingernails

Heat makes itching worse. *Tepid baths* help ease itching. Daily baths help loosen the crusts and prevent infections. To increase the soothing qualities of the bath, put a double handful of plain, dry *oatmeal* with or without a handful of *barley* into an old stocking or pillowcase, tie off the end, and toss it in the bathtub.(Putting the dry oats in a cloth wrap makes cleanup easier.) Alternatively, you can make a watery solution of oatmeal, strain out the oats, and add the leftover water to the bath. Oatmeal is very soothing for all kinds of skin irritations. Commercial oatmeal bathing preparations (such as Aveeno products or Jergens effervescent ActiBath) cost more than breakfast oatmeal and are less messy, but they aren't any more effective than plain old Quaker Oats. Another home remedy is putting a bit of *cornstarch* or *arrowroot* in the bath water to help dry up the blisters. Alternatively, you might add a handful of *baking soda*.

Do *not* add bubble bath to your child's bath water; it can further irritate your child's already suffering skin.

Keep your child *cool*. Do not overdress or bundle him. Dress him in loose-fitting clothing to prevent binding and chafing at sore spots. Cool compresses may help. Let him rub the itchy spots with an ice cube. The ice helps numb the itch and isn't messy.

Keep your child's *fingernails short* to prevent excessive scraping and cuts from vigorous scratching. Keep your child's hands, especially his fingernails, clean to minimize the risk of infection. Consider having your child wear gloves or socks on his hands to keep from scratching himself during sleep.

Mind-Body

Distraction can be helpful in keeping your child from scratching. This is a great time to read stories, play games, and sing songs. Your child will be home from day care or school anyway, and after a day or two will probably have plenty of energy for imaginative games to distract him from itching.

BIOMECHANICAL AND BIOENERGETIC THERAPIES

There are no scientific studies demonstrating the effectiveness of any biomechanical or bioenergetic therapy in treating children suffering from chicken pox.

Several studies have shown that *Therapeutic Touch* is helpful in calming distressed patients, improves wound healing, and is very safe. It may be worthwhile if you would like to try it on your itchy, irritable child, but it has not been specifically evaluated for treating chicken pox. (See Appendix B for simple directions on how to use Therapeutic Touch.)

Rhus tox is the most commonly recommended *homeopathic remedy* for chicken pox—some claim that it is the only remedy needed for this disorder. It has also not been evaluated in comparison trials. Because of their expense and lack of proven effectiveness, I do not recommend homeopathic remedies for chicken pox unless parents are intent on trying them.

WHAT I RECOMMEND FOR CHICKEN POX

PREVENTING CHICKEN POX

1. *Lifestyle—environment.* Avoid contact with other children who have chicken pox.

2. *Biochemical—medications.* Have your child immunized with varicella vaccine.

See Your Health Care Professional If Your Child

- Develops trouble breathing or other signs of pneumonia
- Becomes disoriented, confused, or has other signs of encephalitis
- Develops a high fever (over 102°F)
- Has a weakened immune system from another illness or medication
- Has signs of infection (redness and pain) in or on the pox
- Complains of eye pain or has chicken pox in or around the eyes
- Or if you have any other concerns.

You do *not* need to call or visit your health care professional if your child has a simple case of chicken pox. In fact, visiting a busy waiting room can spread the disease to other children who may not be able to handle it as well as your child. If you want a professional evaluation, please call first and tell the receptionist; there may be a separate waiting room for children with contagious diseases.

TREATING CHICKEN POX

1. *Lifestyle—environment.* For itching:

    a. tepid baths with dry oatmeal, barley, baking soda, arrowroot, or cornstarch,
    b. cool compresses,
    c. keep fingernails short and clean to prevent infection.

2. *Lifestyle—mind-body.* Try to distract your child from itching by reading, singing, playing games, or playing his favorite videos. Be patient. Enjoy your time together as much as you can. This, too, shall pass.

3. *Biochemical—medications.* Consider a nonprescription antihistamine medication to help reduce itching. *Avoid* Caladryl lotion, aspirin, acetaminophen (Tylenol), and steroid creams to reduce the risk of medication side effects.

9

COLDS

Janet Black brought her two-year-old son, Jamal, to see me because he was
congested and had a fever. His temperature had gone up to 103°F the night
before, and at the time of the office visit, it was 101.8°F. He wasn't hungry,
but he was drinking juice and playing just as he usually did. It seemed as if
Jamal had had one cold after another since he started attending his new
day care center. Janet, who smoked about a pack a day of cigarettes, had
suffered from sinus infections all winter; she wanted to make sure Jamal
wasn't getting one too. Jamal's physical exam showed that he didn't have a
sinus infection, bronchitis, or pneumonia. He was simply suffering from the
common cold. She asked me why kids get so many colds, what she could do
to help Jamal get better faster, and what she could do to prevent another
bout with the cold bug.

WHAT CAUSES COLDS?

Sleeping near an open window, getting your feet wet, and being in the wind without a hat do *not* cause colds. *Viruses* cause colds in susceptible children. There are over 200 different kinds of cold-causing viruses. Because so many viruses cause colds, there will probably never be a single vaccine to prevent them.

A person with an experienced, healthy immune system can often resist catching a cold while someone who is physically or emotionally stressed falls ill. When study subjects are intentionally exposed to a cold virus, only about half to two-thirds develop symptoms. The others don't.[1] Although some don't develop symptoms, cultures of their noses indicate that they are infected. That is, the virus takes hold, but symptoms do not develop. Those who remain healthy seem to have an immune system strong enough to keep the virus under control.

A child's immune system is less experienced than an adult's. This is one reason children have more colds than adults. The average preschooler has eight to ten colds a year, school-age children have about five colds a year, and the average adult has only four colds a year. When they do get sick, younger children have cold symptoms longer than older children—an average of nine to ten days for infants less than a year old vs. six to seven days for children one to two years of age.[2]

Although colds are rarely serious or life-threatening, they pack a powerful punch in terms of the *cost* they generate for physician visits, medicines, and absence from normal activities. Colds are the leading reason for doctor visits. Nearly a *billion dollars* a year are spent in the United States on more than 800 varieties of cold medicines. Colds cause children to miss 26 million school days each year. They lead to sinus infections in 5 to 10 percent and ear infections in 30% of children under three years old. Pretty powerful effects from tiny viruses!

At any given moment, 20 to 25 percent of children less than five years old have colds. Children whose *mothers smoke* get 60% more colds than children of nonsmokers. Passive smoking increases the number of infections and the number of symptoms. Children in *day care* experience 70% more colds than children cared for at home.[3] The problem with day care is not the absence of parents so much as the presence of crowds of kids who share viruses.

Could It Be Something Besides a Cold?

There are times when your child's symptoms signal something more serious than a simple cold. A runny nose that lasts for weeks and months is more likely to be an *allergy* than a viral infection. A persistent or worsening cold and fever accompanied by facial pain may be signs of a *sinus* infection.

TAKE YOUR CHILD TO THE DOCTOR IF YOUR CHILD HAS

- A high fever (over 103°F or 39.4°C)
- A sore throat or sore glands in the neck
- Ear pain
- A stiff neck or sore back
- Shortness of breath, wheezing, or trouble breathing
- Cold symptoms for longer than seven to ten days
- Or is too sick to drink

What Are the Best Ways to Prevent and Treat the Common Cold?

"The only way to treat a cold is with contempt."

Sir William Osler, M.D.

Treated or not, most colds resolve on their own within seven to ten days. Let's tour the Therapeutic Mountain to find out the safest symptom relievers. If you want my bottom-line recommendations, skip to the end of the chapter.

Biochemical Therapies: Medications, Herbs, Nutritional Supplements

Medications

The 1833 *Mother's Medical Guide* lists leeches as the preferred treatment for childhood chest colds. Leeches were to be applied to the chest until they dropped off or "until fainting takes place." Modern cold medications may be less gruesome, but most are no more effective at curing colds than leeches were 150 years ago. Children get better over several days *regardless* of whether or not they take a cold medicine. Often parents try a medication in desperation, the child's symptoms eventually improve, and the medication gets the credit.

COMMON COLD MEDICATIONS

- Antihistamines (e.g., Benadryl, Chlortrimeton, Tavist)
- Decongestants (e.g., Sudafed)
- Cough suppressants (e.g., dextromethorphan, DM, codeine)
- Expectorants to loosen dry or thick phlegm or mucus (e.g., guaifenesin)
- Analgesics (e.g., acetaminophen, aspirin, ibuprofen)
- Combinations
- Menthol lozenges
- Antibiotics
- Nedocromil nasal spray
- Ipratropium bromide (Atrovent) nasal spray

Hundreds of nonprescription cold medicines are available, costing desperate consumers nearly $1 billion a year. Most of this money is spent on ineffective remedies. A recent survey indicated that over 50% of three-year-olds had received nonprescription cold remedies within the prior three months.[4]

Though they may be helpful in treating allergies, *antihistamines* are not any more helpful than cherry syrup in relieving children's runny noses.[5] There is no theoretical reason to believe they would be helpful. Unlike the runny nose of allergies, which is due to histamine, the runny nose of colds is caused by a class of chemicals called *kinins.* Antihistamines have NO effect on kinins. They are somewhat helpful for adult cold sufferers, probably because they make people sleepy.[6] The active ingredient in Benadryl, diphenhydramine, is so sedating, it is the active ingredient in many nonprescription sleeping pills. A good night's rest does make people feel better, but kids with colds can do just as well with a dark, quiet room and their favorite stuffed animal. There are some children who have a paradoxical reaction to antihistamines; instead of becoming sleepy, they become awake, active, and irritable. Prescription antihistamines are also *not* effective in treating kids' colds.[7] Unless your child's symptoms are keeping him awake and you want to try a dose of medication at bedtime, I do *not* recommend antihistamines.

Many varieties of *decongestants* are available to help unclog stuffy noses. The best known, pseudoephedrine (Sudafed) and phenylpropanolamine (Rhindecon) decrease nasal congestion and sneezing in adults.[8] Many adults also feel a burst of energy after taking decongestants because decongestants are related to caffeine. However, there are *no* studies documenting decongestants' effectiveness in treating *childhood* colds. Up to 30% of people who take decongestants experience side effects, some of which can be serious: increased heart rate, increased blood pressure, dizziness, hallucinations, psychosis, decreased appetite, and abnormal heart rhythms.[9] I do *not* recommend oral decongestants for children until they reach school age. Even then, they should only be used during the daytime because they may keep children awake at night.

Decongestant nose drops (1/4% Neo-Synephrine) and nose sprays (Afrin, Allerest, Neo-Synephrine 12 Hour) have fewer serious side effects and have proved effective in reducing congestion in adults.[10] However, use for more than a day or two may result in a side effect called rhinitis medicamentosa. This is medicalese for saying the spray eventually causes symptoms that closely mimic the cold itself. The nose becomes dependent on the spray for normal functioning. Within three or four days, the child's nose gets swollen and inflamed inside if the spray is stopped. To relieve the symptoms, more spray is used, but symptoms reappear when it is stopped—a vicious cycle. There are no studies showing that decongestant nose drops or sprays are any more effective than simple saline nose drops (Na-Sal) in young children. I do *not* recommend decongestant drops or sprays unless the child's congestion is so severe that it interferes with drinking or sleeping. Even then, decongestant drops or sprays should be used as little as possible and only for a day or two, to avoid rhinitis medicamentosa. (For more information on breaking your child of the nose spray habit, see Chapter 4, Allergies.)

Saline nose drops are a completely safe way to loosen sticky nasal secretions. You can make your own saline drops:

HOME-MADE SALINE NOSE DROPS

DISSOLVE:

- 1/2 teaspoon of salt in
- 1 cup of tepid water

Put a drop or two of the saline mixture in one nostril. Wait a minute to give the saline a chance to soften and loosen thick or crusted mucus, then remove it with a bulb syringe or nasal aspirator. Repeat on the other side. This process can be safely repeated as often as needed.

Neither of the two most commonly prescribed *cough suppressants*, codeine (prescription only) and dextromethorphan (prescription and nonprescription), are any more effective than placebo cherry syrup in suppressing children's coughs.[11] Save your money. Try a home remedy instead of a cough syrup. (See Chapter 13, Cough).

Expectorants, such as guaifenesin, the active ingredient in Robitussin, supposedly loosen secretions so they are easier to cough out. Expectorants are *no* more helpful than placebo cherry syrup in treating children suffering from coughs and colds.[12, 13]

Analgesics such as Tylenol (acetaminophen), Motrin, or Advil (ibuprofen) help relieve the discomfort of colds and fevers, but despite popular beliefs, they do *not* cure the common cold. A child doesn't need Tylenol for a fever unless the fever is making him uncomfortable (see Chapter 19, Fever). If your child is acting OK, you don't even need to take his temperature. Do not wake your child to give him an analgesic. If he's sleeping, he doesn't need it. Fever may be one of the body's best defenses against infections. Nonprescription analgesic medications tend to suppress the immune system and may worsen cold symptoms over time.[14, 15] Aspirin has been linked to the sometimes fatal illness Reye's syndrome. I do *not* recommend treating a child with analgesics unless he is clearly uncomfortable.

Most cold medications contain *combinations* of antihistamines, decongestants, expectorants, cough suppressants, and analgesics. If the individual ingredients aren't effective in reducing cold symptoms or hastening recovery, there's no reason to think combinations will be any more helpful. Combination cold medicines have proven *not* to be helpful in young children, though teenagers may experience some benefit.[16, 17, 18]

Combining several different medications

increases the risk of side effects. Many children's cold syrups contain alcohol. Most contain sweeteners, artificial colors, artificial flavors, and preservatives as well as the active ingredients.[19] In 1988, three children died from cold medicine overdoses.

Menthol is an ingredient in just about every cough and cold lozenge. Menthol is cooling, soothing, and reduces the sensation of being congested. Adult volunteers who were given menthol lozenges reported marked improvement in their ability to breathe. However, objective measurements of airflow failed to document an effect.[20] On the other hand, menthol is safe, inexpensive, and makes cold sufferers feel better.

Despite their widespread use, *antibiotics* are of no benefit in treating the common cold. Antibiotics kill many bacteria, but they do nothing at all to cold-causing viruses. Nor does taking them prevent a child from developing a more serious infection, such as pneumonia.[21]

A new prescription allergy and asthma medication, *nedocromil*, may benefit children with colds. In a study of adult volunteers who were experimentally infected with two different kinds of cold viruses, nedocromil nasal spray significantly reduced nasal secretions and improved the fuzzy thinking that often accompanies colds.[22] It has not yet been evaluated in children.

Among adults with colds, treatment with *Atrovent* nasal spray reduced runny nose symptoms about 20% compared with placebo spray.[23] Atrovent is not a cure, and it requires a prescription. Atrovent has *not* yet been tested in children.

Although most cold medicines have *not* been demonstrated to be helpful in treating cold symptoms in infants and young children, many parents hopefully purchase them believing that at least they won't do any harm. Wrong. *Even nonprescription cold medicines can have powerful and unpleasant side effects.*[24]

SIDE EFFECTS OF COMMON COLD MEDICATIONS

- *Antihistamines*: drowsiness, irritability, dry mouth, fuzzy thinking, thirst

- *Decongestants*: increased heart rate, increased blood pressure, decreased appetite, dizziness, abnormal heart rhythms, hallucinations, psychosis

- *Cough suppressants*: sleepiness, possible addiction[25]

- *Aspirin/acetaminophen*: suppressed immune function[26]

If medications aren't helpful and may be harmful, why do so many doctors recommend them?

Good question. Some cold medicines *are* useful for adults, and therefore people assume they'll work for children, too. Two-thirds of parents surveyed in one study were convinced that their children *needed* medicine for their symptoms. Because of this strong parental demand, some doctors fear that if they don't give a prescription, their patients will be dissatisfied and go elsewhere.[27] *Please don't pressure your doctor for prescription cold medicines.* These products are *not* any more effective than placebos, but they are costly and do run the risk of substantial side effects.

Herbs

Just as there are a variety of unproven cold medications, there is a similar array of unproven herbal remedies.

HERBS TRADITIONALLY USED TO TREAT COLD SYMPTOMS

- *Calming:* chamomile

- *Decongestant:* ephedra or *Ma Huang*, eucalyptus, pine oil

- *Expectorant* (to loosen dry or thick phlegm or mucus): angelica, lobelia, senega snakeroot, bayberry, hyssop, horehound

- *Anti-inflammatory:* angelica, licorice root, slippery elm bark, hyssop, horehound, bromelain[28]

- *Immune-stimulating:* echinacea, goldenseal, astragalus root

Chamomile tea is safe and calming and may help your child get the rest he needs.

Ephedra or *Ma Huang* is the original source of the medicinal decongestants ephedrine and pseudoephedrine. There is great variability in the potency of different species and different areas of cultivation of ephedra plants.[29] Although ephedra has proved effective in adults, it has *not* been tested in young children. I do *not* recommend it. *Eucalyptus or pine oil* added to a vaporizer or bath adds a soothing smell and may help your child feel less congested.

Angelica was used by both American Indians and Russians as an expectorant. In animal studies (but not in human beings yet), angelica extracts have proved anti-inflammatory activity.[30] *Senega snakeroot* and *bayberry bark* teas are expectorants that cause stomach upset.

Hyssop tea and *horehound* lozenges are safe sore throat soothers. *Licorice root* tea is soothing for sore throats accompanying colds and boosts the body's own virus-fighting

chemical, interferon.[31] Tinctures combining *echinacea* and *goldenseal* are available in many health food stores. These herbs seem to boost the body's own immune defenses rather than attacking cold viruses directly.[32,33] I take the combination of echinacea and goldenseal myself when I feel a cold coming on. However, there are still *no* scientific studies evaluating their effects on children with colds.

Used by several Native American tribes, *slippery elm bark* tea has demulcent or mucilaginous qualities that soothe inflamed throats and noses. I am drinking slippery elm bark tea for a mild sore throat as I write this chapter! There are *no* scientific studies evaluating the effects of these herbs on children with colds.

Spices such as ginger, cinnamon, cloves, allspice, and cardamom may also help your child feel less congested. You can brew 1/8 teaspoon of each of these herbs into 2 cups of water to make a very fragrant tea for your stuffed-up child. Ginger root and cayenne are spicy hot. They may help combat the chills and fatigue of fever. In test-tube studies, ginger extracts successfully combated one of the common cold viruses.[34] No studies have evaluated the effectiveness of raw, cooked, or powdered ginger or ginger ale in easing cold symptoms in children.

Some mothers use old-fashioned cold remedies such as onion, comfrey, and eucalyptus poultices or hot flannel packs of fat and camphor. (See Appendix B for information on how to make poultices.) Hot baths with essential oils of eucalyptus, citrus, thyme, rosemary, or tea tree may be soothing and decongesting. There are no studies on the efficacy of poultices or baths in treating children with colds, but if such things are part of your family's healing tradition, they are certainly worth trying. If they irritate your child's skin, discontinue use immediately and consult your doctor.

Nutritional Supplements

NUTRITIONAL SUPPLEMENTS
FOR COLDS

- Vitamin A—unnecessary
- Vitamin C—yes
- Zinc lozenges—maybe
- Brandy or bee pollen (propolis)—no

Vitamin A deficiency increases susceptibility to severe lung infections such as measles pneumonia. A randomized, double-blind, placebo controlled Australian study showed that in children prone to frequent colds, vitamin A supplements (in doses equivalent to the American Recommended Daily Allowances) decreased the number of colds by about 20%; however, there was *no* effect on the total number of days the children had cold symptoms or on episodes of pneumonia.[35] Studies in Haiti and Indonesia indicate that vitamin A supplements actually *increase* the risk of developing colds.[36, 37] I prefer that children get their vitamins naturally in the foods they eat. To make sure your child gets plenty of natural vitamin A, encourage her to eat vitamin A–rich foods: apricots, cantaloupe, carrots, sweet potatoes, spinach, cheddar cheese, eggs, and fortified milk.

Vitamin C is widely used to prevent and treat colds. A 1975 review of scientific studies concluded that vitamin C reduces symptoms and the length of illness.[38] More recent studies confirm the fact that although high-dose vitamin C doesn't *prevent* colds, it does ease symptoms and shorten the length of the cold.[39, 40] The long-term effects of taking several grams of vitamin C daily starting in childhood are unknown. The doses many people take for colds (several grams a day) are well beyond natural levels found in fruits and vegetables. Children need 1 to 2 grams per day to relieve symptoms.[41, 42] I take vitamin C supplements (500 to 1,000 milligrams four times daily) when I feel a cold coming on, and I recommend it for my patients when they get colds. Each glass of orange juice contains 60 to 80 milligrams of vitamin C. Your child needs to drink *at least* four or five glasses of orange juice throughout the day to boost vitamin C levels.

Zinc lozenges may reduce the severity and length of colds in adults,[43, 44] but they can cause stomach upset, mouth irritation, and an abnormal sense of taste.[45] Zinc lozenges must be sucked rather than swallowed to be effective. Do *not* give zinc for more than ten days; taking high doses for more than two weeks can impair the immune system.[46] Zinc must be started on the first day or two of symptoms to have any effect at all, even in adults. Zinc has *not* been tested or proved effective in children.[47]

What about *brandy?* Brandy has been used by parents for ages to soothe sick children, and it may well put a child to sleep. However, brandy (and all other alcoholic beverages) dilates the blood vessels in the nose, compounding nasal congestion. I do *not* recommend that you give brandy to a sick child.

Several natural health magazines have touted the benefits of *propolis*, a bee product, as an infection fighter because it kills bacteria in test tubes.[48] However, there is *no* scientific evidence in human adults or children that it is helpful in warding off the common cold. Save your money for effective remedies like chicken soup.

LIFESTYLE THERAPIES: NUTRITION, EXERCISE, ENVIRONMENT, MIND-BODY

Nutrition

What about *chicken soup?* Science finally proved that chicken soup is helpful in thinning sticky nasal secretions.[49] Nobody knows what the active ingredient is: the chicken, the vegetables, or love, but chicken soup is definitely good for a cold. For best results, have your child sip the soup slowly rather than gulp it down. Some of the benefit may lie in inhaling the steaming broth. Effects only last for about half an hour, so it's better to have small amounts of soup throughout the day than one big bowl at suppertime.

While chicken soup is known as Jewish penicillin, *garlic* is called Russian penicillin. Garlic is used as a cold remedy around the world. In hundreds of test-tube studies, garlic has proven it can kill cold viruses. It is most potent raw or baked. If your child can't swallow a whole clove of garlic, you might try mincing a raw clove and mixing it with a little mashed potato. Garlic has not been scientifically tested in children with colds, but it is safe and worth trying if your child still has an appetite.

Hot chili peppers, horseradish, mustard, Tabasco sauce, salsa, wasabi (Japanese horseradish), and other spicy foods are also thought to be helpful for cold sufferers. Spicy foods thin nasal secretions, make noses run, and open the sinuses even when you're healthy. Such effects may benefit congested children, too. Although there are no scientific studies evaluating chili peppers in the treatment of colds, when eaten in moderation such foods are certainly safe and are probably worth a try.

When children are afflicted with colds, they tend to breathe through their mouths. This dries out the mouth and results in a water loss. Fevers (which often accompany colds) also increase water loss. All of this means that your child needs extra fluids when he has a cold. This is why physicians and grandmothers alike admonish parents to give their sick children *plenty of fluids*. How much is plenty? A good rule of thumb is that a child is getting plenty of fluids if he needs to urinate at least every two to three hours while he is awake.

Many children lose their appetites temporarily while they're ill. There's no point in forcing a child with a cold to eat. Keep offering foods that are easily digested such as broths, oatmeal, citrus fruits and juices, pears, plums, or peaches, lettuce, celery, and carrots.

Exercise

Make sure your child is well rested during cold and flu season so that his immune system is at full power to fight off attacks by viruses. Fatigue is one of the most common symptoms of the common cold. Some kids seem immune to this particular effect and continue to play normally. You don't need to force your child to go to bed when he has a cold, but do let him know it's OK to take an extra nap. Sleeping frees some of the body's energy up to mend itself. It also reduces your child's exposure to other people he might infect.

Moderate exercise may help ward off colds. Several studies indicate that those at the highest risk of colds are couch potatoes and exercise addicts.[50] Moderation is the key.

Sleeping with his head elevated may help reduce your child's congestion. You might try an extra pillow or letting an infant sleep in his car seat.

Environment

Keep your child warm and out of drafts, but don't let the bedroom get too stuffy. Eucalyptus, menthol, pennyroyal, pine, rosemary, wintergreen, and tea tree oils placed in the medicine cup of a hot air vaporizer or as part of a steam bath are believed to be helpful by millions of parents, but there is not a single scientific study evaluating their effectiveness. They are safe (if you keep your toddler away from the hot vaporizer itself to avoid burns) and worth a try. *Warning:* Do *not* take eucalyptus oil internally or apply it to the skin; it is for inhalation only.

Tobacco smoke paralyzes the cilia that sweep cold viruses out of the nose and throat. Exposure to cigarette smoke increases the chance that your child will get a cold and makes it more difficult for him to fight it off. Please, do *not* smoke and do not allow others to smoke around your child.

Steam has been used by countless people to combat congestion. In a recent study, a one-hour treatment with very hot steam had no impact on adults' cold symptoms.[51] Previous studies had suggested that steam treatment was helpful.[52, 53] None of these studies tells us about the effect of steam or mist on children's colds, whether repeated (as opposed to the one-time treatments tested in the studies) steam treatments are helpful, or how much time a child must spend with the vaporizer or steam treatment to benefit from it. A cool mist vaporizer is probably just as helpful and is less likely to cause unintentional burns.[54] At this point the jury is still out. Until it comes in, give vaporizers a try. If your child benefits, keep it up; if not, discontinue treatment.

A word about vaporizers and humidifiers. If you use one, clean it daily. Mold and bacteria love the moist environment in a vaporizer and will quickly grow inside. Follow the manufacturer's instructions for regular cleaning.

Most kids under four years old just can't blow their noses the way adults can. To help infants and toddlers clear their secretions, use a bulb syringe or nasal aspirator. Squeeze the syringe, then insert the small end in the child's nostril. Release the bulb and allow the suction to draw the mucus out. If the mucus is dry or thick, you can loosen it with a drop or two of water or saline drops (Na-Sal). Wait for the mucus to soften and then use the bulb syringe. Do one nostril at a time.

Wash your hands! Washing your hands and having your child wash his hands are the best ways to cut down the spread of colds and other infectious illnesses.

Mind-Body

Psychological stress lowers resistance to colds. The more stress, the higher the risk of catching a cold.[55] Among volunteers who were intentionally infected with cold viruses, those with the most stress were the most likely to develop symptoms; those with less stress had almost no symptoms.[56] Interestingly, the chance of getting symptoms was most strongly related to what the subjects actually experienced rather than whether they interpreted these experiences as stressful. One easily avoided stress is lack of sleep. Cuddling and reassuring your child that you love him are great antidotes to stress.

The power of a variety of placebos to improve cold symptoms also suggests that our minds have powerful effects on both getting colds and the amount we suffer from them once infected. Given these facts, it is important to reinforce the idea that the child is strong and has the power and ability to overcome his cold symptoms. If you give your child the message that he is weak or susceptible to illness, you may be creating a self-fulfilling prophecy.

BIOMECHANICAL THERAPIES: MASSAGE, SPINAL MANIPULATION

Massage

One of my fondest memories of childhood is of receiving a Vicks Vaporub massage when I had a cold. I have been unable to find a single study evaluating the efficacy of this time-tested technique, but I'm sure that the combination or parental love, a warm bed, and Vicks has made colds more bearable for thousands of children, and I heartily recommend them. Other massage oils that help open up a clogged nose include camphor, camphorated olive oil, eucalyptus, menthol, and pine. Tiger Balm, a fragrant balm found in many health food stores, contains a combination of camphor, menthol, cajeput, and clove oils.

Massage the face, pressing on cheekbones, following the contours of the bone in a downward movement. Also massage feet, especially the big toe. Massage the back of the child's head, downward over the base of the skull, the spine, chest, and abdomen. This can be done on infants as young as one month old. If the lymph glands in the neck are enlarged, gently massage the glands downward (to help them drain toward the heart). Folk remedies include massaging the soles of the feet with mustard powder. If you try this, you must be careful to wash off the mustard afterward to avoid burns.

Spinal Manipulation

Osteopathic manipulation of the neck and upper back to aid the lymphatic drainage of the head and neck has been recommended but has *not* been scientifically evaluated. I do *not* recommend spinal adjustments as cold remedies.

BIOENERGETIC THERAPIES:
ACUPUNCTURE, HOMEOPATHY

Acupuncture

There are no studies comparing acupuncture to any other treatment in children with colds. One series of adults treated with acupuncture for respiratory illnesses reported improved symptoms, but there was no untreated comparison group, so it's hard to tell how many would have improved without treatment.[57] I do *not* recommend acupuncture therapy for children with colds.

Homeopathy

Homeopathic remedies for the common cold include Aconitum, Allium, Arsenicum, Belladonna, Bryonia, Euphrasia, Gelsemium, Kali bichromium, Nux vomica, Phosphorus, and Pulsatilla. A recent study of individually prescribed homeopathic remedies for children with frequent colds showed *no* significant improvement compared with placebo treatments.[58] I do *not* recommend homeopathic remedies for children with colds.

WHAT ABOUT JANET AND JAMAL?

Janet had just enrolled Jamal in his new day care and didn't think she could transfer him any time soon. The first thing I advised her to do was to quit smoking. Quitting now would help reduce Jamal's frequent colds and minimize her recurrent bouts with bronchitis and sinusitis. I had her choose a date she would quit, gave her the name of an internist who could prescribe a nicotine patch to battle her cravings, and called her in a week to see how it was going. I recommended that until her quit date, she avoid smoking in Jamal's presence— especially indoors or in the car.

Second, I recommended that she make a big pot of chicken soup that she and Jamal could sip over the next few days. While she was at the grocery store, she decided to try the ready-made chamomile and slippery elm bark herbal teas.

Third, we discussed the home vaporizer. Janet wanted to try adding eucalyptus oil to the medicine cup to see if that helped. She said that when she was a little girl, her mother rubbed Mentholatum on her chest and that it made her feel much better. She decided to continue the family tradition.

Both Janet and Jamal were back to normal within three days. Janet quit smoking, but she relapsed two weeks later. I reassured her that

relapses are common and that one slip did not mean she was doomed to failure. Three tries later, she has finally quit for good. She and Jamal enjoy making their cold remedy (chicken soup) together and have had fewer colds every year for the last three years.

WHAT I RECOMMEND FOR COLDS

PREVENTING COLDS

1. *Lifestyle—environment.* Do *not* smoke and do *not* allow others to smoke around your child. If your child must be in day care, try to make sure he is in a setting with small groups of children or in small classes in separate rooms to minimize his exposure to cold viruses. Wash your hands, and make sure your child washes his.

2. *Lifestyle—exercise.* Regular moderate exercise helps to keep the immune system in top shape.

See Your Health Care Provider If Your Child Has

- A high fever (over 103°F or 39.4°C)
- A sore throat or sore glands in the neck
- Ear pain
- A stiff neck or sore back
- Shortness of breath, wheezing, or trouble breathing
- Cold symptoms for longer than seven to ten days
- Or is too sick to drink

TREATING COLDS

1. *Biochemical—home remedy.* Use saline nose drops.

2. Do *not* use antihistamines, cough syrups, decongestants, or expectorants in children less than five years old. Older children may benefit from decongestants. Avoid decongestant nasal sprays unless your child is having so much trouble breathing that he can't eat or sleep. Use analgesics only to treat discomfort. Treat the child, not the thermometer.

3. *Biochemical—nutritional supplements.* Give vitamin C, 1 to 2 grams divided into several doses over the course of the day.

4. *Lifestyle—nutrition.* Give plenty of fluids, chicken soup (sipped slowly through the day), raw or baked garlic, ginger, spicy foods.

5. *Lifestyle—exercise.* Ensure sufficient rest, encourage extra naps.

6. *Lifestyle—environment.* Use a steam or cool mist vaporizer, especially with menthol or eucalyptus oils in the medicine cup.

7. *Lifestyle—mind-body.* Give extra hugs and encouragement, and encourage positive thoughts.

8. *Biomechanical—massage.* Give massages using Mentholatum, Tiger Balm, or Vicks Vaporub.

10

COLIC

Ken Johnson called one evening about his baby girl, Nancy. He had just arrived home after a hard day at the office; his wife, Erica, was cooking dinner, and six-week-old Nancy was crying again. He had tried feeding her, rocking her, singing to her, carrying her, and bouncing her. Nothing seemed to work for more than a minute before she started crying again, and she looked as if her tummy hurt. He wondered how Erica had coped with this all day, but she said that Nancy was not that fussy until about the time he came home. He wondered if the baby didn't like him, if he did something to cause the crying, or if she had a medical problem. He called his mother for advice; she said it sounded like colic. He wanted to know what I thought, whether he should bring her in for an evaluation and if there were any natural remedies that would help.

All babies cry. By the time she's six weeks old, the average baby (even without colic) cries for one and a half to two-and-a-half hours a day. Colic is intense or excessive (more than three hours a day for three or more days a week) crying between the ages of three weeks and three months. It is *not* a sign of serious illness, bad temperament, mis-behavior, or inadequate parenting, but it *is* distressing for parents.

Most parents quickly learn the difference between a hungry cry, a pain cry, an angry cry, and a bored cry. Colic is different. It sounds like a cry of pain—intense, high-pitched, and continuous. Colic is usually worse in the evenings when parents are getting home, trying to fix dinner and unwind from the day.[1] Colic usually peaks around the time the baby is six weeks old and is almost always over by three months. Sometimes the screaming and crying are accompanied by vigorous kicking, and the baby is difficult to console. While crying, babies with colic often pull their legs up, make tight fists, have swollen or distended tummies, appear to be in pain, and burp or pass gas.

About 15 to 20 percent of babies develop colic. Colic is more common in first-born babies than in subsequent siblings. It is most common among babies whose parents are professionals and least common among babies whose parents are unskilled laborers. It may be that these babies really have different amounts of colic, or it could be that their parents just have different expectations about how much babies should cry.

Babies with colic may appear to be totally miserable, but they are generally very healthy from every other standpoint. They eat well and gain weight; they don't have fevers or diarrhea or any other symptoms.

WHEN TO TAKE A COLICKY BABY TO A HEALTH CARE PROFESSIONAL

- Poor feeding, diarrhea, or weight loss
- Fever
- Crying is unusually severe or more than three hours daily
- Colic starts before two weeks of age or persists beyond three months of age

If your child has any of these signs, take her to her doctor for an evaluation. She may be suffering from another problem such as a

bladder infection, ear infection, or other serious health problem.[2]

What causes colic? No one has come up with one right answer for what causes colic in all babies, but there are lots of theories.

COLIC CAUSES?

- Developmental stage
- Emotions and family stress
- Differences in infant temperament and physiology
- Food intolerance

Infants continue to develop rapidly after birth. For example, the coordination between swallowing, digestion, and peristalsis (movement through the intestines) is still developing. The nervous system is also developing, and the baby may be plain old worn out or overstimulated by the time evening comes—at least until she has learned to pace her arousal and sleep cycles over the course of the day.

Emotions also affect digestion and gas formation. Family tensions often precipitate increased infant crying. Parents who feel they have plenty of help and support and who feel they had a good childbirth experience are less likely to have colicky babies.[3] Confident mothers are less likely to have colicky babies than mothers who are anxious about their parenting abilities.[4] On the other hand, having a colicky baby can make even a calm, happy mother lose confidence and feel anxious and depressed.[5] (Sorry, dads, there just aren't very many studies about how fathers' moods and expectations affect infant colic.) Having a baby with colic doesn't mean you are a bad parent, but it can surely make you feel like a failure.

Even very young babies definitely have different temperaments and physical make-ups. Some babies are just fussier and have different digestive dynamics than others. Babies who have difficult temperaments (for example, irregular sleep patterns, oversensitive, more squirmy) in the first two weeks of life cry and fuss more at six weeks than other babies.[6] Higher levels of motilin (a molecule that increases intestinal activity) are present in newborn babies who eventually develop colic than in those who do not.[7] Colicky babies also produce more gas and digest milk sugar (lactose) more poorly than babies who are not colicky.[8] Some colicky babies seem to be suffering from reflux or heartburn.[9] Having colic doesn't necessarily mean that the child will have a difficult disposition later on. One of my former mentors, Dr. Peter Karofsky, frequently assures parents that the fussiest babies become the sweetest toddlers.

DOES DIET CAUSE COLIC?

- Formula vs. breast milk—no
- Iron-fortified vs. low-iron formulas—iron is better
- Infrequent vs. frequent feeding—frequent is better
- Cow's milk sensitivity—in some cases
- Diet of the nursing mother—in some cases
- Solid evidence against solids

There is no difference in the risk of developing colic between babies who are *breast-fed* (20%) and those who drink *formula* (20%).[10] Breast-fed babies tend to cry and fuss more often than babies who are fed formula, but they do not cry more total hours overall. Breast-fed babies' stomachs empty faster after a feeding, and they are hungry again sooner. Once their hunger is attended to, they usually stop crying.

The risk of having colic is twice as high among infants fed *low-iron formula* as among the babies fed *iron-fortified formula*.[11] Several studies have shown that iron supplementation does *not* make colic (or spitting up or diarrhea or gas) worse, old folklore notwithstanding.[12]

Breast-fed babies who are fed *less often* (every three to four hours) tend to cry more than babies who are fed *more often* (every two hours). Feeding your baby every two hours may seem exhausting, but over the first few weeks of life it may result in less crying.

Babies whose parents *respond to their cries* more *quickly* fret much less than babies whose parents wait a bit longer to see if the baby will stop crying on its own.[13] You can't spoil a young baby! In fact, you may make your life easier if you respond to the baby quickly and feed the baby more often in the first two to three months of life.

There is a small group of babies whose colic improves when they no longer drink *cow's milk* formulas or their breast-feeding mothers abstain from drinking cow's milk.[14, 15, 16] Among breast-fed babies, there is no overall difference in the risk of colic between babies whose mothers drink cow's milk and those whose mothers do not drink cow's milk. Cow's milk proteins are absorbed by mothers and concentrated in breast milk; there can be even higher concentrations in the breast milk of mothers who drink cow's milk than there are in cow's milk itself.[17] A randomized, controlled trial among formula-fed infants who seemed to be sensitive to cow's milk showed that colic disappeared when infants were fed a formula free of cow's milk protein; when the protein was reintroduced, the babies became colicky again.[18] *For most babies, what the mother drinks makes no difference at all.* If you decide to stop drinking cow's milk, be prepared to wait a week or more to see an improvement in your baby's symptoms; it may take that long for all of the cow's milk proteins to be totally flushed out of your system. And make sure you're getting enough protein and calcium from other foods.

Some *nursing mothers* notice that when they *eat certain foods*, their baby has more colic. A New Zealand study showed that the only foods eaten by nursing mothers that were consistently associated with colic in their babies were fruit and chocolate.[19] Chocolate, as well as coffee, tea, and cola, contains caffeine. Some babies are sensitive to other foods in the nursing mother's diet, such as soy, corn, wheat, and eggs. These foods are also the most common food allergens in infants and young children (see Chapter 4, Allergies). Other foods that find their way into breast milk and seem to distress some babies are cabbage, broccoli, onions, peppers, and beans. On the other hand, many babies like the taste of their mothers' milk better if she's eaten garlic.

You can probably do well without some of these items in your diet, but if you omit milk, be sure you get enough calcium from other sources. It is important that the nursing mother's diet be well balanced, with plenty of green vegetables and other sources of calcium, vitamin D, and protein (such as calcium-fortified orange juice, canned fish, or tofu). If you decide to omit or restrict your intake of dairy or other major food groups, please check with your health care professional to make sure you are getting all of the nutrients you and your baby need.

Feeding a baby a *variety of foods early* in life is a definite risk factor for developing food allergies as well as colic.[20] Do *not* try to treat your child's colic by offering her solids. Solids (such as rice cereal) have been proven *not* to be helpful in treating colic. Hold off on solids until your baby is at least four months old to minimize her chances of developing food allergies.

CAN COLIC BE PREVENTED?

Some babies get colic no matter what you do. However, there are things you can try to reduce the chances that your baby will develop colic. All of the effective prevention techniques are from the lifestyle side of the Therapeutic Mountain.

Nutrition

If you are *nursing* your baby, *feed at least every two hours* rather than every three to four hours. If you are feeding your baby *formula*, choose one that is *iron-fortified* to reduce the risk of colic and anemia. Do *not* introduce solids in your baby's diet until she is at least four to six months old.

Behavior

Carry your baby as much as possible. Several years ago, a Canadian study showed that parents who carried their babies four to five hours a day were rewarded by a 50% reduction in infant crying at six weeks of age compared with parents who carried their babies two to three hours a day.[21] The improvement was especially noticeable in the evening hours when colic tends to be worse. Unfortunately, more recent studies have been unable to duplicate the benefits of increased carrying on infant colic.[22, 23, 24] Despite these studies, I still advocate carrying your baby at least three hours daily because I believe it helps promote bonding between parents and infants and facilitates quicker responses to babies' needs.

Respond to your young baby's cry quickly (within ninety seconds). This reduces crying both in the short term and in the long term as your baby learns that you are ready, willing, and able to meet her needs. "Spoiling" the young baby (under four months old) actually improves his behavior. You don't make a two-month-old tougher or stronger or more self-sufficient by expecting him to cry it out; you just get more crying.

Don't smoke. Smoking parents are more likely to have babies who cry a lot during infancy, and their children are more likely to suffer from colds, ear infections, and other problems later on.[25]

Relax. The more you and your spouse can do to remain calm, to gain the support and confidence you feel you need to be good parents, and to nurture your own relationship, the less likely you are to have a baby who develops colic, and the better you will be able to cope with colic or any other problem that comes along. Make sure you get enough *sleep* and support to cope with a crying baby. Many parents find it helpful to join a *parent support group* so they can hear how other parents deal with the same issues they face and so they can feel less alone in learning how to be good parents.

WHAT CAN YOU DO TO TREAT COLIC?

All babies outgrow colic. Colic doesn't do any long-term or serious damage to babies unless the parents become very frustrated and lash out at the defenseless child. Colic is definitely distressing for the baby and the baby's family. The best remedies involve *lifestyle therapies*. If you don't feel you can cope, get help. Let's go around the Therapeutic Mountain to find out what works in treating colic. If you want to skip to the bottom-line summary, flip to the end of the chapter.

BIOCHEMICAL THERAPIES: MEDICATIONS, HERBS, NUTRITIONAL SUPPLEMENTS

Medications

MEDICATIONS—NONE PROVED SAFE AND EFFECTIVE

- Simethicone: (nonprescription Mylicon)
- Lactase
- Sedatives (prescription), antihistamines, alcohol
- Dicyclomine: (Bentyl)

One of the most commonly used medications to treat infant colic is *simethicone* (Mylicon), which seems to reduce gas. Simethicone reduced the number of crying attacks and was preferred by twenty of twenty-six parents in one study.[26] However, a European study showed *no* benefits of simethicone compared with placebo,[27] and a large study conducted in pediatric clinics from North Carolina to Utah showed that simethicone was not more helpful than placebo in reducing infant colic.[28] Babies improve at the same rate regardless of whether they receive placebo or simethicone. I do *not* routinely recommend simethicone for treating colic. Save your money; don't buy it.

Because some babies seem to be sensitive to lactose (milk sugar), some folks recommend using supplemental *lactase* (the enzyme that helps us digest lactose) for treating colic. Unfortunately, two studies have failed to show that lactase is any more helpful than a placebo.[29, 30] I do *not* routinely recommend it.

Sedatives, antihistamines, and motion-sickness medications, including dicyclomine (Bentyl), are outdated and potentially harmful colic remedies.[31] These treatments have some potentially serious side effects, including Sudden Infant Death Syndrome.[32, 33] Like these old-fashioned medications, old-fashioned remedies such as giving the baby wine or another *alcoholic beverage* are dangerous and are now discouraged by most pediatricians. I do *not* recommend *any* medications as colic remedies.

Herbs

HERBAL REMEDIES FOR COLIC

- Effective: combination of balm-mint, chamomile, fennel, licorice, vervain
- Other traditional remedies: mint family, anise, caraway, catnip, chamomile, cumin, dill, fennel, ginger

A 1993 study documented that 3 to 4 ounces per day of an herbal tea (containing chamomile, fennel, vervain, licorice, and balm-mint) was significantly more effective than a placebo (a tea with simple sugar and flavoring but no herbs) in eliminating infant colic.[34] It is not known which of the herbs in the herbal tea is the effective ingredient. Many of my Eastern European and Mexican parents bring chamomile tea with them, asking if it is safe to give the baby. Chamomile is a traditional tummy-settling tea in many parts of the world. Although no babies in this study had any side effects, it is possible that some babies might. Some babies are even allergic to chamomile. A California baby developed botulism from contaminated home-grown chamomile tea.

Other traditional herbal recommendations for colic and indigestion include anise, catnip, peppermint leaf, fennel, caraway seed, dill seed, chamomile, and ginger root. The old remedy gripe water, which is still available in Britain and Canada, was made from dill. Dill, fennel, and caraway are all from the same family of plants. Although these herbs are probably safe, they have not undergone extensive, rigorous scientific study.

> *Warning*: Do *not* give your baby more than 4 to 6 ounces per day of herbal tea. Filling up on tea means there is less room for the milk your baby needs to grow. Start slowly, say one ounce at first, and watch the baby for several hours for any side effects or reactions before trying more. Also, do *not* give your baby noncommercial preparations. The side effects of contaminated herbs can be deadly.[35]

Nutritional Supplements

A favorite British remedy for colic is onion tea. Slice one or two yellow onions into 2 cups of water. Bring to a boil and simmer for fifteen minutes. Strain the onion. Cool the tea to room temperature. Try giving it a teaspoon at a time. Many babies do not like the flavor of onion tea, but some respond immediately. Although I like the idea of this simple home remedy, it has *not* been evaluated in a formal study. No other nutritional supplements have been scientifically evaluated as colic treatments.

LIFESTYLE THERAPIES: NUTRITION, ENVIRONMENT, MIND-BODY

Nutrition

NUTRITIONAL APPROACHES TO COLIC

- Formula: cow's milk–free
- Rice cereal
- Fiber
- Frequent burping

Although there is no difference in the rate of colic between breast-fed and formula-fed infants, a few formula-fed babies' colic improves if they are switched to a formula that does not contain cow's milk, such as soy formula or Nutramigen.[36, 37] A favorable response to a diet free of cow's milk does *not* necessarily mean that your baby is allergic to cow's milk; she may tolerate it easily when she gets a little older. After a month or two on an alternative formula, many babies can return to their previous (less expensive) formula without difficulty.

For years, parents have believed that giving the baby a little *rice cereal* helps with crying. A recent study from Johns Hopkins disproved this common myth.[38] It turns out that most parents started the solids about the time their baby was getting over colic anyway, and the cereal got the credit for the improvement. There's no scientific evidence that cereal cures colic.

Because babies with colic look as if they're in the same kind of pain as adults with irritable bowel syndrome (who are often helped by increased fiber), some people have tried treating colicky babies with *fiber*. However, a comparison study showed that adding fiber does *not* improve colic.[39] Another nice-sounding theory bites the dust!

Another old-fashioned, safe (and still scientifically untested) therapy is *frequent burping*. Some babies eat very fast and swallow a lot of air. All that gas in the tummy may make colic worse. Try burping your baby every five to ten minutes during feeding.

Environment

A *warm pack* or *hot water bottle* on the baby's tummy is a well-known colic remedy. Others recommend a *warm bath* as a way to relax an upset baby. There are also lots of recommendations in old medical texts about placing the baby on her tummy over your knees or over a rolled-up towel to increase pressure on the abdomen. Some parents put the baby's tummy across their knees and then gently bounce her to help break up gas bubbles and relieve pressure. There are no scientific studies evaluating the effectiveness of these time-honored remedies. Because they are safe, you may want to try them. If you use a warm pack or hot water bottle, test the temperature to make sure it is not too hot for a baby's sensitive skin.

Music has also proven useful in treating infant colic. In one study, psychologists trained parents to do classical conditioning. When the colicky baby was quiet, calm, and not crying, the parents played a recording of the baby's favorite music and paid extra attention to the baby. When the infant started to cry, the parents turned off the tape and left the room briefly. This procedure was followed throughout the day. Within days, crying and colic had significantly decreased. When the parents returned to their old way of dealing with crying, the crying again increased.[40] Music therapy is definitely safe and worth trying.

Mind-Body

Behavioral strategies are the keys to effective colic management. Many parents have found it useful to get into a rhythm of responses to a colicky baby.[41]

BEHAVIORAL RESPONSES TO COLIC

1. Check to make sure that she isn't hungry (has she fed in the last two hours?).

2. Check to make sure nothing is causing pain (an open diaper pin or a hair wrapped around a finger, toe, etc.).

3. Check to see if the diaper needs changing.

4. Think about her level of stimulation and activity:

a. Is she bored? Does she need more attention and activity?

b. Is she overstimulated? Too much playing, singing, rocking, or any other stimulation can overwhelm a baby.

Still no luck? After you have checked these things, you may find the following helpful[42]:

- Slow, rhythmic rocking (not jiggling or shaking)
- Going for a walk in a stroller
- Swaddling or wrapping her snugly and placing her in a dark, quiet room
- Letting her suck her fist or fingers
- Going for a ride in the car
- Putting her in her car seat and putting the car seat on top of the dryer while it is running on "fluff" (no heat). This provides vibration and white noise that soothes many babies. Make sure someone stays with the baby to see that the car seat doesn't vibrate right off the dryer!
- Running the vacuum cleaner or a hair dryer next to the baby while she's in the car seat. This is simply a source of white noise, which some babies find strangely soothing.

Because so many parents have found a car ride an effective way to soothe their babies, manufacturers have devised a product to simulate the effects of going on a car ride. This device, called *SleepTight,* can be attached to the infant's crib, and reduces crying in many infants.[43] Because you are likely to use such a device for only a short time, I recom-

mend that you talk with other parents or your child care provider about buying one together and then renting it out as families need it. Some insurance companies will help with reimbursement for part of the cost if you have a physician's prescription. You can reach the manufacturer at 1(800)662–6542 (1–800 NO COLIC). SleepTight is available on a fifteen-day trial basis from the manufacturer.

As a last resort, you can let your baby cry himself to sleep. This is very hard for most parents to do. Most parents feel guilty and also worry that the neighbors will be annoyed or think they are bad parents. You may want to take turns being responsible for the baby for an hour or two so you can get a break. If you are a single parent, try to find a trustworthy family member, neighbor, or friend to care for the baby for an hour so you can take the time to recenter yourself.

Take some time to *relax.* This is very difficult when you are exhausted and overwhelmed with all of the chores and responsibilities involved in taking care of a new baby, but it is very important for you *and* the baby. The best thing you can do for your baby is to take care of yourself. Find some things that make you feel good–a bubble bath, relaxing music, a brisk walk, a talk with a friend, meditation, or breathing exercises. Do at least one nice thing for yourself every day! Ask for help from someone you trust.

BIOMECHANICAL THERAPIES: MASSAGE, SPINAL MANIPULATION

Massage

Danish custom includes massage treatment for infant colic.[44] The baby is held on his side, supported by the parent's arm, with the head somewhat down and the bottom elevated. The tummy is then massaged in a cir-

cular, clockwise fashion, starting with small circles at the belly button and gradually increasing the size of the circles outward. You can do the tummy rub through the baby's clothes, or if he is naked, use warmed olive oil, almond oil, castor oil, or cocoa butter. Massage oils that include chamomile, lavender, or geranium are thought to be especially soothing. The massage should be given about twenty to thirty minutes after a meal so the baby's stomach has had a little time to empty (and she doesn't spit up all over you). You can extend the massage to include the baby's whole body. Other massage therapists recommend variations on this technique.[45] Although I think massage is terrific, feels wonderful, helps bonding between parents and babies, and probably does not have a single bad side effect when it is done gently and lovingly, I cannot in all honesty say that I've run across any studies that document its effectiveness in treating infants with colic.

Spinal Manipulation

You may have heard that *chiropractic* helps babies with colic. In one study, six-week-old babies treated with three sessions of chiropractic manipulation cried less over the course of the next two weeks.[46] However, treatment started just when colic was at its worst and would have improved over time without any treatment. Since this study did not include a group of babies who were not treated (control group), we can't say that chiropractic was any more helpful than no treatment. Don't waste your money on chiropractic for colic; invest in patience. It pays far bigger dividends in the long run.

BIOENERGETIC THERAPIES: THERAPEUTIC TOUCH, HOMEOPATHY

Therapeutic Touch

Therapeutic Touch *is* helpful for crying babies and children.[47] Although there are no studies on colic specifically, I know from my own clinical experience that TT relaxes and calms both the giver and receiver, and I use it in the clinic when confronted with a baby who is crying for any reason. (See Appendix A and Appendix B for more information on Therapeutic Touch.)

Homeopathy

The most common homeopathic remedies for colic are *Chamomilla*, *Colocynth* (from the herb bitter apple), *Dioscorea* (wild yam), *Magnesia phosphorica*, *Nux vomica*, and *Pulsatilla*. There are no scientific studies evaluating the effectiveness of these remedies in treating infant colic. I do *not* recommend them.

WHAT I RECOMMEND FOR COLIC

PREVENTING COLIC

1. *Lifestyle—nutrition.* If you are nursing your baby, nurse often (every two to three hours). If you are formula feeding, use iron-fortified formula.
2. *Lifestyle—mind-body.* Respond to your baby's cries quickly. Surround yourself with supportive family and friends. Take care of yourself, too.
3. *Lifestyle—environment.* Don't smoke.

When to See Your Doctor

- If the colic persists or recurs daily, talk with your doctor about a temporary change in formulas to one that does not contain cow's milk; if you are nursing, consider altering your diet to omit suspect foods.
- If home remedies do not work, if your baby has other symptoms, or if she is over three months old and still has colic, see your health care professional. Severe, persistent crying may be a sign that your child has an infection (like an ear, bladder, or kidney infection) or other treatable condition. Other worrisome symptoms include black or bloody stools, vomiting, diarrhea, or fever in an infant less than two months old.

TREATING COLIC

1. *Lifestyle—mind-body.* Check to make sure she's not hungry, not in pain, not in a wet or dirty diaper, and not bored or overstimulated.

Try a ride in the car seat, five to ten minutes in a swing or rocker, or try SleepTight.

If you've done all of the above and the baby is still crying, ask for help, put the baby in her crib for ten minutes, close the door, and take time to get calm and regroup before you try again.

2. *Biomechanical—massage.* Consider a tummy massage or a warm hot water bottle.

3. *Lifestyle—environment.* Try music therapy: when she's quiet, play her favorite music and praise her; when she starts crying, stop the music and ignore her for a minute or two.

4. *Biochemical—herbs.* Try *herbal tea* containing chamomile, mint, fennel, licorice, and vervain.

11
CONJUNCTIVITIS
(PINKEYE)

Jose Fernandez came into the clinic on a Thursday afternoon with his three-year-old daughter, Maria, bearing a note from her day care center. He'd been called at work to come pick her up and take her to the doctor because she had pinkeye; they wanted her to be seen and treated before she returned to the center. Maria had been fine except for a runny nose. She awoke that morning with some yellowish crusting that matted her eyelashes together, but she was happy and playful. She had also begun tugging at her left ear. Jose wanted to know how to help Maria get well soon and how to prevent the disease from spreading to his infant son, George.

Pinkeye or conjunctivitis is an inflammation of the conjunctiva, the transparent covering that lines the inner surface of the eyelids and the front of the eyeball. It is very common. Conjunctivitis can cause several symptoms, although affected children usually feel fine except for their eyes.

Different things cause conjunctivitis at different ages. Newborns can catch bacteria going through the birth canal during delivery; their eyes can also be irritated by the antibi-

SYMPTOMS OF CONJUNCTIVITIS

- Red or pink eye with watery discharge
- Dry matter in eyelashes or gooey yellowish-green discharge
- Swollen eyelid
- Itchy feeling or irritation that feels like sand in the eye
- Swollen lymph nodes under the chin or in front of the ear

otic drops used to prevent infections. Conjunctivitis in older children and adults can be caused by allergies (see Chapter 4) and irritants as well as infections. Occasionally red eyes can be a sign of a serious illness affecting other parts of the body, such as measles.

CAUSES OF CONJUNCTIVITIS IN CHILDREN

- Infection
- Irritants or allergies
- Injuries
- Other illnesses

Conjunctivitis in the *newborn* may be caused by gonorrhea or chlamydia (the two most common sexually transmitted diseases in mothers). These infections are serious. Gonorrhea conjunctivitis can cause blindness if it is not recognized and treated quickly. Chlamydia infections can spread to the lungs, causing pneumonia. Symptoms starting on the third or fourth day of life are usually due to gonorrhea, and those that start when the baby is a week or two old are more likely to be due to chlamydia.

The eye drops given at birth help prevent newborn eye infections; they are given routinely (and in some states by law) to all babies. The eye medicines given to most newborns (erythromycin, tetracycline, or povidone-iodine[1]) are safe, effective, and nonirritating.[2] However, silver nitrate drops can sometimes cause irritation. It usually clears within two to three days. Conjunctivitis on the first day of life is usually due to eye drops.

Among *older children*, the bacteria that cause conjunctivitis are the same culprits that cause ear infections, sinus infections, and pneumonia. One bacteria, *Hemophilus*, is notorious for causing the combination of conjunctivitis and ear infection (see Chapter 17, Ear Infections). Most eye infections in older children resolve on their own without treatment in seven to ten days, although antibiotics can speed healing by three to five days.

The viruses that cause conjunctivitis in older children are the same bad actors that cause colds, sore throats, and bronchitis. Viral infections tend to last a bit longer—up to two to four weeks. Two viruses deserves special mention—*herpes virus* and *adenovirus*. Herpes virus causes cold sores and genital infections. If it spreads to the eye, it can cause serious damage. If your child has signs of a herpes infection (tiny blisters on red skin) near the eye, the eyelid, or the tip of the nose, take her to be evaluated immediately so appropriate treatment can be started promptly. Adenovirus is a common summertime viral infection that causes conjunctivitis and a sore throat.

The most common eye *irritants* in older children and adults are cigarette smoke, wood smoke, and pollution. Swimmers' eyes often become irritated with chlorine. Allergies such as hay fever commonly cause red, irritated, itchy, watery eyes during pollen season. Allergies usually cause other symptoms as well, such as runny nose, cough, and an itchy mouth (see Chapter 4, Allergies).

The most common causes of minor eye *injuries* are insect bites, accidental pokes from stray fingers, and scratches from overuse of contact lenses. Rarely, children get glue in their eyes. SuperGlue is one of the worst offenders. Chemical injuries from bleach splashes, lye, or other cleaning agents can cause serious damage.

More serious eye diseases, such as glaucoma, are also characterized by red, painful eyes, but they don't cause as much discharge or matting as with infectious conjunctivitis. If your child's eyes are not getting better after a few days of treatment, if the eye is painful, or your child is having trouble seeing, don't wait around trying home remedies. Seek professional help. Conjunctivitis can also be a symptom of more serious illness such as measles, Lyme disease, or rheumatoid arthritis. In these cases, your child will have other symptoms besides an irritated eye.

DIAGNOSING CONJUNCTIVITIS

Usually, diagnosing the different causes of pinkeye is pretty straightforward based on the child's symptoms and a physical examination. For example, itching is usually due to allergies. Insect bites usually affect the eyelid around the eye rather than the eye itself. Infectious conjunctivitis caused by viruses is usually accompanied by cold symptoms. Viral and bacterial eye infections can occur in one or both eyes at the same time and are sometimes difficult to distinguish from each other without additional tests.

Laboratory tests can help sort out the cause of conjunctivitis. These tests include taking a swab of the inner eyelid for a culture, measuring the pressure inside the eye, checking the eye's reaction to light, using a special stain to look for scratches on the eyeball, and looking deep inside the eye with a special instrument. Newborns require a culture to help distinguish between different kinds of serious infections. Children who have red, painful eyes need to have their vision tested and to have the pressure inside their eyes measured to make sure they don't have glaucoma.

On physical examination, Maria had an infected left ear as well as a gooey, yellow discharge and redness in both eyes. Because she had signs of another infection (ear), it was most likely that bacteria were the cause of her conjunctivitis. No other tests were necessary.

SEE YOUR HEALTH CARE PROFESSIONAL IF YOUR CHILD HAS

- Eye symptoms any time in the first two months of life
- Any injury to the eye
- Pinkeye and ear pain
- Severe pain in the eye
- Trouble seeing from the eye
- Cloudy spots on the eyeball
- Abnormal or irregular pupil (the black disk in the middle of the eye)
- A bulging eye

These symptoms may signify a more serious condition requiring immediate medical care.

WHAT CAN YOU DO TO PREVENT CONJUNCTIVITIS?

There are several things you can do to reduce the chances that your child will develop conjunctivitis.

PREVENTING CONJUNCTIVITIS

- Regular prenatal care
- Avoid eye irritants: *no smoking around children*
- Avoid allergens
- Minimize exposure to other ill children
- Practice good hygiene
- Plenty of sleep

Mothers who receive regular *prenatal care* are less likely to have an infection when they deliver their babies. This reduces the chance that the baby will become infected during delivery.

Don't smoke and don't let others smoke around your child. Cigarette smoke not only irritates the eyes but also predisposes to colds, ear infections, and asthma. *Avoid allergens.* If your child has hay fever or other allergies to pollen, keep the windows closed between 5 a.m. and 10 a.m. when pollen counts are highest. (See Chapter 4 for more tips on preventing allergic symptoms.)

Most children who have infectious conjunctivitis catch it from *other kids*. Crowding is one of the surest ways to spread infectious illnesses. If you have options in your day care provider, choose one that has fewer children or smaller classrooms rather than a large, crowded environment. If your child has infectious conjunctivitis, try to keep her away from other kids so she doesn't spread it to them.

Good hygiene helps prevent the spread of infectious conjunctivitis. Don't let your youngsters share towels, washcloths, pillows, or bedding with each other. Wash your hands frequently. Have your child wash her hands after each trip to the bathroom, before every meal, and before bed.

Make sure your child gets *plenty of sleep.* Sleep helps boost immunity to infections and calms allergic reactions. Sleeping also rests the eyes and gives them a chance to heal if they become irritated.

WHAT IS THE BEST WAY TO TREAT CONJUNCTIVITIS?

Even without treatment, infectious conjunctivitis usually resolves on its own in seven to ten days. Let's tour the Therapeutic Mountain to find out what works and what doesn't. If you want to skip to my bottom-line recommendations, flip to the end of this chapter.

BIOCHEMICAL THERAPIES: MEDICATIONS, HERBS

Medications

Different medications are indicated for different kinds of conjunctivitis. The medicine used to treat a potentially serious infection in the newborn is different from that used to soothe irritated or allergic eyes in older children.

MEDICATIONS FOR CONJUNCTIVITIS

- Newborns: antibiotics
- Infectious conjunctivitis: antibiotics
- Irritated eyes: nonprescription drops or eye washes
- Allergies: several types of medication

Newborns who have infectious conjunctivitis must be treated with antibiotics by mouth or injection to prevent serious complications such as blindness and pneumonia. All of these medications require a prescription. They include ceftriaxone (injection or intravenous), cefotaxime (intravenous), and erythromycin (by mouth).

Ceftriaxone is a powerful antibiotic that can be given as a single dose by vein or by injection to eliminate gonorrhea conjunctivitis.[3] An alternative antibiotic, cefotaxime, is used for jaundiced babies in whom ceftriaxone is contraindicated. If there is a lot of discharge, the infant's eyes need to be thoroughly washed several times daily to eliminate all of the infectious goo. This should be done by professionals. Erythromycin kills chlamydia and helps prevent the infected infant from developing pneumonia. If a child is diagnosed with either gonorrhea or chlamydia conjunctivitis, both parents should be tested and treated as well. *Eye drops alone are insufficient treatment for a newborn with conjunctivitis* unless cultures have proved that neither gonorrhea nor chlamydia are to blame for the symptoms.

If an older child has an ear infection, sinus infection, or pneumonia at the same time she has pinkeye, the culprit is almost certainly *bacteria*. The combination of an ear infection and pinkeye, known as the *otitis-conjunctivitis* syndrome, is especially common in the winter months.[4] It can be effectively treated with prescription antibiotics such as amoxicillin.

Because Maria had an ear infection plus conjunctivitis, I gave her a prescription for amoxicillin to cover both infections. After twenty-four hours of antibiotic therapy, Maria could return to her day care center without the risk of infecting other children.

Prescription antibiotic eye medications work well for conjunctivitis caused by bacteria in children beyond the newborn period. The antibiotics are placed into the affected eye three to four times daily. Eye drops can be tricky to give young children. Eye ointments are easier and last longer but can cause blurry vision. I recommend eye ointments to treat infants and toddlers and eye drops to treat school-age children and teenagers. My nurse always demonstrates the best technique for giving eye drops and ointment for parents who have never done it before. Pull down the lower eyelid and place the medication in the dip between the eyeball and the eyelid, as close to the outer corner of the eye as you can. The body's natural tears will spread the medication over the eye

before flushing it through the tear duct located at the inner eye near the nose. Antibiotic eye drops often sting when they are first applied. The stinging usually stops within sixty seconds. You should start to see some improvement within twenty-four hours.

If your child has been sent home from day care, as Maria was, she can return to school after she has completed twenty-four hours of treatment for a bacterial conjunctivitis.

There are also prescription antiviral medications to treat the serious eye infections caused by the herpes virus. These medications work only against herpes, not pinkeye due to other viruses. Herpes is serious and should be monitored by an eye specialist (ophthalmologist).

For children and teenagers whose eyes are simply irritated due to smoke or overuse, several nonprescription medications are available. If your child's eyes are not better after three days of nonprescription medication, take her to a health care professional to make sure the problem doesn't require prescription medication.

EYE DROPS FOR IRRITATED EYES		
GENERIC NAME	BRAND NAME	DURATION OF EFFECT
Phenylephrine	AK-Nephrin, Isopto-Frin, Prefrin	30–90 minutes
Tetrahydrozyline	Visine, Mallazine, Murine Plus	1–4 hours
Naphazoline	Allerest, Clear Eyes, Naphcon	2–3 hours
Oxymetazoline	OcuClear, Visine LR	up to 6 hours

These eye drops can make your child feel better while the body is healing the underlying problem, but they do *not* cure the problem. They shrink the blood vessels and dilate the pupil, reducing the swelling and irritation. If your child has blurry or painful vision, have her examined first by a physician before using any eye drops; these symptoms could signal a more serious condition, and you do *not* want to simply cover them up. Drops should also *not* be used if there has been an injury (such as a cut or scrape) to the eye, because they can slow the blood flow needed for healing; in children suffering from glaucoma or high blood pressure; or in children under two years old. Do not use any eye drops for more than three days in a row without seeing a health care professional. Using them longer could result in dependence on the medication; that is, when you stop the drops, the eyes will become even redder than before.[5] Read the package directions carefully and do not exceed the recommended doses.

Artificial tears are simply saline solutions that help wash irritants out of the eye and help keep eyes moisturized when they feel dry. There are numerous brands. They are very safe. Rarely, children are allergic to one of the buffers or preservatives used to maintain the shelf life or sterility of these products. Many nonprescription eye washes contain boric acid and salt. Even though acid sounds scary, boric acid solutions are very gentle and have been used safely for many years. Check the label for precise directions.

Several kinds of prescription medication can help ease the discomfort of allergic conjunctivitis, easing the itching, tearing, and redness triggered by pets or pollens.

Eye drops containing *nedocromil* (Tilade) or *lodoxamide* (Alomide) reduce sensitivity to allergens such as ragweed. They are most helpful when used to *prevent* allergic symptoms; they are less effective after your child has already developed red, itchy eyes. They are also useful for treating conjunctivitis due to chronic irritation, such as irritation from contact lenses. Nedocromil drops are effective even when used as little as twice daily to prevent allergic conjunctivitis.[6] They are my first choice for preventing allergic conjunctivitis.

PRESCRIPTION EYE MEDICATION FOR ALLERGIC CONJUNCTIVITIS

- Nedocromil, lodoxamide (Tilade, Alomide)
- Anti-irritant plus antihistamine (Naphcon-A, Vasocon-A)
- Ketorolac (Acular)
- Steroids

If your child already has symptoms, eye drops containing *antihistamines* may help ease the itching and watering. Most antihistamine eye drops also contain phenylephrine or naphazoline, which help shrink swollen blood vessels and dilate the pupil, thereby reducing redness and swelling. The strong prescription anti-inflammatory and pain medicine *ketorolac* (Acular) relieves eye itching caused by allergies. It is expensive and may cause quite a bit of stinging, but it lasts up to six hours.

Prescription *steroid eye drops* reduce inflammation. However, they may increase the risk of developing an eye infection, so you must be very sure that symptoms aren't really due to an infection before using them. I never prescribe steroid eyedrops without consulting an eye specialist.

Herbs

There are *no* scientific studies evaluating herbs as treatment for children with conjunctivitis. None have been proven effective, and some are dangerous. Natural remedies are not necessarily safe. There is one case report of a child who had a severe allergic reaction to chamomile tea wash.[7] Common house and garden plants can cause severe irritation. The Euphorbia family (poinsettia, mole plant, and others) produces an irritating milky sap that actually causes conjunctivitis if it comes in contact with the eye.[8] I do *not* recommend homegrown herbal remedies for children's eye problems.

Common traditional herbal remedies for conjunctivitis are chamomile flowers, eyebright, and pot marigold (calendula). Less commonly recommended are complex concoctions containing chickweed, comfrey, elderflowers, goldenseal, marsh mallow, plantain, raspberry leaves, and/or rosemary. Rose water or a compress or poultice made of rose petals, witch hazel, and oil of chamomile is believed to be soothing and cooling to irritated eyes. In test tube and animal studies, goldenseal (Hydrastis canadensis) has antibacterial and anti-inflammatory properties, but it has *not* yet been studied in children. Folk remedies for conjunctivitis include poultices made from castor oil, grated raw Irish potato, cucumber slices, violet leaves, or yogurt. If your child's eyes do not improve within three days of home remedies, consult your health care professional.

Some herbalists also recommend drinking certain herbal teas such as eyebright, chrysanthemum (available in many Chinese groceries), goldenseal, and marsh mallow. Again, there are *no* studies evaluating their effectiveness in treating conjunctivitis. I do *not* recommend them.

LIFESTYLE THERAPIES: NUTRITION, EXERCISE, ENVIRONMENT, MIND-BODY

Nutrition

No particular diet has proved helpful in preventing or treating conjunctivitis. Many parents feed extra carrots to children with eye problems because carrots are good for the eyes. Most of carrots' benefit comes from their high concentration of vitamin A, which is important in preventing blindness. Eating a well-balanced diet with an emphasis on fresh, organic fruits, vegetables, and grains is helpful in maintaining health and overcoming illness, no matter what the cause. But extra carrots will *not* help your child heal her conjunctivitis any faster.

Exercise

It's almost impossible to keep a child from rubbing his eyes when they're irritated, but this is one time it's helpful to support your child's efforts to exercise some restraint. Rubbing and itching aggravate the irritation and increase the risk of spreading an infection.

Help your child *rest her eyes*. Turn off the television. Turn on the radio. Read her a story. Sing her a song. Have her close her eyes, and go on an imaginary journey together.

Environment

Wash your hands every time you touch the area around your child's eye. Encourage her to wash her hands frequently. She will inevitably touch her irritated eyes frequently. Handwashing helps stop the spread of disease, and is a good habit in general. Infectious conjunctivitis is *very contagious*, so be sure that no one else uses the washcloths, pillowcases, and towels used by the child with pinkeye. Don't let a teenager with conjunctivitis share cosmetics with anyone else. It's a good idea to refrain from sharing eye makeup even when your child and her friends are completely well; viruses can hang around on makeup for long periods just waiting for someone to place them near a vulnerable eye.

Washing the eye with warm water, salt

water, or artificial tears is soothing and helps loosen the crusts that adhere to eyelashes. Warm, wet compresses applied four or five times a day will help increase circulation to the eye, hastening healing. For children who have pinkeye because of exposure to a caustic chemical such as bleach, lye, or SuperGlue, the most important treatment is to flush the eye with plenty of water (several quarts), followed by immediate evaluation by an eye specialist.

Contact lenses should *not* be worn until pinkeye has completely resolved.

Mind-Body

In any illness, the child can be helped to feel more comfortable by calm, reassuring parents. I encourage parents to spend extra time with their child when she is ill. This helps the child rest, so other treatments and the body's own regenerative powers can work.

BIOMECHANICAL THERAPIES: MASSAGE, SURGERY

Massage

Although massage is great for most conditions, rubbing the eyes just aggravates the irritation. Do *not* massage irritated eyes.

Surgery

Surgery is not necessary for simple pinkeye. If your child has suffered an eye injury, especially if a sharp object has penetrated the eye, see an ophthalmologist (eye specialist) immediately.

BIOENERGETIC THERAPIES

There are no studies documenting the effectiveness of any bioenergetic therapy in preventing or treating conjunctivitis. The most commonly used homeopathic remedies for pinkeye are Apis, Belladonna (homeopathic doses *only*), a combination of Calendula and Hypericum (Hypercal), Euphrasia (eyebright), Mercurius, and Pulsatilla. Until studies document their effectiveness, I do *not* recommend them for children suffering from conjunctivitis.

WHAT I RECOMMEND FOR CONJUNCTIVITIS

PREVENTING CONJUNCTIVITIS

1. Prospective mothers should receive regular prenatal care to detect and treat any infections early and avoid passing them on to their infants.

2. *Lifestyle—environment.* Do not smoke and do not allow others to smoke around your child to prevent eye irritation.

Avoid allergens or seek professional help to prevent allergic symptoms (see Chapter 4).

Maintain good hygiene to avoid catching conjunctivitis. Wash hands frequently. Do *not* share eye makeup.

Seek Professional Help Immediately For

- Redness or discharge from the eye in the first two months of life
- Eye pain
- Loss of vision in either eye
- A history of injury to the eye or chemical contact with the eye
- Pain in the eye with exposure to light
- Bleeding from the eye
- A swollen or bulging eye
- A pupil (the black disk in center of eye) that is irregular or does not get smaller when a light is shined in the eye

---

TREATING CONJUNCTIVITIS

1. If you suspect that the symptoms are due to an *infection,* see your health care provider to consider using an antibiotic.

2. If the symptoms are due to *allergies,* avoid the allergen, use cool compresses, and consider nonprescription eye drops to help reduce symptoms. If your child's eyes are still irritated, see your physician about prescription medications.

3. *Lifestyle—exercise.* Rest the eyes; avoid rubbing them.

4. *Lifestyle—environment.* Gently wash the crusty or gooey matter around the eyes and eyelashes with warm water, sterile saline, or a boric acid solution using a clean washcloth or cotton ball.

Try warm compresses several times daily. Read a story or sing to your child while the compresses are in place.

Remove contact lenses and do not use them again until symptoms have resolved.

12

CONSTIPATION

Belle Zagorski called about her four-week-old grandson, Walter, who was having a bowel movement only every two days. She thought a breast-fed baby should have a stool every time he nursed. She was worried that Walter was constipated, although his stools were soft and he wasn't straining to have them. Belle's daughter wasn't worried, but Belle wanted my opinion about what was normal and whether she should be concerned.

Penny Brandenburg, a local nurse-practitioner, called me to ask my advice about Karo Syrup. She had been taught that adding a little corn syrup to a bottle of formula was a good remedy for constipation in babies; recently she'd seen a child suffering from botulism contracted from eating honey. She knew that honey could harbor botulism spores, and she wondered if corn syrup, a similar sweetener, held the same hazard.

Eric Kay came in with his three-year-old daughter, Susan, because of her severe constipation. Susan had been doing fine until she was being toilet trained, but then she'd started having less frequent stools. Because she'd held them so long, they were hard and painful when they passed, so she was even more reluctant to sit on the potty. Eric wanted to know what to do.

Occasional constipation is a fairly frequent childhood complaint; it becomes even more common during adulthood and is practically epidemic among those over sixty-five. Chronic constipation increases the risk of colon cancer in later life. There is an inverse association between the intake of fruits and vegetables and the risk of developing colon cancer[1]; the more fruits and vegetables you eat, the lower the risk of cancer.[2]

There's a great deal of variability in the normal frequency of bowel movements. Almost all babies (98.5%) have their first bowel movement within the first day of life; those that don't may have a bowel blockage rather than simple constipation.[3] Breast-fed babies can have a stool every time they nurse. Others have a stool every day or two. Most toddlers have one or two bowel movements daily.[4] Others can go three days between bowel movements without any ill effects. Anything less often than every five days calls for a professional evaluation.

Constipation simply means that your child is having stools less frequently than is normal for her, has hard or dry stools, or is having difficulty passing them. Encopresis is the technical term for prolonged, severe constipation with stool buildup (impaction) in the rectum and occasional leaking of stool into the underwear (soiling).

WHAT ARE THE COMMON CAUSES OF CONSTIPATION?

COMMON CAUSES OF CONSTIPATION

- Insufficient fiber in the diet
- Insufficient water or other fluids, especially in hot weather or with a fever
- Changes in diet or routine
- Ignoring the urge to defecate, postponing defecation
- Prolonged bed rest
- Severe dieting, anorexia nervosa
- Medication side effects

The commonest cause of constipation is *insufficient fiber* in the diet. Americans and Western Europeans eat the least fiber of any group in the world and have the highest rates of constipation and bowel cancer. Fast foods are typically low-fiber foods. If Americans doubled the amount of fiber in the diet, we could dramatically reduce problems with constipation and colon cancer.

Constipation is a more common complaint in the summertime because children sweat more and may get dehydrated. *Dehydration* makes stools dry and harder to pass. Feverish children also lose more fluid than normal, increasing their risk of dehydration and constipation. Faced with dehydration, the body starts to draw on water wherever it can, including the bowels, resulting in drier, smaller stools and constipation. Another reason to give plenty of fluids to a feverish child!

Dietary changes are often accompanied by changes in stool frequency. Many babies who are switched from mother's milk to formula have a temporary period of constipation before their bowels adjust to the new food. Breaks in the regular routine of eating, sleeping, and playing, such as traveling, moving, or the arrival of a new baby in the house frequently provoke temporary constipation. The bowels usually return to normal when the child becomes adjusted to the new routine or life returns to normal.

Some children are just so busy and preoccupied that they *postpone* going to the toilet until after the urge has passed. The stool remains in the rectum, and the body gradually reabsorbs more and more water from it until the stool becomes hard and dry. Dry, hard stool is more difficult to pass, and it may be uncomfortable or even cause tiny tears in the delicate skin around the anus. A vicious cycle sets in, wherein the child postpones defecating, the stool becomes hard, defecation becomes painful, and the child delays further. It's best to avoid this cycle altogether by having a regular toilet time every day during which the child sits for five minutes, regardless of the outcome.

Bed rest slows down many bodily functions. Sedentary or wheelchair-bound children are more prone to constipation than their active peers. Even a little mild to moderate exercise keeps blood flowing to all the organs. Don't let your child spend hours glued to the television. Have her get up and play.

Teenage girls who *diet* intensively or have *anorexia nervosa* frequently have problems with constipation. Interestingly, teenage girls are more prone to constipation during certain phases of their menstrual cycle; they are most likely to suffer from constipation about sixteen to twenty-one days from the start of their periods.[5]

Widely used *medications* such as antacids containing aluminum (Amphogel, for example) and prescription painkillers containing codeine also slow down the intestinal flow. Overuse of laxatives results in dependence on them; when the child stops taking the laxative (even natural ones such as senna and cascara), the bowels slow down.

Unusual causes of constipation in children are Hirschprung's disease (in which part of the bowel does not have a proper nerve supply and doesn't move the stool along), botulism, spinal cord tumor, and hypothyroidism. Milk allergy may present as constipation during the toddler years.[6] If you suspect any of these problems, see your doctor for a definitive diagnosis.

Constipated children often suffer from other symptoms such as irritability, tiredness, headaches, depression, and just feeling out of sorts. The ongoing pressure from large amounts of stool in the colon irritates the bladder[7]; children who suffer from chronic constipation are prone to bedwetting and bladder infections too.[8,9] (See Chapter 6, Bedwetting.)

WHEN TO SEEK PROFESSIONAL HELP FOR A CONSTIPATED CHILD

- No stools for four or more days
- Swollen, distended, or painful abdomen
- Vomiting as well as constipation
- Pain when passing a stool
- Blood in the stool
- Dark black stools
- Constipation alternating with diarrhea
- Frequent, painful, or rushed urination

These symptoms may indicate a more serious problem such as an intestinal blockage, intestinal bleeding, impaction, irritable bowel syndrome, or a bladder infection.

How Can You Prevent Constipation?

FIVE TIPS FOR PREVENTING CONSTIPATION

- Begin by breast-feeding
- High-fiber diet (whole grains, fruits, and vegetables)
- Plenty of fluids (six to eight glasses per day)
- Exercise
- Regular routine

Breast-fed babies tend to have softer, more frequent stools than babies who are fed formula. Formula-fed babies do just fine in general, but they are slightly more prone to constipation. Babies on soy formulas in particular tend to have harder, less frequent stools than babies who are nursed or who are fed cow's milk–based formulas.[10] In the summertime, formula-fed babies may benefit from water supplements between feedings.

For older infants and children whose diet includes solids, the top remedy for preventing constipation is eating a diet high in natural *fiber* or roughage. Fiber increases the bulk of stools, draws water into the bowel, softening stools and making them easier to pass, and stimulates contractions in the colon that move the stool along. Eating a diet that is high in whole grains, fruits, and vegetables is the best way to prevent constipation.

Drinking plenty of *fluids* is also important for maintaining healthy bowels. Fiber draws water into the intestines, softening the stool. If there is not enough water in the system, the fiber can just clog up and make things worse. Water helps soften stools so they are easier to pass.

Regular *exercise* also helps keep things flowing. Children who are confined to bed for long periods (such as after surgery) have more trouble with constipation than children who are up and running around.

Keeping a *regular schedule* is helpful in preventing constipation. Most adults have experienced the temporary constipation that accompanies a trip in which the normal daily routine is disrupted. Children who are being potty trained benefit from having a scheduled time on the toilet. It is best to schedule potty time after a meal to take advantage of the gastrocolic reflex. This is a physiological reflex: when the stomach is full, a nerve reflex stimulates the bowels. This is why so many babies have a bowel movement right after they nurse. Children who are so constipated they no longer feel the urge to go need a routine time in which they sit on the toilet no matter whether they feel they have to go or not. Just sitting on the toilet stimulates thoughts and reflexes that enhance regular bowel movements.

WHAT IS THE BEST WAY TO TREAT CONSTIPATION?

The best way to treat constipation is to prevent it by having a healthy lifestyle—high-fiber diet, fluids, exercise, and a regular routine. If the problem persists, there are additional proven remedies. Let's circle the Therapeutic Mountain to find out what works. If you want my bottom-line recommendations (so to speak), flip to the end of the chapter.

BIOCHEMICAL THERAPIES: MEDICATIONS, HERBS, NUTRITIONAL SUPPLEMENTS

Medications

Though many medications are effective, do *not* use them until you've tried dietary changes first. A variety of nonprescription medications are available to treat constipation. Do *not* use any of them for more than a week without checking with your child's doctor. Do *not* use them if your child has severe abdominal pain, nausea, vomiting, blood in the stools, or cramping, because they could worsen a serious underlying condition.

The mainstay of prevention and treatment for constipation is increased *fiber*. Fiber is the safest, most natural treatment for constipation. The two principal natural types of fiber medications are based on *psyllium* (from psyllium seeds) and *methylcellulose* (plant fiber). There is also an effective synthetic fiber, *polycarbophil*.

The fiber in Metamucil and many other bulk laxatives is psyllium. These medications come in a variety of forms: fruit-flavored, sweetened, or unsweetened powder to mix with water or juice, or wafers. Allergic reactions to psyllium are rare. Each teaspoon of Metamucil contains about 2.2 grams of fiber.

This is the same amount of fiber found in one dark Finn Crisp cracker (2.5 grams) and less than the amount in two Fiber Rich Bran crackers (6 grams).[11] Methylcellulose is the fiber in Citrucel. Each rounded teaspoon of Citrucel contains approximately 2 grams of fiber. *Read labels* to find out how much fiber each remedy contains.

NONPRESCRIPTION MEDICATIONS TO TREAT CONSTIPATION

- *Fiber or bulk agents:* Psyllium (Metamucil and others)

- Methylcellulose (Citrucel)

- Polycarbophil (Fiberall chewable tablets and others)

- *Stool softeners:* Docusate (Colace)

- *Lubricants*: Mineral oil

- *Stimulants*: Bisacodyl (Dulcolax)

  Yellow phenolphthalein (Ex-Lax and others)

  Cascara (Nature's Remedy Natural Vegetable Laxatives)

  Senna (Senokot, Fletcher's Castoria)

  Castor oil

- *Magnesium salts (*Milk of magnesia, epsom salts)

- *Others:* Maltsupex, Glycerin suppositories (Babylax), Lactulose (Cephulac)

Fiber works best if it is taken with lots of *fluid*. The liquid combines with the fiber, swelling up and creating the bulking effect that expands the colon and softens the stool. You may need to repeat doses two to three times daily for one to three days before you see results. Fiber-containing laxatives should *not* be used by children who have blocked bowels, because they can make the blockage worse. Fiber laxatives are too harsh for children under three years old.

Docusate (Colace) is one of the most frequently used stool softeners in hospitals. Colace draws water into the bowel, softening the stool and making it easier to pass. Aspirin, ibuprofen, and other anti-inflammatory medicines may interfere with it.[12] Colace is helpful when stools are hard and dry or when passage of a firm stool is painful, as in children suffering from anal fissures (tiny tears in the skin around the anus from passing hard stools). Colace is available as capsules, syrup, and infant drops. It is one of the safest medicines around, though some children do not like the taste and complain of nausea when they are forced to swallow the liquid form.

Mineral oil has long been used to "grease the skids" of children suffering from severe, chronic constipation. The dose for children with mild constipation is 1 teaspoon to 1 tablespoon given at bedtime. For children with severe encopresis, higher doses can be used; check with your doctor for the proper amount for your child. It generally works in six to eight hours. Mineral oil tastes awful, but please do *not* hold your child's nose while getting him to swallow it. If it is accidentally inhaled, it produces a nasty pneumonia, and you may end up with a gasping, choking child whose symptoms are far worse than simple constipation. Mineral oil is much more palatable if it is cold, emulsified, or mixed with frozen yogurt or ice cream, peanut butter, or chocolate syrup. Despite concerns that prolonged use of mineral oil may lead to loss of vitamins and minerals in the stool, a study that actually measured the levels of beta-carotene, vitamin A, and vitamin E showed that even prolonged (four months) use of mineral oil did not lower blood levels of these vitamins.[13] If your child has severe, chronic constipation, mineral oil can be safely given for several months to get things back on track.

Bowel stimulants work directly on the intestines to stimulate peristalsis, the waves of contractions that move food and waste through the bowel. Stimulants generally produce results in six to ten hours when taken by mouth. They can work in as little as an hour if given as suppositories. Bowel stimulants can lead to dependence if they are used on a regular basis. They can be very powerful and cause cramping pain and diarrhea if too much is given. Several kinds are available.

Bisacodyl (Dulcolax) is the most widely used bowel stimulant in hospitals. It is available as tablets or suppositories. Like fiber, it should *not* be used in children who may have blocked bowels or appendicitis, because it could aggravate these conditions.

Yellow phenolphthalein is a bowel stimulant contained in several widely used nonprescription stool softeners such as *Ex-Lax*. It softens stools and stimulates bowel movements. Don't be surprised if it turns your child's stool from brown to red or purple! Some children have a severe allergic skin reaction to it; if your child develops a reaction to any medication, discontinue its use and see your doctor. Keep chocolate Ex-Lax out of reach of small children because they can mistake it for candy, with predictable results.

Cascara sagrada (Nature's Remedy Natural Vegetable Laxative) is a natural bowel stimulant. Cascara is secreted in breast milk, so if you take it while you are nursing, your baby may get diarrhea. *Senna (Senokot, Fletcher's Castoria,* and others) is another potent natural bowel stimulant, which is safe even for nursing mothers. *Castor oil* is an old-fashioned natural bowel stimulant extracted from castor beans; several brands contain sweeteners and flavorings that may make castor oil more palatable. Frequent use of these natural bowel stimulants may result in dependence on them. Do *not* use them for more than two or three days in a row without professional consultation.

Magnesium salts are the active ingredient in *Milk of Magnesia and epsom salts.* Many families keep them on hand to treat indigestion, heartburn, and upset stomach. By drawing water into the intestines, magnesium salts soften the stool and increase peristalsis.[14] They generally work in one to three hours. The dose of epsom salts for children is 1 to 2 teaspoons in a glass of water. Magnesium salts can impair the absorption of some prescription medicines. If your child is taking a prescription medicine, check with your doctor or pharmacist to make sure that Milk of Magnesia will not interfere with it. Ibuprofen and aspirin can interfere with magnesium's effect on the bowel.

Maltsupex is a natural extract of barley malt, which helps draw water into the bowel, softening stools. Like fiber laxatives, Maltsupex should be taken with plenty of liquids. *Glycerin suppositories (Fleet Babylax)* are among the safest remedies for constipated infants. They work within half an hour by stimulating the defecation reflex. *Lactulose (Cephulac* and other brands) is an artificial sugar that is not digested by humans. It is broken down by the normal gut bacteria, resulting in carbon dioxide and other compounds that stimulate bowel movements. Lactulose can cause gas, belching, nausea, and discomfort. It should *not* be used with other laxatives.

There are many varieties of nonprescription laxatives. The similarities in names can be confusing. Some products made by the same manufacturer contain different kinds of ingredients. *Read labels carefully.* To treat mild constipation start with fiber; consider Maltsupex or Milk of Magnesia because they have great safety records. Do not use bowel stimulants (synthetic or natural) without professional consultation; relying on bowel stimulants for more than a week could result in dependence.

Enemas

The vast majority of constipated children can be effectively treated without resorting to enemas. However, children who have severe stool buildup or impaction may need enema therapy to clean out the problem before starting on other treatments to restore normal bowel patterns. Enemas are *not* helpful for children who have a decrease in bowel movements because they have not eaten. Once impacted stool has been evacuated from the rectum, enemas do not have any advantage over oral laxatives in maintaining normal bowel function.[15] I do *not* recommend them except for children whose severe constipation has not responded to other therapies.

Pediatric enemas contain a variety of ingredients. The most widely used are *Pediatric Fleet* products. Do not use phosphate enemas repeatedly except under the supervision of a health care professional, because they can result in abnormalities in the body's normal salt and water balance.[16] Home-made enema solutions include milk and molasses, detergent, milk alone, coffee, and a variety of other substances. These solutions have *not* undergone rigorous safety evaluations and may cause severe side effects. Do *not* give your child coffee enemas, because they can upset the body's delicate balance of salt and water.

Many specialists in treating severe constipation recommend a combined approach: enemas initially to clean out impacted stool, followed by a high-fiber diet, daily mineral oil, a stool softener (such as Colace) to help retrain the bowel, and counseling to address possible causes and consequences of this problem. Despite concerns that this regimen might deplete blood levels of vitamins and impair growth, recent studies have shown that with proper medical supervision, these combination regimens are safe and effective.[17]

Herbs

HERBS TO TREAT CONSTIPATION

- Cascara sagrada (buckthorn)
- Senna
- Aloe
- Dong quai
- Others

Do not rely on herbs or medicines that are bowel stimulants until after you've tried dietary therapy, increased water, increased exercise, and regular time on the toilet. Do *not* use herbal laxatives for more than two days without consulting your health care professional. Chronic use can lead to dependence on the laxative for normal function and disturbances in blood chemistry.

Cascara and *senna* are powerful laxatives. Senna is one of the safest and most physiological of all laxatives.[18] It generally works in eight to ten hours; bedtime doses should achieve results by breakfast. You can find these herbs in the grocery store or health food store as commercially prepared teas. They are sometimes combined with fennel and peppermint—two traditional tummy soothers that may soothe the cramps provoked by strong bowel stimulants. *Aloe juice,* prepared from the inner surface of aloe leaves, is a more potent cathartic (bowel stimulator) than *aloe gel,* yet the gel does have some laxative qualities. It is not as effective as senna and cascara and tends to cause more cramping. Overuse of aloe and cascara has been linked with bowel cancer.[19] Treatments are not necessarily safer just because they're natural.

Dong quai (from the root of Angelica sinensis), which is often used to treat menstrual cramps, is also a mild laxative. Other herbs that may help relieve the intestinal spasms that sometimes accompany constipation are chamomile, ginger, lemon balm, licorice root, mulberry, and wild yam.[20] Herbs that may help soothe an irritated intestine are comfrey, goldenseal, marsh mallow root, and slippery elm bark tea. (See Chapter 16, Diarrhea.) None have been tested as constipation remedies for children.

Nutritional Supplements

Vitamin C overdoses can cause diarrhea. You can safely give vitamin C supplements to a child who is constipated, but the primary treatment for constipation should be diet, not supplements.

Avoid aluminum. Aluminum can make constipation worse. Aluminum is found in some antacids such as Amphogel in the form of aluminum hydroxide. Read labels before you give your child an antacid for an upset stomach related to constipation. Also avoid cooking acidic foods (such as tomato sauce) in aluminum saucepans, as the acid tends to leach aluminum into the food.

LIFESTYLE THERAPIES: NUTRITION, EXERCISE, MIND-BODY

A healthy lifestyle is the cornerstone of therapy for constipation.

Nutrition

What are the top three remedies to prevent and treat constipation? Fiber, fiber, and more fiber! Fiber also decreases blood cholesterol and evens out blood sugar levels. An Australian community education effort to increase the intake of whole grain bread led to a 58% increase in the sale of whole grain bread and a 49% decrease in laxative sales![21] It takes about a week for increased fiber intake to show results.[22] There are several different kinds of dietary fiber. You may want to combine different kinds to achieve the most balanced effect.

TYPE OF FIBER	FOOD SOURCE
Cellulose and hemicellulose	Wheat, rice, or oat bran
Mucilages	Psyllium seeds, legumes, guar
Pectin	Apple peel
Others	Food thickeners and additives: gum arabic, xanthan gum, algin, carrageenan

Fiber is not digested by humans but is partially broken down by the bacteria that normally live in the intestines. The bacterial breakdown releases chemicals that help stimulate peristalsis. *Cellulose* (the fiber in bran) is present in all plants. It helps draw water into the intestine, making stools larger, softer, and easier to pass. Wheat bran increases the volume of stool and decreases the time it takes to move through the intestines.[23] *Psyllium seed* (Plantago ovata) is one of the most powerful laxatives from the plant kingdom. *Guar* and *pectin* are good for the bowel and help to lower cholesterol. *Gums*, such as xanthan gum, gum arabic, algin, and carrageenan, are used in many prepared foods to help stabilize them and give them substance; they are also mild laxatives.[24]

Start slowly and gradually increase your child's fiber intake. For kids who are used to a steady diet of white flour, fat, and sugar (such as doughnuts for breakfast), suddenly switching to a high-fiber menu can spell flatulence, cramping, and diarrhea. Start by replacing doughnuts or white bread with whole grain bread or bran cereal. Then add one or two fresh fruits or vegetables a day. If foods alone don't do the trick, consider adding wheat or rice bran to your child's cereal or sprinkled on top of toast. Go slowly. Try adding one high-fiber food every few days. Do *not* give bran supplements to children under three years old without a doctor's advice. It could cause bowel blockages in young children who don't drink enough fluid.

HIGH-FIBER FOODS

- Bran: wheat or rice
- Bran cereals, puffed whole grain cereals, muesli
- Bran muffins, bran cookies, bran crackers, whole grain pancakes
- Beans, peas, lentils
- Dried fruit (prunes are best; figs, apricots, raisins, and dates are also good)
- Fresh fruit and vegetables, especially cabbage, carrots, apples, and celery
- Seeds and nuts (for children over four who are unlikely to choke)
- Popcorn

Prunes have a well-deserved reputation as laxative food. Other excellent dried fruits include figs and dates. You can make a yummy jam that will help keep your child regular:

RIGHT AND REGULAR JAM

- 2 cups water
- 1 ¼ cup dried, chopped, pitted dates
- 1 ¼ cup dried, chopped figs
- 1 tablespoon corn meal

Combine all ingredients in a glass, ceramic, or stainless steel pot. Bring to a boil. Simmer and stir until thickened. Cool to room temperature before serving. Keep refrigerated. Use as desired on whole grain toast, pancakes, waffles, or sandwiches.

Most kids love fruit, and fresh fruits and vegetables are excellent sources of fiber. The most fiber is provided by bran, followed by cabbage, carrots, and apples—cole slaw anyone?[25] Rhubarb is a traditional remedy for constipation, but there are no scientific studies evaluating the effectiveness of plain old garden rhubarb. If your kids like it, go ahead and let them have it, but it is probably no more potent than any other fresh fruit or vegetable. If your child doesn't like eating fruit, you can make a delicious fruit smoothie.

FRUIT SMOOTHIE FOR EXTRA FIBER

IN A BLENDER COMBINE:

- 1 banana
- ½ apple (with peel but without seeds or core)
- ½ cup of yogurt with active cultures
- ½–1 teaspoon of wheat or rice bran (optional)
- ½ cup of pear, apple, or black cherry juice

You can add other fruits as you wish and adjust the amount of fruit and juice until you achieve the consistency your child prefers. This makes a delicious shake, and it contains all the fiber and fruit sugar your child needs to get going in the morning.

Psyllium seeds are the source of several laxative medications. Rather than give your child a medication, look for psyllium seeds at the health food store. Try small amounts (1/4 teaspoon) sprinkled on breakfast cereal. Alternatively, to make sure your child gets fluid along with the seeds, soak the seeds in a cup of water to soften them and allow them to start to swell; have your child swallow the whole thing—water and seeds. Some children develop severe allergic reactions to psyllium seed. If your child develops a rash, hives, or any other symptoms, stop the psyllium. Alternative seeds are linseed or flax seed. Flax seed is one ingredient in Uncle Sam cereal, which also contains bran flakes. This is an excellent cereal for children prone to constipation. You can find flax seed in most health food stores. It tastes fine. You can add 1/2 teaspoon to your child's regular cereal or sprinkle it on toast.

Plain popcorn is an excellent and fun source of fiber. Don't wipe out the nutritional benefits by adding butter or salt. Stick to plain popcorn, flavored with a bit of your favorite herbs, Brewer's yeast, or Parmesan cheese.

Following fiber, the most important dietary component is *water*. Fiber draws water into the bowel to increase its bulk, stretch the colon, stimulate bowel action, and soften the stools. If there is not enough water, the fiber can become hardened and stuck, causing complete bowel blockage.[26] On the other hand, pushing fluids beyond the body's basic needs doesn't offer any particular advantage.[27] Offer your child fluids, but don't hound her into drinking more than she is comfortable with.

Fruit juice helps promote regular bowel movements. Fruit juices contain the fruit sugar fructose, and another sugar that is not well absorbed by the body, sorbitol. Fruit juice is so good at loosening the bowels, it is often an unsuspected cause of chronic diarrhea.[28] The most potent fruit juices are pear, apple, black cherry, prune, and syrup of figs. Fruit juices in moderation are safe even for children less than three years old, but too much fruit juice can lead to diarrhea and poor growth.

Many "sugar-free" candies and gums also contain fructose and sorbitol as sweeteners. Both of these sugar substitutes are poorly absorbed by many children and adults.[29] Because they are not well absorbed, they draw water into the intestines, softening the stool and making it easier to pass. They are also broken down by normal gut bacteria, creating gas and further stimulating the bowel. Sorbitol is so good at moving things along it is used in an emergency medication to help speed the elimination of poisons.[30] Thus, children with sloppy stools may benefit from cutting back on sugarless foods, while constipated kids might benefit from having a few more "sugar-free" sweets.

Like Penny Brandenburg, I was taught to add 1 to 2 tablespoons of Karo corn syrup to each bottle of formula for babies suffering from constipation. Since we now know that infant botulism is associated with being fed honey or corn syrup, many practitioners strenuously recommended *avoiding* these products for infants under a year of age.[31]

I advised Penny Brandenburg not to recommend Karo Syrup but to stick with syrup made from simmering dried figs, dates, raisins, and prunes in plain water: 1 to 2 teaspoons with each meal. She was relieved to have an alternative remedy.

Many adults notice that their morning cup of *coffee* can really get things moving. Coffee stimulates the bowel, and it does so quickly. Even decaffeinated coffee can provoke increased bowel action in as little as four minutes.[32] I am *not* advocating coffee as a regular beverage for children; but for occasional use when a child is constipated due to travel or a disruption in schedule, a small cup of coffee just might do the trick.

Cheese is frequently blamed for constipation, and many practitioners recommend avoiding cheese if a child is constipated. Despite widespread injunctions against cheese, a recent study in older adults showed that even a tenfold increase in cheese intake had no effect on stool volume or frequency.[33] In fact one dairy product, yogurt, may actually be helpful in restoring healthy bowel bacteria and reducing constipation.[34] Try adding yogurt (with active cultures) to your child's regular diet.

Exercise

Bed rest slows down bowel activity. Mild to moderate exercise helps keep things moving.[35] Exercise also helps reduce stress. Strenuous endurance sports such as long-distance running and cycling are associated with an increased risk of diarrhea, especially in girls.[36] The best idea for maintaining balance and regularity is to keep moderately active—neither too much time in bed or in front of the TV nor marathon running. Make sure that your child has access to plenty of fluid during exercise to avoid dehydration.

Mind-Body

Stress upsets the stomach and aggravates all kinds of bowel problems. Some children react to stress with headaches, some have diarrhea, some have sleep problems, and some suffer from constipation. Anticipate the possible consequences of unavoidable stress (such as starting school, moving, death of a pet or family member) by increasing your child's intake of fiber-rich foods during stressful periods.

To keep the gastrointestinal system functioning smoothly, try to keep meal times and toileting times low key. Make sure that your child's time on the toilet is pleasant; don't demand performance. Simply allow it to happen naturally. When your child has the desired results, positive reinforcement such as praise and stickers can work wonders. Behavior management techniques are most effective when combined with fiber and stool softeners.[37]

Much of childhood constipation is a result of the child ignoring the urge to defecate because she is preoccupied with something else. Ignoring the urge to go allows the colon time to reabsorb more water from the stool, making it dry and difficult to pass. Habitually suppressing the urge to defecate actually changes the bowel's normal dynamics and makes it more difficult to go once the child is willing.[38] Remind your child *not* to postpone the urge to defecate.

Hypnosis and *biofeedback* have proven effectiveness in treating chronic, severe constipation and encopresis.[39] They are *unnecessary* for the vast majority of children with short-term or mild constipation. Biofeedback helps retrain the defecation reflex, leading to improved control of bowel function that can last for months after the training is completed.[40, 41, 42] It is most effective if used in the context of increased fiber, stool softeners, and behavioral techniques such as regular toilet-sitting times.[43] Biofeedback therapy should be reserved for children with severe constipation who have not benefited from other lifestyle therapies. (See Appendix A for more information on how to contact a biofeedback therapist.)

BIOMECHANICAL THERAPIES: MASSAGE, SURGERY

Massage

Despite its widespread use, massage did *not* prove helpful in the only scientific study of its effectiveness in treating constipation.[44] Still, massage is safe and can improve communication and attachment between parents and their children. As long as you are gentle, there is probably no harm in giving your child a tummy rub when she is constipated.

Surgery

Surgery is *not* needed to treat garden-variety constipation.[45] It *is* necessary for illnesses such as Hirschprung's disease, in which part of the bowel has an abnormal nerve supply. It is also lifesaving in cases of intestinal obstruction. If you suspect either of these problems, see your doctor.

BIOENERGETIC THERAPIES: ACUPUNCTURE, HOMEOPATHY

Acupuncture

Acupuncture was *not* found to be effective in the only scientific study evaluating it.[46] This study was done on adults; no studies have been done on children. Until such studies have been done, I do *not* recommend acupuncture as a constipation remedy.

Homeopathy

There are *no* scientific studies evaluating the effectiveness of homeopathic remedies in treating adults or children suffering from constipation. Commonly used remedies include *Alumina, Bryonia, Calcarea carb, Lycopodium,* and *Nux vomica* (especially if the child has vomiting as well as constipation). Until they have been scientifically tested, I do *not* recommend them.

WHAT I RECOMMEND FOR CONSTIPATION

PREVENTING CONSTIPATION

1. *Lifestyle—nutrition.* Start your infant's life out right by breast-feeding. If you are feeding your baby formula, you may need to give him water supplements in the summer. Feed your toddler or older child a diet rich in whole grains, fresh fruits, vegetables, yogurt, and plenty of water.

2. *Lifestyle—exercise.* Encourage your child to get some exercise or outdoor play. Keep a regular scheduled potty time (after meals works best) every day.

3. *Lifestyle—mind-body.* Give positive rewards for positive results.

4. *Biochemical—medications.* Avoid codeine-containing pain relievers and antacids that contain aluminum.

When to Seek Professional Help for Constipation

- No stools for four or more days despite lifestyle therapies described below
- Swollen or distended belly
- Vomiting as well as constipation
- Pain with passing a stool or pain in the abdomen, especially on the lower right side
- Blood in the stool
- Dark black stools
- Constipation alternating with diarrhea
- Frequent, painful, or rushed urination

TREATING CONSTIPATION

1. *Lifestyle—nutrition.* For constipated *infants* try a little extra water, fruit juice (apple, pear, black cherry, or prune juice), or the juice from stewed figs, dates, raisins, or prunes. For constipated *toddlers* or *older children,* increase fiber intake: high-fiber crackers and cookies, more fruits, vegetables, dried fruit, beans, popcorn, flax or psyllium seeds; add pear, apple, prune, or black cherry juice; consider sugarless gums or candies that contain sorbitol as treats; try a teaspoon of flax seeds on bran cereal or whole grain toast; make sure she's getting plenty of fluids.

2. *Lifestyle—exercise.* Encourage regular exercise. Have a regular time to sit on the toilet after meals.

3. *Lifestyle—mind-body.* Give positive rewards (such as stickers) for positive results. For severe encopresis with soiling that has not responded to other treatments, consider biofeedback therapy.

4. *Biochemical—medications.* Try fiber-based medications (Metamucil), stool softeners (Colace), mineral oil, milk of magnesia, or epsom salts. For infants, try a glycerin suppository. Try one or two days of a mild laxative such as Ex-Lax. If all else fails and your child is severely blocked up, consider a Fleet's enema to clear out the impaction in the rectum initially.

5. *Biochemical—herbs.* Try laxatives such as cascara or senna (Fletcher's Castoria or Senokot) given in divided doses over the course of the day. Do *not* use for more than two days without seeing your health care professional.

Susan had impacted stool in her rectum. Eric began giving her 2 tablespoons of mineral oil at night (mixed with chocolate frozen yogurt) and in the morning (followed by pear juice). We gave her Colace to take twice daily as well to soften her stools. Her mom also began making fruit-bran-yogurt smoothies for breakfast and sending Susan to day care with a container of pear juice and bran crackers for snacks. Susan had a sticker chart that she filled in with a new sticker each time she had a bowel movement. Six months later, she was regular as a clock on her new high-fiber diet without any medications or herbal treatments. She never needed another enema or referral for biofeedback. Her parents were delighted and felt that the changes in Susan's diet had spilled over to theirs, benefiting the whole family.

13
COUGH

Nine-month-old Philip Koshi started coughing two days ago when he developed a cold. He sounded like a seal barking, and his cough was worse at night. His parents started to bring him to the emergency room at 2 a.m., but on the way, he improved so much they thought the doctors would think they were crazy, so they sheepishly returned home. Philip seemed better this morning, but his parents wanted to make sure he didn't have another night like that one.

Terri Nguyen was a pale, tired-looking fourteen-year-old who had been coughing for several days. She had recently returned from a trip to visit her grandmother in Vietnam. The last two days she had noticed more phlegm and had developed a fever. This morning she had coughed up some yellow-green mucus, flecked with blood. She wanted a shot of antibiotics so she could participate in a swim meet the next day.

Kris Masterson brought in his fourteen-month-old daughter, Emily, who had been coughing off and on for weeks, ever since she had bronchiolitis. Emily's lungs seemed to be extra sensitive; every cold she caught brought on more coughing spasms. Chris wanted to know if this was normal or if he should worry about cystic fibrosis.

Coughing is the body's natural method for clearing the airway. Anything that irritates or blocks the air passages stimulates a cough reflex. Generally the cough happens for a good reason. It is a mistake to suppress a cough unless you know for certain what is causing it and that it is not serving a useful function.

TAKE YOUR CHILD TO A HEALTH CARE PROFESSIONAL IF SHE IS

- Persistently coughing for more than a week despite home therapies
- Coughing so hard she can't catch her breath
- Coughing up blood
- Wheezing
- Breathing very fast
- Turning blue in lips or fingernails
- Lethargic
- Complaining of pain in the chest
- Complaining of headache or facial pain as well as coughing
- Or has a fever over 103.9°F

Coughs have many causes.

CAUSES OF COUGH

- Infections (see Chapter 9, Colds)
- Reflux or aspiration
- Allergies, smoke, irritants (see Chapter 4, Allergies)
- Asthma (see Chapter 5)
- Cold air
- Heart failure
- Reflex, nerves, habit
- Serious illness–cystic fibrosis

Most coughs in children are due to colds and tend to get better over the course of a few days (see Chapter 9). However, some viruses such as pertussis, influenza, and respiratory synctitial virus (RSV) cause coughs that last for weeks or even months. Other cough-causing infections include croup, sinus infection, bronchitis, and pneumonia.

Coughs in infants may be due to a condition called gastroesophageal reflux. Reflux means that some of the baby's stomach (gastric) contents come back up the esophagus and a little is inhaled into the airway, causing cough and irritation. *Aspiration* is when a piece of food goes down the wrong way and gets in the lungs.

Other cough causers are allergies (Chapter 4), cigarette smoke and other irritants, asthma (Chapter 5), cold air, and even heart failure (when fluid from the heart backs up into the lungs). Sometimes tickling the ear canal (when we look inside to see if there is an ear infection) provokes the cough reflex. Most adults have experienced a nervous cough. Children can develop a chronic coughing habit following an illness in which their cough was rewarded by extra attention. Serious illnesses such as cystic fibrosis are also characterized by recurrent coughing.

Despite modern myths to the contrary, immunizations do *not* weaken the immune system or cause coughing. Literally hundreds of studies on millions of children have shown that while immunizations are often uncomfortable, they actually boost immunity and prevent many serious illnesses such as whooping cough.

Dry coughs are usually due to irritants, allergies, a foreign body (such as a piece of food that got stuck going down the wrong way), or asthma. *Rattlelike coughs* stem from phlegm in the back of the nose or throat and are usually due to simple colds. *Productive coughs* indicate that mucus is present in the airways and needs to be cleared. Most children under the age of eight swallow their mucus instead of spitting it out. The swallowed mucus usually passes through the intestines uneventfully. However, if a lot of mucus is swallowed, it can irritate the stomach, producing nausea and even vomiting.

DIAGNOSING COUGHS

- Symptoms
- Physical examination
- Chest X rays
- Other: blood tests, skin tests

Most of the time, the reason for the cough can be determined by its characteristics, other symptoms (such as fever and wheezing), and a physical examination. *Croup* coughs are dry, worse at night, and usually affect children between the ages of six months and three years during the fall and winter.[1] Croup is usually caused by a virus. The cough sounds like a seal barking. It is relieved by mist, steam, or going out in the cool night air. Croup sounds terrible as the child struggles for breath and then coughs and coughs and coughs. The child's sudden improvement on the way to the emergency room is embarrassing for many parents who were sure their child was on the brink of death, but it is a completely normal response to the cool night air. If the child doesn't improve on the way to the doctor's office or hospital, medical treatments are effective. Croup usually lasts for three to four days and is worse on the second and third nights of the illness.

Philip Koshi's cough was due to croup. Emily Masterson had the typical, unfortunate, prolonged cough that follows a bout with respiratory synctitial virus. Though you might think that a cough from bacterial pneumonia would be worse, it usually resolves with a few days of antibiotics. Viruses, on the other hand, can damage the cells lining the air passages, leaving the child's lungs weakened for weeks or months. Kris was right to think about cystic fibrosis (CF). Infants with recurrent coughs or pneumonia (especially infants who are not growing well) should be tested for CF. Emily's tests turned out to be negative; she did not have CF. Emily eventually overcame her cough.

Sometimes an X ray of the chest or sinuses is helpful. Less commonly, blood tests (to check for white blood cells fighting pneumonia) and skin tests (to check for tuberculosis [TB]) are needed. If the child is old enough to spit out the phlegm he coughs up, it can be checked for bacteria and TB.

Terri Nguyen's cough sounded like pneumonia because of her fever, cough, fatigue, and blood-flecked sputum. We did an X ray of her chest, took some of her sputum to the laboratory for a culture, and did a skin test for tuberculosis before starting her treatment.

WHAT'S THE BEST WAY TO PREVENT COUGHS?

PREVENTING COUGHS

- Avoid cigarette smoke
- Immunize against pertussis (whooping cough)
- Treat underlying illnesses
- Minimize exposure to sick children

Avoid exposure to cigarette smoke. Smoke irritates the airways and makes even healthy kids cough. Do not smoke and do not allow others to smoke around your child, especially in enclosed spaces such as your home or car.

Make sure your child is *immunized against pertussis* (whooping cough). Despite its detractors, the highly effective pertussis vaccine has practically eliminated the old scourge of whooping cough. Whooping cough epidemics have reemerged in countries where governments stopped pertussis immunization programs due to public fears about the vaccine. Immunization is very effective in preventing this potentially fatal illness during childhood. Protection wanes over the years. By twenty years of age, 90% of those who were fully immunized as children are again susceptible to pertussis. Most adults who get pertussis are only moderately ill and never even go to the doctor. This is why pertussis will probably never be completely eradicated and why childhood immunization programs must continue.

I caught pertussis from one-month-old Dedra Shapiro (who hadn't yet received her first immunizations) during my residency training. Dedra was hospitalized with a severe cough. Soon after admission she stopped breathing. I immediately began mouth-to-mouth resuscitation. She did well, but an hour later her laboratory tests came back positive for pertussis. Two days later, I was coughing and had positive tests for pertussis, too. I took antibiotics for a week and continued to cough for six months. Even years later, my lungs were extra sensitive to infection. Like most young infants, Dedra caught pertussis from a parent who was sick with what he thought was simple bronchitis.

Treat any underlying allergies and asthma (see Chapters 4 and 5) to reduce the risk of asthma attacks and the coughing that accompanies them.

As much as you can, minimize your child's exposure to other children who are *sick*. The more time spent with young children, the more exposure to infections. If your child is in day care, select a situation with fewer rather than more children, if possible.

What Is the Best Way to Treat a Cough?

Treatment should always aim at helping the child's body heal the underlying illness rather than just suppressing the cough. Coughs can indicate a serious problem that should be treated (such as asthma or pneumonia); they can also be very annoying and lead to sleep loss for the whole family if the child coughs at night. On the other hand, coughing may be the body's best defense and protection against pneumonia. Let's tour the Therapeutic Mountain to find out what works for most coughs; if you want to skip to my bottom-line recommendations, flip to the end of the chapter.

Biochemical Therapies: Medications, Herbs, Nutritional Supplements

Medications

There are three main types of cough medicines: cough suppressants, expectorants (to help loosen secretions), and throat soothers such as cough drops.

There is good news and bad news about *cough suppressants*. The good news is that you can save a lot of money. The bad news is that none of them are very helpful, which is why you can save your money.[2] The two most commonly used cough medicines (dextromethorphan, the DM ingredient in many nonprescription cough medicines, and codeine, the most common prescription cough medicine) are no more effective than placebo syrup in reducing coughs in children under twelve years old.[3] Placebos make us feel that we are doing something to help ourselves; some children (and adults) feel better and have fewer symptoms even with a placebo. Cough medicines are *not* any better than placebos, and they may have serious side effects such as irritability, fussiness, lethargy, and high blood pressure. *The American Academy of Pediatrics Committee on Drugs says that cough medicines should not be used for children.*[4]

Expectorants supposedly loosen secretions so they are easier to cough out. The most common one is guaifenesin (Robitussin). Although guaifenesin helps thin secretions, it is no more helpful than placebo syrup in reducing the frequency or severity of coughs.[5,6] I do *not* recommend expectorants for treating children with coughs.

Cough drops work mostly by stimulating saliva, coating and soothing an irritated throat. Any hard candy will do the same thing; lemon and other citrus flavors are particularly potent saliva stimulators. Do *not* give cough drops or hard candy to children under four years old who might choke on them. Cough drops with menthol or eucalyptus oils also help a congested nose feel less stuffy. Sucking on a vitamin C lozenge also stimulates saliva and may help fight the cold behind your child's cough.

The ineffectiveness of cough suppressants and expectorants does not mean that other medicines for specific types of cough are not helpful. *If your child is coughing because of croup, asthma, or allergies, use the treatments your health care professional has recommended and any others you have found to be helpful.*

For example, children suffering from severe croup that has not responded to home therapies can be helped by two prescription medications.

CROUP MEDICATIONS

- Racemic epinephrine (epi)
- Steroids

Racemic epinephrine is given by a mist machine (called a nebulizer) in a doctor's office or emergency room. Racemic epinephrine helps shrink the swollen and inflamed blood vessels. Racemic epinephrine can be lifesaving. It works within minutes, providing rapid relief of breathing difficulties, but it only works for one to two hours, so it may need to be repeated several times.[7] Rather than risk sending home a child who may need another treatment within an hour, many doctors automatically hospitalize a child who needs one racemic epinephrine treatment to be sure additional treatments are readily available if needed. Like caffeine (to which it is related), racemic epinephrine can cause a rapid heartbeat, shaky hands, agitation, and trembling. These side effects quickly disappear as the medicine wears off.

Steroids help reduce inflammation and swelling. Although they can have serious side effects when used over long periods of time (weeks or months), steroids are safe when used for less than five days for temporary problems such as croup. The steroids that are used for children's illnesses are *not* the same kind of steroids athletes use to build muscles. Steroids given by mist machine (nebulizer) provide significant symptomatic improvement for several hours.[8] They could eliminate some hospitalizations for children with croup. Steroids are also effective when given by injection.[9] Though a shot is more painful than a mist treatment, you can be sure your child is actually receiving the medication; some children do not cooperate with the mist machine, and the parent ends up getting most of the dose! Steroid syrups taken by mouth are also helpful,[10] even in children suffering from severe, life-threatening croup.[11]

We gave Philip Koshi a three-day course of a steroid syrup to help prevent more serious symptoms and a possible hospitalization. His parents were pleased to tell me at his next checkup that his croup symptoms rapidly improved, and there were no more midnight trips to the hospital.

Antibiotics have *no* role in the treatment of coughs due to viruses. However, if your child's cough is caused by bacterial pneumonia, bronchitis, or a sinus infection, antibiotics can help clear the underlying cause.[12, 13] If you suspect that your child has one of these illnesses, have her evaluated by a health care professional.

Herbs

Different kinds of herbs are used for different kinds of cough, but there are *no* studies evaluating their effectiveness in common childhood coughs. There are infection-fighting herbs, expectorants, herbs that soothe an irritated throat, herbs to warm and stimulate a child who is fatigued and chilled, and herbs to sedate a child who has been kept awake by a cough. Herbal remedies are usually taken as tea (see Appendix B for directions on how to make an herbal tea). Doses vary by age.

DOSES OF HERBAL TEA FOR COUGHS

- Children *under a year:* no more than 1 teaspoon three to four times daily
- Children *one to three years old:* up to 1 ounce four times daily
- Children *four to six years old:* up to 2 ounces four times daily
- Children *seven to twelve years old:* up to 3 ounces four times daily
- *Teenagers and adults:* 3 to 4 ounces every four to six hours

The heat from hot tea helps increase circulation to the throat, hastening healing to the whole area. *There have not been any studies confirming that any herbal remedies are useful treatments for coughing children.*

HERBAL COUGH REMEDIES

- *Infection-fighting herbs*: echinacea, eucalyptus, garlic, hyssop, plantain, thyme
- *Herbs to stimulate the immune system*: borage, dandelion root, echinacea, garlic, marigold, nettles, wild indigo
- *Herbs to help loosen mucus so that it is easier to cough up (expectorants)*: angelica root, anise seed, cowslip, elecampane, fennel, white horehound, hyssop, lobelia, mullein, plantain, sage, senega snakeroot, thyme
- *Herbs to soothe a dry cough (demulcents)*: anise, comfrey, elecampane, horehound, licorice, lobelia, marsh mallow root, mugwort, mullein, slippery elm bark, wild cherry bark
- *Herbs to stimulate and warm a weak and chilled child*: anise, cinnamon, cloves, fennel, ginger, ginseng, hyssop, sarsaparilla root, thyme
- *Relaxing herbs to help a coughing child sleep*: chamomile, catnip, lime flowers

Warning: Although coltsfoot has been used in Europe, Asia, and America for many years as an herbal remedy for coughs, recent studies indicate that coltsfoot flowers (the most commonly used part of the plant) are toxic to the liver and may cause cancer.[14] Senega snakeroot can cause severe stomach upset. Overdoses of licorice tea can adversely affect the body's salt and water balance. No scientific studies document the effectiveness of any of these remedies in treating children with coughs.

POULTICES FOR COUGHS

- Mustard, garlic, or onion
- Turpentine or camphor
- Castor oil

A time-honored treatment for chest colds is the *mustard poultice.* Mustard poultices apparently increase circulation to your child's chest, creating a soothing sense of warmth. Do not let the mustard come in direct contact with your child's skin. It is irritating and could cause a burn. This same sense of heat and increased circulation can be achieved with a *garlic* or *onion poultice.* Do not use a garlic poultice for more than twenty minutes at a time. Some herbalists recommend that the garlic poultice be placed over the soles of the feet to draw heat downward.

Other folk remedies placed on the feet to draw the circulation downward are *turpentine* and *camphor.* A North Carolina woman who was my patient during medical school swore that her homemade turpentine poultices were what was really curing her but asked me not to tell her doctor, because she didn't want him to be disappointed in his antibiotics!

Castor oil poultices are also used in many parts of the country and were recommended by the psychic Edgar Cayce as a remedy for many illnesses. Castor oil is very soothing, so it can be applied directly to the skin or as a

poultice for the chest, abdomen, or back. (See Appendix B for directions on how to make a castor oil poultice.)

None of these folk remedies has undergone scientific evaluation. If your child fails to improve in a day or two or becomes more ill, consult your health care professional to make sure there is not a serious and easily treated condition causing the cough.

Nutritional Supplements

Vitamin A protects the mucous membranes of the nose, throat, and lungs, but it is *not* helpful against ordinary coughs. Among malnourished children, vitamin A supplements are helpful for treating measles pneumonia.[15] However, vitamin A supplements do *not* reduce the risk of cough or pneumonia in well-nourished children.[16] Too much vitamin A may *increase* the risk of respiratory infections.[17] If your child eats a healthy diet, he does *not* need supplemental vitamin A.

Vitamin C has proved effective in reducing the symptoms of the common cold (see Chapter 9). Vitamin C decreases the sensitivity of adults' lungs during a cold, making coughing and wheezing less likely.[18] Studies on children have not yet been done.

Garlic-honey is a combination of two common folk remedies. It is made by combining four to five cloves of minced garlic with 3 ounces of honey in a blender. You can give a teaspoon several times daily. Both garlic and honey have antibacterial properties, but there are *no* scientific studies evaluating their effectiveness in treating coughs. Both ingredients are safe, readily available, and have a long history of use.

A favorite British remedy is *onion-honey* cough syrup. This is made by combining 2 to 3 cups of chopped onions with 1/2 cup of honey and cooking slowly for two or three hours over low heat. This combination is safe and can be given by teaspoon every one to two hours as needed. To avoid the risk of botulism, do *not* give honey remedies to children less than one year old. Honey remedies have *not* been scientifically tested for treating coughing children.

A better-tasting combination for dry, tickly coughs is *honey and lemon*. You can combine them as a syrup or add a bit of each (to taste) to hot water or an herbal tea.

Red pepper, hot pepper, and curries that make your eyes water will also make your nose water and loosen secretions. If your child feels like eating, try spicy foods to help thin the phlegm in the lungs and throat.

LIFESTYLE THERAPIES: NUTRITION, EXERCISE, ENVIRONMENT, MIND-BODY

Nutrition

Kris was frustrated with Emily's chronic cough. He'd read that milk made mucus worse and should be avoided when a child has a cough or cold. Millions of Americans avoid dairy products when they have a cough or cold. Does milk make mucus thicker?

An Australian study divided 169 adults into two groups: one was given a milk drink, and the other was given a soy drink disguised so as to be indistinguishable in appearance or taste from the cow's-milk drink. Before the study started, nearly half of the adults believed that milk made mucus worse. *Both* test drinks (cow's milk and soy) made some subjects' tongues and throats feel "coated" and made their saliva feel thicker.[19] So the culprit may not be the cow's milk itself so much as any beverage that is thicker than juice or water. Milk does *not* increase mucus produc-

tion in adults with colds.[20] I have not found a single scientific study that answers the question of whether milk increases lung secretions or makes coughing worse.

Do give your child plenty of *fluids* when she has a cough. Fluids help soothe irritated airways and help clear the bacteria, viruses, or irritants that are causing the cough. Fluids also help keep phlegm loose so it is easier to cough out.

Exercise

Despite her fatigue, Terri wanted to participate in a swim meet the following day.

When the body is fighting a serious infection, it needs all of its reserves to win the battle. I generally recommend that kids take it easy until their fever and cough have been gone for twenty-four hours before resuming their normal activities. Even then they should take it slow and be gentle with themselves. They may feel well enough to walk around the house but find that they tire and their cough returns when they resume more vigorous activities. Children tend to cough more with exercise, especially when exercising in cold, dry air (such as speed skating or sledding).[21]

I advised Terri to sleep in and take naps rather than push herself to compete the following day.

If your child has a wet, productive cough, you can help secretions drain with a simple exercise. Have your child lie face down on a bed and slide forward until the head and chest are hanging down off the bed. Your child can rest her head and arms on the floor or on a pillow on the floor. Being upside down helps the mucus drain out. In medicine, this is called *postural drainage* because it is the hanging-down posture that helps the lungs drain. It may also make your child feel light-headed, so don't do it for more than five to ten minutes at a time. After the child has been upside down for a minute or two, encourage her to cough to help bring out the mucus and phlegm.[22] Studies of children with severe coughing due to cystic fibrosis have shown that this simple exercise results in a fivefold increase in the amount of mucus cleared compared with simply resting.[23] In children with asthma or bronchitis, this exercise is even more effective when it follows treatment with inhaled medications such as albuterol.

When your child is resting, prop her head on a pillow. Propping the head up minimizes postnasal drip, the source of many a night-time cough.

Environment

Environmental Therapies

- Avoid smoke.
- Avoid damp, moldy environments.
- Try mist or steam.
- Suction nose with bulb syringe.

Do not smoke and do not allow others to smoke around your child. Tobacco smoke, wood smoke, and air pollution aggravate respiratory problems such as coughing. Keep your child warm, away from cold drafts. If you keep the window open in your child's bedroom to provide fresh air, make sure she has plenty of covers to prevent her from feeling chilled.

Although mist or steam may be helpful in treating a child with a cough, living in a damp house with mold growing on the walls is not.

Coughs are 80 to 90 percent more common among children living in homes parents describe as *damp or moldy* than among children in homes parents say are without damp or mold.[24, 25] Nasty mold and irritating dust mites prefer to live in damp environments.[26] Remove mold thoroughly with a 10% bleach solution. To discourage mold and dust mites from living in your home, consider using a dehumidifier, vacuum regularly, and use an electrostatic air filter.

On the other hand, dry air aggravates most coughs because it dries the secretions that normally soothe the air passages in the throat and lungs. *Mist, steam, and vaporizers* increase the moisture in the air passages and help loosen secretions. Despite the lack of controlled trials evaluating its effectiveness,[27] mist is recommended by most health care providers because of its history of helping children with croup. One of my favorite home remedies for croupy kids is to run the hot water in the shower until the bathroom is very steamy. Then sit with the child on your lap in the steam and tell him stories or sing songs.

Despite years of use, *cool mist* has not proved helpful in treating croupy coughs.[28] The cool mist tents previously used in hospitals caused chills and made it difficult for parents to cuddle their child. If you use a vaporizer, please make sure you clean it regularly to prevent a buildup of mold or fungus in the unit. A seldom-cleaned print shop humidifier harboring fungi and bacteria was responsible for a serious coughing illness in sixteen out of twenty-eight workers in the shop.[29] Be careful with steam vaporizers to avoid accidental burns to curious toddlers.

If your child's cough is due to a runny nose (postnasal drip) and he is too young to blow his nose, you can try *suctioning* his nose *with a bulb syringe*. Suctioning may need to be repeated every few hours. If your child's secretions are too thick to be removed easily with a bulb syringe, place a few drops of salt-water solution (1/2 teaspoon of salt in 8 ounces of water) in each nostril before suctioning. Do one nostril at a time so your child doesn't feel as if he's drowning.

Mind-Body

As with any illness, it is helpful for the parent to remain calm and stay with the child to reassure him. Extra attention, such as reading stories, will help distract your child from whatever is ailing him and remind him that he is loved. Crying and being upset increase your child's need for oxygen. This is not a problem under normal circumstances, but if your child is having trouble breathing, crying may make matters worse.

Coughs often keep everyone in the house awake, especially as parents lie in bed wondering if their child is going to stop coughing or even stop breathing. If your child is having a hard time breathing, you and your spouse might want to take turns staying up with him. If you know that someone is responsible, you can more easily relax and sleep yourself, so that you are better able to care for your child when your "shift" comes.

Some coughs are simply a kind of bad *habit*, which lingers on long after the initial cause for the cough is gone. This kind of cough is dry, harsh, and *very* frequent; it usually stops when the child falls asleep. Children who have these coughs don't usually have any other behavioral problems or emotional problems, but they can often be helped with behavioral therapies, such as the *bedsheet technique*.[30] The child is told that the coughing has weakened his chest muscles and that a bedsheet tied around his chest will help support the muscles. The sheet is tied firmly around the chest, the child is told to stop

coughing, and that the bedsheet will not be removed until the cough has resolved. Physicians who recommend the bedsheet technique report a greater than 90% success rate within a day. Despite its rapid, proven effectiveness for treating children with chronic cough habits, this technique horrifies many parents and is not widely used.

Hypnosis has also proven useful in treating the child with a habitual cough. An eleven-year-old boy who had such a severe, persistent cough that he missed a month of school was able to stop coughing with the help of a psychologist who taught him to use mental imagery and self-hypnosis.[31] The imagery involved characters from Star Wars who had a special medicine that would eliminate the cough. His cough quickly subsided, and he was able to return to school. When coughing recurred, he returned to his Star Wars companions, whose imaginary ministrations restored his health.

Another behavioral technique is to simply *count and record* the number of coughs per half hour. This is done several times over the course of the day. Sometimes the coughing will decrease with counting alone. You can also give your child stickers or other rewards for reducing the number of times she coughs per hour. As she achieves the goal, praise her, reward her, and set a new goal.[32]

BIOMECHANICAL THERAPIES: MASSAGE, SURGERY

Massage

Millions of parents and children around the world can attest to the healing power of a chest rub when a child has a cough or cold. If you haven't tried it yet, do. The old standards are Vicks Vaporub and Mentholatum. Alternatively, consider mixing vegetable oil (5 teaspoons) with two to three drops of essential oils of eucalyptus, lavender, pine, or thyme for a pleasant-smelling rub. Place a bit of the oil in your palm, and rub your hands together until they are warm. Massage your child's chest, neck, and upper back with this mixture.

Several studies have shown that thumping, shaking, and pounding a child's back (known as *percussion* in medicalese) are *not* helpful in loosening up mucus or making it easier to cough up.[33] Beating on your child will not make him better!

Surgery

Surgery is rarely necessary *unless* your child has gotten food (such as a peanut, raisin, or piece of hot dog) or a toy down the wrong pipe (aspirated it), and it has landed in the lungs. In this case, bronchoscopic surgery (in which a fiberoptic tube is placed down the airway so that the object can be seen and removed) might be necessary. *If your child aspirates (chokes on) something, take him to an emergency room immediately.*

BIOENERGETIC THERAPIES: ACUPUNCTURE, HOMEOPATHY

Acupuncture

In China, coughs have been treated with acupuncture for many years. In one series of patients with different kinds of cough, cupping (a variation of acupuncture treatment) for five to ten minutes was helpful.[34] However, this study did not include a control (comparison) group of untreated patients, so it is impossible to tell how many would have improved anyway. I do *not* recommend acupuncture as therapy for common coughs.

Homeopathy

Commonly recommended homeopathic treatments for *dry, barky coughs* (such as croup) are Aconitum, Belladonna (use homeopathic doses only; more concentrated doses can be poisonous), Ipecac, Phosphorous, Rumex, and Spongia. For *productive (wet) coughs* with much mucus: Euphrasia (eyebright) and Natrum sulfuricum (sodium sulfate) are used. For *coughs with colds*: Allium cepa (common red onion) and Bryonia (white bryony) are used. Pulsatilla is recommended for several types of childhood coughs. None has undergone comparison studies in children with coughs. I do *not* recommend them.

WHAT I RECOMMEND FOR COUGHS

PREVENTING COUGHS

1. *Lifestyle—environment.* Avoid exposure to cigarette smoke and other irritants. Avoid exposure to sick, coughing children. Discourage cough-causing mold and dust mites by keeping the humidity under 50% and thoroughly cleaning your home weekly.

2. *Biochemical—medications.* Have your child immunized against pertussis (whooping cough). Treat underlying illnesses such as asthma and allergies (see Chapters 4 and 5).

Take Your Child to a Health Care Provider If She Is

- Coughing so hard that she can't catch her breath
- Coughing up blood
- Wheezing
- Breathing very fast
- Turning blue in lips or fingernails
- Lethargic

Or If She Has

- Pain in the chest for more than a day
- Headache or facial pain as well as coughing
- A fever over 103.9°F
- A persistent cough that has not improved with home remedies

---

TREATING COUGHS

1. *Lifestyle—nutrition.* Encourage your child to drink plenty of fluids to keep the mucus and phlegm loose so it is easier to cough up.

2. *Lifestyle—exercise.* Encourage your child to rest. To help drain phlegm from the lungs of a child with a wet cough, have her lie with her head and chest hanging down off the edge of the bed for five to ten minutes. Then have her cough hard to clear the phlegm.

TREATING COUGHS (cont.)

3. *Lifestyle—environment.* Try a humidifier, vaporizer, or steam treatment. Consider adding essential oils of eucalyptus, menthol, tea tree, and thyme.

4. *Biochemical—medications, herbs.* Hard candy, herbal cough syrups, cough drops, and hot tea with honey may help soothe a throat irritated by coughing. Antibiotics may be necessary for pneumonia. Other medications as needed depending on the underlying cause. No need for guaifenesin, dextromethorphan, or codeine in kids less than 12 years old.

14

CRADLE CAP

Joan Andrews brought in her son, Jeremy, for a two-month checkup, frantic at his appearance. "He's being christened next week, and just look at his head," she lamented. Jeremy had a large patch of cradle cap on his scalp. Joan wanted to know if there was anything she could do or if he would have to wear a hat until he was school age.

Cradle cap is a thick, greasy-looking yellow or white crusting rash on the baby's scalp. The skin underneath is often red and irritated looking. It is also known as infantile seborrheic dermatitis—red, flaking skin on the forehead, scalp, behind the ears, under the armpits, and in the groin. As awful as it looks, it is not itchy or painful. It usually bothers parents much more than it bothers the baby!

Cradle cap often begins unnoticed behind the ears and spreads to the scalp and eyebrows. It usually starts when the baby is two weeks to three months old and can last into the toddler years. Seborrhea is caused by an overactivity of the skin's sebum glands and sometimes by a yeast called *Pityrosporum*

ovale.[1] It is *not* caused by poor hygiene or poor parenting, and it is *not* caused by vitamin deficiencies.[2,3] Washing more frequently or with harsh soaps often just makes seborrhea worse.

Rare children have cradle cap as a symptom of a severe defect in their immune system.[4] These babies also grow poorly and have diarrhea. If your baby has other problems besides cradle cap, please have him evaluated by a health care professional.

TREATMENT FOR CRADLE CAP

Cradle cap eventually resolves on its own regardless of what you do. Though there are a few time-honored home remedies, the primary modern treatments are medicated shampoos, moisturizers, oils, and patience. Let's tour the Therapeutic Mountain to find out what works and what doesn't. If you want to skip to my bottom-line recommendations, flip to the end of the chapter.

BIOCHEMICAL THERAPIES: MEDICATIONS, HERBS, NUTRITIONAL SUPPLEMENTS

Medications

The main medical therapies are medicated shampoos, hydrocortisone cream, and antiyeast medications.

MEDICATED SHAMPOOS AND CREAMS

- Selenium sulfide (Selsun Blue and others)
- Pyrithione zinc (Danex and others)
- Coal tar derivatives (Tegrin Medicated and others)
- Combinations (Sebulex [sulfur and salicylic acid], Neutrogena T/Sal [coal tar and salicylic acid], Sebex T [coal tar, colloidal sulfur, salicylic acid]

Selenium sulfide shampoo (such as Selsun Blue) and pyrithione zinc (Danex) slow down skin turnover on the scalp, reducing the flaking and scaling symptoms. Coal tar derivatives (such as pine tar soap) are commonly used folk remedies for scaling skin conditions such as seborrhea, but they can irritate the skin and may make it more sun sensitive. Coal tar is *not* recommended for children under two years old. Coal tar and sulfur products have a disagreeable odor, which makes them unacceptable to some

families. Be careful not to get any of these products in your child's eyes. If they make the scalp more irritated, discontinue use and consult your health care professional.

For infants whose cradle cap does not respond to medicated shampoos, a mild hydrocortisone cream often does the trick. You don't need anything stronger than 0.5% or 1% hydrocortisone (available without a prescription) applied two or three times daily.

Because the yeast *P. ovale* is more common on the scalps of babies with cradle cap, some dermatologists recommend prescription antiyeast medications such as ketoconazole (Nizoral) cream or shampoo.

Herbs

Some herbalists recommend washing the baby's scalp with a tepid tea made from burdock, chamomile, comfrey root, meadow sweet, slippery elm bark, or plain tea. Others put goldenseal tincture directly on the rash. Cocoa butter is another old-fashioned home remedy to rub into the scalp of babies suffering from cradle cap; cocoa butter may soften the crusting so it is easier to remove. There are *no* studies evaluating the effectiveness of any of these herbal preparations in treating cradle cap. If you have some on hand and are so inclined, go ahead, but if your baby develops any increased irritation, stop the remedy and see your health care professional.

Nutritional Supplements

Years ago it was believed that biotin deficiency was a contributing factor in developing cradle cap. The biotin theory has been proved false. Some practitioners also recommend supplementing the diet with essential fatty acids such as evening primrose oil. This has also *not* proven helpful. If your baby is growing well and does not have other symptoms, he does *not* need nutritional supplements for cradle cap.

LIFESTYLE THERAPIES: ENVIRONMENT, MIND-BODY

Environment

My favorite treatment for seborrhea was taught me by an Italian pediatrician. After washing the baby's scalp with plain water, massage in a little extra virgin olive oil. The olive oil softens the scales so they are easier to remove. Gently comb out the loose scales or flakes of skin. Do *not* try to remove scales that still adhere to the skin, because you could cause further irritation and bleeding. There are no scientific studies of this time-honored treatment, and I honestly can't say that extra virgin oil is more effective than plain olive oil, but I have recommended this traditional treatment for years. It is safe, relatively inexpensive, and readily available. Other practitioners recommend wheat germ oil or other oils. Use what you have on hand; discontinue any treatment if your baby's rash becomes worse or looks irritated.

Mind-Body

The only effective mind-body therapy for cradle cap is patience!

BIOMECHANICAL THERAPIES: MASSAGE

Aromatherapists recommend adding a drop or two of essential oil of lavender to 1 teaspoon of vegetable oil as a massage oil for the scalp. There are no scientific studies evaluating the effectiveness of essential oils in treating this or any other pediatric problem, but lavender oil is probably safe and is easily obtained from health food stores. If you would like to give it a try, go ahead, but discontinue use if your baby's scalp gets worse or becomes irritated.

BIOENERGETIC THERAPIES

There are no studies evaluating the effectiveness of any of these therapies in treating babies suffering from cradle cap.

WHAT I RECOMMEND TO TREAT CRADLE CAP

See Your Health Care Professional If

- The rash does not improve with home remedies
- The rash gets worse, spreads, or looks infected
- Your baby has other symptoms such as poor growth or diarrhea
- You are concerned about the rash or other symptoms

1. *Lifestyle—environment.* Use only water to wash your baby's scalp. Avoid irritating soaps.

2. *Biomechanical—massage.* Massage the scalp with pure olive oil or other vegetable oil. Consider adding a drop of lavender oil to 1 teaspoon of vegetable oil. Then gently comb out the loosened flakes, or rub them loose with a soft toothbrush.

3. *Biochemical—medications.* Consider using a medicated shampoo such as Sebulex. Be careful not to get it in the baby's eyes. If there's no improvement in two weeks, consider a trial of nonprescription 0.5% or 1% hydrocortisone cream. If there's no improvement after two weeks, see your health care practitioner about the possibility of prescription medications such as ketoconazole cream or shampoo.

15
DIAPER RASH

Carmen Morales brought her son, Marco, in for his twelve-month checkup and asked about a new diaper rash. He had been on antibiotics for an ear infection for the past week and had developed a bright red, irritated rash that was worst on his scrotum and the creases in his thighs. Red patches and spots led up to his belly button. Carmen had been using cloth diapers, changing them five or six times a day. Carmen's mother thought Marco had a yeast infection on his bottom. Carmen wanted to know if the antibiotics caused Marco's yeast infection, if she should avoid giving Marco bread and other foods containing yeast, and what was the best way to prevent and treat a diaper rash.

Very few babies escape infancy without at least one bout of diaper rash.

WHAT CAUSES DIAPER RASH

- Irritation from contact with stool and urine
- Yeast (*Candida albicans*)
- Less commonly—allergy, eczema, seborrhea, infection

Irritation diaper rashes are pink or red; they look a bit like a sunburn. They do not extend beyond the diaper area and are usually less severe in the skin creases than on the flat skin that directly touches the diaper. Irritation rashes occur when the bacteria that are normally present in stool break down the chemicals present in urine, forming ammonia—an alkaline (high pH) irritant to babies' delicate skin.[1] Prolonged exposure to wet, dirty diapers is the chief cause of irritation diaper rashes; many are also complicated by yeast infections.

Yeast diaper rashes are usually bright or dark red and are worst in warm, damp skin folds or creases. Typically, yeast diaper rashes extend out from the main rash in red spots. The yeast that cause these rashes, *Candida albicans*, is *not* the same as brewer's yeast, nutritional yeast, or baking yeast. Yeast infections are *not* aggravated by eating yeast. Food yeast and infectious yeast are completely different organisms. *Candida* also causes infant thrush (a white rash in the mouth) and vaginal yeast infections in teenagers and adult women. *Candida* yeast can be carried on mothers' nipples, reinfecting the baby every time he nurses.[2]

Candida yeast are usually kept in check by the normal bacteria that reside in babies' stool, intestines, and skin. When a child takes antibiotics, the normal bacteria are reduced, making way for *Candida* to take over. Thus, children who take antibiotics are at increased risk of developing thrush and *Candida* diaper rashes.

Less commonly, diaper rashes are caused by allergy to soaps, detergents, diaper wipe chemicals, or fabric softeners. Eczema (see Chapter 18), seborrhea (see Chapter 14, Cradle Cap), or bacterial infections can also cause diaper rashes. Bacterial infections usually start at either the umbilical cord or the anus and spread from there. They tend to be painful and red, and the skin is tight-looking. If you think your baby has one of these unusual causes of diaper rash, see your health care professional.

Several things increase the odds of developing diaper rashes.[3]

Diaper rashes are more common among babies who drink formula than those who breast-feed. Rashes are most common in nine-to twelve-month-olds. They are very common when babies have diarrhea because there are more stools and they frequently contain more irritants. Diaper rashes are most common in babies who are kept in cloth diapers (especially if plastic covers are used) and least common in babies kept in super-absorbent disposable diapers. Babies who have more *Candida* yeast in their stool tend to have more frequent and severe rashes. Antibiotics such as amoxicillin suppress the body's normal protective bacteria, allowing yeast to multiply and precipitating diaper rashes.[4] Diarrhea-inducing antibiotics (such as Augmentin) are double jeopardy—reduced protective bacteria and increased dirty diapers.[5]

DIAPER RASH RISKS

- Feeding formula instead of nursing
- Age: nine to twelve months old
- Diarrhea
- Cloth diapers with plastic covers
- Antibiotics

Carmen's mother was right. Marco had a typical yeast diaper rash, which may have been precipitated by the antibiotics he was taking for his ear infection. Carmen did not have to withhold yeast-containing foods.

TREATMENTS FOR DIAPER RASH

Irritant diaper rashes usually resolve within two to three days if treated promptly. *The best treatment for diaper rash is environmental: keeping the diaper changed regularly.* Let's tour the Therapeutic Mountain to find out what works. If you want to skip to my bottom-line recommendations (so to speak), flip to the end of the chapter.

BIOCHEMICAL THERAPIES: MEDICATIONS, HERBS, NUTRITIONAL SUPPLEMENTS

Medications

Medications help heal yeast diaper rashes faster.

NONPRESCRIPTION OINTMENTS FOR *IRRITANT* DIAPER RASH

- Barrier ointments: petrolatum (A&D, Vaseline), lanolin
- Drying agents: zinc oxide (Desitin, Dyprotex)
- Antibacterial: methylbenzethonium chloride (Diaparene, A&D Medicated)
- *Don't use*: clioquinol (Vioform) or iodoquinol (Vytone, Yodoxin)

I recommend ointments rather than powders or creams because they are less likely to wash off when the baby urinates. Barrier ointments, such as A&D ointment, help keep urine and stool away from the baby's skin. If the baby's diaper is changed regularly, a barrier ointment such as A&D ointment or Vaseline may be all you need to prevent diaper rashes. Drying agents such as zinc oxide, the active ingredient in Desitin, help dry up weepy, oozing skin. The active ingredient in Diaparene is mild to babies, but it kills the bacteria that break down urine's chemicals into ammonia. Thoroughly clean and dry the baby's bottom before applying any medication.

Do *not* apply any products containing clioquinol or iodoquinol to your baby's skin. These two compounds have severe toxic effects on the brain and nervous system. Both the World Health Organization and the American Academy of Pediatrics recommend that they *not* be used to treat diaper rashes.[6]

Antifungal medications can help cure diaper rashes caused by yeast.

NONPRESCRIPTION CREAMS AND OINTMENTS FOR *YEAST* DIAPER RASH

- Nystatin: generic brands, Mycostatin, Nilstat
- Undecylenic acid: Caldesene, Desenex
- Miconazole: Micatin, Monistat
- Clotrimazole: Lotrimin
- Gentian violet

I recommend *nystatin* ointment as the first medical treatment for yeast infections. Nystatin is a natural yeast killer derived from *Streptomyces* bacteria. It is safe, effective, and inexpensive; it has been used for over forty years to treat yeast infections of the mouth (thrush), vagina, and diaper area. Side effects are extremely rare, even if it is used recurrently or for long periods of time. Nystatin can be given by mouth to eradicate thrush and to kill the yeast hiding in the intestines, preventing reinfection and repeated diaper rashes.

Undecylenic acid (Caldesene) is effective against yeast diaper rash, prickly heat, and jock itch (which is also caused by a fungus). *Miconazole and clotrimazole* ointments kill many common fungi and yeast, including *Candida*. They are generally safe, but allergic reactions and mild irritation, burning, and stinging have been reported. Symptoms tend to improve within two to three days, but it takes a full two weeks of treatment to completely eradicate the yeast.

Gentian violet has long been used to treat yeast infections. It is very effective for both oral yeast (thrush) and diaper yeast infections. Because it is so messy, stains clothing a deep purple, and can cause skin and mouth sores, it is no longer widely used.[7] Still, because it is so effective, many grandmothers request gentian violet when more modern treatments fail.

More powerful (and more expensive) antifungal medications are available with a prescription. If none of the above nonprescription treatments have worked within two to four weeks, take your child to be evaluated by a health care professional to make sure you are not dealing with something more complicated than a simple irritation or yeast. And consider more potent, prescription medication.

Be cautious about what you put on your baby's skin. Infants' skin is very thin and can easily absorb medicines. For example, an Indiana baby treated with a veterinary salve, Phillip's Corona Ointment, absorbed enough of the active ingredient (a hormone) through her skin to develop early puberty, with pubic hair and breast development.[8]

Herbs

Many grandmothers, some herbalists, and even some physicians recommend chamomile tea as a wash for the diaper area.[9] Other herbal teas sometimes used to wash an irritated bottom include chickweed, comfrey, elder flowers, lavender, marigold, marsh mallow root, and rosemary. These herbs can also be mixed with almond oil (then strained out) to make a soothing bottom rub. Other herbal remedies for diaper rash are tinctures of calendula, goldenseal, or myrrh (available in health food stores and some pharmacies). Ointments containing calendula, comfrey, or marsh mallow (found in many health food stores and herbal catalogs) are also used to soothe irritated skin such as diaper rashes. This is another case where there are *no* scien-

tific studies, but herbal remedies are generally inexpensive. There are rare children who are allergic to chamomile and other herbs. If any treatment makes your child worse, discontinue it and seek the help of a health care professional.

Another old-fashioned bottom wash is witch hazel (which is drying, as is rubbing alcohol). You can find witch hazel in your local pharmacy. Apple cider vinegar and lemon juice are also used as washes for the diaper area to create a more acid (lower pH) environment, which is less hospitable to yeast infection. Although lowering pH to reduce yeast infection is a good theory, there are no studies evaluating the effectiveness of these home remedies; they may cause stinging if applied to broken or irritated skin.

Garlic has antifungal properties in test tubes and animal studies.[10, 11, 12, 13, 14, 15] However, garlic is irritating, and putting a garlic poultice on too long can cause allergic reactions, irritation, and even minor burns.[16] Do *not* put garlic on a baby's bottom. Berberine, the active ingredient in goldenseal, has also been shown to have antifungal effects in test-tube studies.[17] None of these herbal remedies have been evaluated for their safety or effectiveness in human infants suffering from diaper rashes.

Beware of applying egg white to your baby's bottom as a treatment for diaper rash. Although this home remedy is widely used in Britain, it has caused severe egg allergies.[18] Eggs are a fairly common allergen among infants under one year old; it is not surprising that applying a potential allergen to broken skin causes problems.

Nutritional Supplements

Babies with frequent diaper rashes have lower levels of zinc in their systems than infants with less frequent rashes.[19] This has led to trials of zinc supplements to reduce the risk of diaper rash. Zinc supplements (10 milligrams per day) may prevent yeast diaper rashes in some formula-fed babies, but they are *not* helpful in preventing diaper rashes in nursing babies.[20] Breast-fed babies get all the zinc they need from mother's milk. If your baby drinks formula and has already had several yeast infections, you might want to give zinc a try to prevent future episodes.

Vitamin A is used to treat a number of skin conditions. In a Spanish study, vitamin A cream (such as that used in A&D ointment) was evaluated as a preventive therapy for diaper rash.[21] It failed to reduce the number or severity of diaper rashes compared with placebo cream. Although it is widely used and recommended, vitamin A is no more effective than simple ointments such as Vaseline.

Some parents simply break open a vitamin E capsule and rub the oil on their baby's irritated skin. This may be worth a try if you have vitamin E capsules on hand; there are *no* studies evaluating its effectiveness or safety.

LIFESTYLE THERAPIES: NUTRITION, ENVIRONMENT

Nutrition

For babies over six months old, some mothers supplement their child's diet with yogurt (with active cultures) when he is taking antibiotics. The live acidophilus bacteria in the yogurt are thought to help replace the yeast on the baby's skin, preventing diaper rashes. The yogurt must contain active cultures to have any chance of being helpful. Check the label; many commercial brands do *not* contain active cultures. Some mothers apply the acidophilus or yogurt directly to

the baby's bottom. I have not heard of any side effects from this treatment, nor are there any actual studies of its effectiveness.

Many parents have heard that excessive sugar in the diet predisposes to yeast infections such as diaper rash. While it is true that diabetic adults are more prone to yeast infections, it is not clear that altering a child's diet changes his risk of having a diaper rash. Most nine- to twelve-month-old babies do not need and do not eat sugar, yet this is the peak age of diaper rashes. Sugar is unlikely to be a major factor in diaper rashes. On the other hand, sugar intake *does* increase the risk of tooth decay.

Environment

The most effective treatment for diaper rashes is to keep the baby's bottom clean and dry. The best ways to accomplish this are by:

- changing the diaper frequently (at least eight times daily),
- avoiding plastic pants, which reduce air circulation to the diaper area, and
- allowing the baby's bottom to be exposed to air.

Change your baby's diaper immediately after he has a bowel movement or urinates to minimize the time his tender skin is in contact with urine or stool. If he already has a diaper rash, check his diaper every hour, and change it immediately if it is wet or soiled. After cleaning his bottom with plain water (nothing else is really needed, and soap may be irritating), allow him to air dry before you put the next diaper on him. You can lay a diaper or towel under him so he doesn't wet his bed or the floor or wherever he is lying. The best times for air drying are during naps and right after diaper changes. Some parents make sure their baby's bottom is really dry by using a hair dryer (set on low) to blow-dry the bottom. Be very careful; unintentionally, overzealous parents have severely burned their baby's bottom with hair dryers.[22]

Be careful with the *diaper wipes*. Many of them contain alcohol, which can sting broken or irritated skin. Some wipes also contain perfumes and other chemicals that could further irritate your baby's tender skin. Stick with plain water and mild soap. Nothing else is necessary, and everything else is more expensive.

There is conflict between the values of health, convenience, and ecology over which is better—*cloth vs. disposable diapers*. There are fewer and less severe rashes in babies diapered exclusively in disposable diapers than in those using cloth diapers.[23] The new super-absorbent diapers are even more effective in keeping babies dry and reducing diaper rash.[24, 25, 26] The main thing is to keep the baby clean and dry with frequent changes rather than worrying about what the diaper is made of. If you use cloth diapers and wash them at home, use chlorine bleach to sterilize them and double-rinse them to make sure all of the potentially irritating detergent, bleach, and softener residues are removed before putting them in the dryer.

You can add 1/4 cup of *vinegar* to the final rinse to make the diaper more acidic (discouraging the growth of yeast), but remember that vinegar does not kill germs as effectively as bleach.

Long-time home remedies for diaper rash include the use of *cornstarch or arrowroot powder* sprinkled on the baby at diaper changes. There are many testimonials to the effectiveness of cornstarch (including some from physician-parents)[27], but there are *no* scientific studies showing that it is any more effective than simply changing the diaper frequently and keeping the baby clean and dry. Still, it's inexpensive and readily available and may be worth a try.

Do not use talcum powder; talc creates a dust cloud when it is applied, and inhaling the powder has caused serious lung problems in some babies.

Biomechanical Therapies

None has any proved benefit in treating infants with diaper rash.

Bioenergetic Therapies: Homeopathy

Commonly used homeopathic remedies include creams, ointments, and sprays made from calendula and arnica. Extremely dilute homeopathic remedies given by mouth for yeast diaper rashes are Arsenicum, Belladonna, Chamomile, Graphites, Hepar sulfur, Symphytum, and the combination of Hypericum and Calendula known as Hypercal. There are *no* scientific studies showing that these remedies are any more effective than other creams or ointments. There are also no reported side effects.

WHAT I RECOMMEND FOR DIAPER RASH

PREVENTING DIAPER RASH

1. *Lifestyle—nutrition.* Breast-feed your baby.

2. *Lifestyle—environment.* Change your baby's diapers at least eight times a day, more often if he has diarrhea. Keep the baby's bottom clean and dry. Consider using disposable diapers, especially the super-absorbent brands. If you use cloth diapers, double-rinse them. Use vinegar in the last rinse to make them mildly acidic and discourage yeast from living there. Do not use plastic diaper covers. It is better to allow some air circulation.

3. *Biochemical—medications.* Consider using a barrier ointment (such as Desitin, A&D ointment, or Vaseline) with each diaper change, especially when your child has diarrhea, to protect his skin from stool and urine.

Take Your Child to a Health Care Professional If

- The rash looks as if it may be infected (blisters or open sores)
- The rash spreads outside the diaper area
- Your child has a fever, decreased appetite, or other symptoms
- The rash is not improving or is getting worse with home treatment
- You are concerned about the rash or any other symptoms

TREATING DIAPER RASH

1. *Lifestyle—environment.* As above. Allow your baby to go for a period without any diapers on at all to allow the bottom to dry completely. Do not use commercial baby wipes containing alcohol, fragrances, or other chemicals, because these may further irritate your baby's skin. Use a clean washcloth and plain water. Do *not* use talcum powder; inhaling it can cause lung problems.

2. *Lifestyle—nutrition.* If you are feeding your baby formula, consider supplementing his diet with 10 milligrams per day of zinc. Consider using yogurt with live cultures to restore the "good" bacteria to the diaper area. Try giving it by mouth (1/2 cup daily for children over one year old), or apply directly to the baby's bottom.

3. *Biochemical—medications.* For yeast diaper rashes, try nonprescription medications containing nystatin (Mycostatin, Nilstat), undecylenic acid (Caldesene), clotrimazole (Lotrimin), or miconazole (Monistat). If none of these are helpful, see your health care professional about prescription medications.

16

DIARRHEA

The morning after her family's picnic, Suzanne Cooper awoke with diarrhea. Her stools were so watery they ran out of her diaper and down her leg. What a mess! No one else was sick, and she wasn't vomiting. Her parents wondered if it was something she ate or one of those viruses that made weekly rounds at her day care center. Her grandmother encouraged them to feed her flat soda. Their neighbor said to stop all milk products. Her aunt said to feed her whatever she wanted. Her father, Joe, had several questions for me:

- *Did Suzanne need to come in to the office to be seen?*
- *How would he know if she was dehydrated?*
- *Besides food poisoning and the flu, why do children get diarrhea?*
- *How could he prevent Suzanne from getting it again?*
- *What was the best way to treat her now that she was sick?*

Sooner or later all parents deal with diarrhea. The average child younger than five years old has two to three episodes a year. Diarrhea is simply when children have more stools than is normal for them, especially if the stools are runny or watery. The normal number of stools varies from child to child; it also varies with the child's diet. Breast-fed babies can have a bowel movement as often as after every meal.

Diarrhea is the body's way of getting rid of toxins, bacteria, and parasites. It usually lasts a day or two, but it may last for a week. Diarrhea is not life-threatening unless the child becomes severely dehydrated or the diarrhea is a symptom of an underlying problem.

This chapter is about *acute diarrhea* (diarrhea that lasts less than ten days). If your child has *chronic diarrhea* (diarrhea that has lasted weeks to months) and is not growing well or gaining weight, please take her to a health care provider for a complete evaluation.

Worldwide, diarrhea is the leading cause of death during childhood; fatal cases almost always occur in malnourished children under five years old. As many children die of diarrhea each *day* as the number of persons who die from AIDS each *year*.[1] Almost all diarrhea deaths are due to dehydration. What are the most worrisome symptoms?

WHEN TO CALL YOUR CHILD'S HEALTH CARE PROVIDER

- The diarrhea lasts longer than a week or there are more than ten stools per day.
- Your child has a fever higher than 101°F for more than one day.
- She has pain in the lower right part of her abdomen.
- There is blood in the stools.
- Your child is less than six weeks old.
- She is losing weight.
- She is vomiting for more than one day.
- She is lethargic, disoriented, confused, or doesn't recognize you.
- She is not acting like herself.
- She has a high fever (over 103°F) at any time or has a seizure.
- She refuses to drink or isn't thirsty. (*Note*: It's normal for children to refuse solids when they're sick, but they should still be thirsty.)
- She looks dehydrated.

These may be signs that your child has something other than simple diarrhea or needs more therapy than you can provide at home.

HOW DO YOU KNOW IF YOUR CHILD IS BECOMING DEHYDRATED?

- She voids (pees/urinates) less than four times per day or less than half of what is normal for her.
- She doesn't have tears when she cries.
- She loses weight.
- She has sunken eyes, sunken fontanel (soft spot on baby's head).
- Her lips and tongue are dry; she has stringy saliva.
- Her hands and feet are much cooler than her arms and legs.

If your child has any of these signs, she needs more fluid. Children who are *vomiting* (see Chapter 26) are more likely to become dehydrated than children who have diarrhea alone.

Suzanne did not have any signs of dehydration; she could be treated safely at home.

WHAT CAUSES DIARRHEA?

There are many causes for diarrhea. The table below lists the most common ones.

The leading cause of diarrhea in young children is a *viral infection*, most commonly rotavirus. Rotavirus is the number one cause of diarrhea worldwide among children who are between three and fifteen months old. Every year, rotavirus infections among American children cost approximately $1 billion in parents' missed work, doctor visits, laboratory tests, treatments, and extra diapers.[2]

COMMON CAUSES OF DIARRHEA

- Infections with viruses, bacteria, or parasites
- Reactions to food
  — Food poisoning (e.g., *Staphylococcus* bacteria)
  — Food intolerance, sensitivities, allergies
  — Excessive intake of fruit or "sugarless" gum
- Reactions to vitamins or medications
  — Excessive vitamin C
  — Excessive use of laxatives
  — Side effect of antibiotics, antacids, or other medications
- Other causes
  — Nervous diarrhea
  — Miscellaneous: teething, ear and bladder infections

Bacteria cause diarrhea in several ways. A few bacteria, such as cholera, attack the intestinal walls, while others, such as *Staphylococcus* (the cause of most food poisoning), indirectly cause symptoms by producing toxins that poison the gut. Other common diarrhea-causing bacteria include *Salmonella, Shigella,* and *E. coli.* Viruses and bacteria are usually passed from person to person, but they can also be transmitted by contaminated meat, poultry, and water. When you go camping and drink from a stream, you risk picking up a diarrhea-causing parasite, *Giardia. Giardia* can also be passed from person to person, especially in day care centers with insufficient handwashing and children in diapers.

Suzanne could easily have caught rotavirus at her day care. Food poisoning was a less likely cause of her diarrhea because no one else was sick who ate the same foods.

Overindulgence in hot dogs and other greasy *foods* accounts for post–ball game diarrhea, but even healthy foods can cause diarrhea if consumed in excess. Lactose (milk sugar) intolerance is a common cause of crampy abdominal pain, bloating, and diarrhea in those who lack the enzyme necessary to digest it (lactase). Cow's milk, eggs, soy protein, and other allergenic foods cause diarrhea in fewer than 10 percent of children.[3] Children who are sensitive to cow's milk usually develop symptoms within the first six months of life.[4] Undercooked hamburgers resulted in a deadly epidemic of *E. coli* diarrhea in Washington state in 1993.[5] Drinking too much pear or apple juice accounts for astonishing amounts of toddler diarrhea; these fruit juices contain the stool-loosening sugars sorbitol and fructose. A recent outbreak of infectious diarrhea from fresh-pressed apple cider emphasizes the importance of good hygiene even in natural products.[6] Chewing a lot of sorbitol-containing "sugarless" gum can also induce diarrhea. In fact, constipation can be treated by ingesting extra sugarless snacks and pear juice.

Diarrhea is one of the early signs of a *vitamin C* overdose. Children or adults who suddenly start taking 500 to 1,000 milligrams of vitamin C several times a day to prevent illness may find they are having more frequent and looser stools. Children can tolerate higher doses of vitamin C when they are ill or if they gradually build up tolerance.

Many *medications* cause diarrhea, either as a direct effect (e.g., chocolate-flavored Ex-Lax, which children may mistake for candy) or as a side effect. The antibiotics prescribed for many ear infections kill the normal bacteria in the gut as well as the bacteria in the ear, resulting in diarrhea. Sugar-free medications such as sugar-free theophylline are sometimes sweetened with sorbitol, which can cause diarrhea.[7] Antacids can also cause diarrhea by drawing water into the intestines.

Several other unrelated factors can also trigger diarrhea. Diarrhea due to *stress* is exemplified by the long lines to the bathroom right before a test in school. For reasons we do not fully understand, some children also get diarrhea when they are cutting *teeth* and when they get *ear infections. Bladder infections* cause sympathetic bowel irritation, occasionally resulting in diarrhea. Unusual, serious bowel diseases and enzyme deficiencies can also cause diarrhea, but this diarrhea is usually chronic (long-term) rather than acute (short-term).

The best treatment for your child's diarrhea depends on what is causing it. Regardless of the cause, give your child extra fluids to replace what she is losing with all those runny stools.

HOW TO PREVENT DIARRHEA

TO PREVENT YOUR CHILD FROM GETTING DIARRHEA

- Use good hygiene: frequent hand-washing, especially after diaper changes, when cooking poultry, and with toddlers who are toilet-training.
- Thoroughly cook all meat, poultry, and eggs.
- Breast-feed for at least three months.
- Make sure your drinking water is pure.
- Be on the lookout for future vaccines.

Because most diarrhea is caused by viruses that are passed from person to person, the best prevention strategy is *frequent handwashing*. Toilet-training toddlers need reminders to wash their hands after using the potty and before eating. Frequent handwashing is absolutely essential in day care centers where there are children in diapers. Diarrhea outbreaks are more common in crowded day care settings than in those with fewer children. Handwashing is also important in the home before, during, and after food preparation. Much of the poultry in this country is contaminated with diarrhea-causing *Salmonella* bacteria. *Salmonella* is killed when the poultry is thoroughly cooked (eliminating the risk from the meat itself), but be sure to clean your cutting board, counter, knife, and hands before preparing other foods, especially raw salads.

Breast-feed your baby for at least the first three months of life.[8] Formula feeding markedly increases an infant's chances of getting diarrhea. In one study, formula-fed babies had ten times the risk of getting rotavirus diarrhea compared with breast-fed babies.[9] Breast-feeding can also decrease the duration of diarrhea if your child does get sick.[10] Nursing effectively reduces the risk and severity of diarrhea from outbreaks of even very aggressive bacteria[11] and parasites.[12] Breast milk contains immune factors (immunoglobulin A) that help prevent bacteria from attacking the intestines and help reduce symptoms of diarrhea even when bacteria and parasites do get into the system.[13,14]

Consider feeding yogurt to your child regularly to prevent diarrhea. A study at Johns Hopkins showed that regularly giving infants from five to twenty-four months old the "good bacteria" contained in yogurt markedly reduced their chances of getting rotavirus diarrhea.[15] You can get these benefits only with yogurt containing live cultures or by giving supplements of *Bifidobacteria* or *Strep thermophilus* (available at health food stores).

Always *boil your water* or use a special filter when you go camping. When you travel abroad, use bottled, boiled, or filtered water if there is any question about its purity.

Researchers are working on a *vaccine* to prevent diarrhea due to rotavirus.[16] Scientists are also evaluating the effectiveness of rotavirus immune globulin (molecules that fight rotavirus). Preliminary studies show that immune globulin cuts in half the number of days children suffer from diarrhea.[17]

WHAT'S THE BEST WAY TO TREAT DIARRHEA?

The two principles of treatment are:

1. Address the underlying cause

2. Give fluids to prevent dehydration

If your child has diarrhea from drinking too much pear juice, the obvious treatment is to cut back on the juice. Even if the cause is not so obvious, you can still help prevent dehydration by making sure your child drinks plenty of fluids. Offer something to drink every fifteen to thirty minutes while she is awake. Over the course of a day the frequent fluids add up, preventing dehydration. Let's circle the Therapeutic Mountain to find out what works best. If you want to skip to the bottom line, flip to the end of the chapter.

BIOCHEMICAL THERAPIES: MEDICATIONS, HERBS, NUTRITIONAL SUPPLEMENTS

Medications

MEDICATIONS FOR DIARRHEA

Do use: bismuth subsalicylate (Pepto-Bismol)

Don't use: kaolin-pectin (Kao-Pectate), paregoric, loperamide (Imodium), diphenoxylate (Lomotil)

Sometimes use: antibiotics, immune globulin

Good old-fashioned *Pepto-Bismol* (bismuth subsalicylate) given every four hours has been shown to be a helpful treatment for sudden watery diarrhea, even when the diarrhea is caused by a bacterial infection.[18] Bismuth subsalicylate contains the active ingredient in aspirin (salicylate); to minimize the risk of developing the serious complication Reye's syndrome, do *not* give Pepto-Bismol or other aspirin-containing remedies when your child has influenza. Although their names are similar, influenza is not the same as intestinal flu. Influenza symptoms are usually high fever, exhaustion, weakness, headache, muscle aches, and coughing. Diarrhea is not a typical part of the influenza picture, but there's no guarantee that a child can't get influenza and a rotavirus infection at the same time. When in doubt, skip the Pepto-Bismol or consult a health care professional.

Another commonly used medication is *kaolin-pectin (Kao-Pectate)*. Pectin is found in apple peels and is used to thicken jams and jellies. Pectin thickens stools and makes them less sloppy, but it does *not* decrease the overall amount of fluid lost or speed up the child's recovery from diarrhea.

Joe had already given Suzanne some Kao-Pectate by the time he called me. Kao-Pectate is not actually harmful, but the improved consistency of the stools can be deceiving. I urged Joe to continue to offer Suzanne frequent sips of fluid to avoid dehydration even though her stools appeared to be less watery.

Avoid the adult diarrhea medicines *paregoric, loperamide* (Imodium), and *diphenoxylate* (Lomotil). These medicines are from the same drug family as codeine and morphine. Although one of their main effects is constipation, their side effects include sleepiness, nausea, and distended bellies. Some children have become comatose and died from taking loperamide (Imodium).

The vast majority of American children with diarrhea do not need and do not benefit from *antibiotics*. Many antibiotics actually cause diarrhea because they wipe out the "good" bacteria that normally live in the intestines as well as the "bad" bacteria that cause ear infections, sore throats, and other infections. Antibiotic treatment for diarrhea is only indicated for children who have diarrhea due to certain bacteria or parasites, such as cholera, *Shigella*, amebiasis, or persistent *Giardia*. If your child is severely dehydrated or has bloody stools, a stool test is necessary to determine if she needs antibiotics.

Herbs

HERBAL REMEDIES FOR DIARRHEA

Do not use: carob, other tannin-containing herbs

Maybe use: goldenseal, barberry, oregon grape, chamomile, cinnamon, garlic, ginger, mint, raspberry leaf, slippery elm bark

There are no comparison studies demonstrating that any herbal remedies safely reduce the length or severity of childhood diarrhea. Nonetheless, many herbal remedies have been used for generations. Their main benefit is probably due to the fact that they are taken as tea, which helps prevent dehydration.

Carob powder is an old-time Mediterranean folk remedy for diarrhea, but it contains a possible cancer-causer, *tannin*. Carob reduces the growth of bacteria and binds some of the toxins produced by bacteria. In a Dutch study, carob pod powder was significantly better than placebo in shortening the course of diarrhea.[19] Dosages in different studies vary up to tenfold. Because carob is a biological substance, its potency varies. Despite its documented effectiveness, I will *not* recommend carob treatment for diarrhea until there are better studies documenting its safety.

Many of the other herbal remedies commonly recommended for treating mild diarrhea also contain a substantial (5 to 8 percent) amount of cancer-causing tannin. Herbal remedies that have a high tannin content include agrimony or cocklebur, alder, and the leaves and tops of betony. Avoid herbal diarrhea remedies that contain these herbs.

Goldenseal, barberry and *Oregon grape* all contain the chemical berberine. Berberine kills many of the bacteria and parasites that cause diarrhea.[20] Goldenseal was used by Native Americans to treat diarrhea. Goldenseal is generally the easiest of the berberine-containing plants to obtain. You can give either the tincture or the fluid extract mixed in 4 ounces of water, three times daily while your child has diarrhea:

- Tincture (strength of 1:5): 1/4 to 1/2 teaspoon
- Fluid extract (strength of 1:1): 1/8 teaspoon

Higher doses can create problems with metabolizing B vitamins.

Other herbal remedies that do *not* rely on tannin include *chamomile tea and red raspberry leaf tea,* widely used in Europe as an aid to digestion, and *cinnamon,* which is commonly recommended for digestive disturbances. You can add a pinch of cinnamon to yogurt to help soothe the intestines of a child suffering from diarrhea. *Garlic* is believed to help the immune system fight whatever bacteria or virus is causing the diarrhea. You can flavor rice with a bit of garlic. *Ginger* (the basis for old-fashioned ginger ale) is recommended worldwide for treating upset stomachs. Ginger (1/4 teaspoon chopped or grated), combined with the juice of half a lemon and 1 teaspoon of honey in a cup of hot water, makes a lovely tea for children with an upset stomach.

Peppermint leaf tea and catnip tea are also recommended for all sorts of stomach pains, cramps, indigestion, and diarrhea. (See Appendix B for instructions on making herbal teas.) You can also add a leaf or two of mint to flavor yogurt and calm the stomach.

Nutritional Supplements

NUTRITIONAL SUPPLEMENTS FOR CHILDREN WITH DIARRHEA

Do use: zinc if you suspect zinc deficiency or the diarrhea is protracted

Don't use: vitamin C, copper

Maybe use: vitamin A

When children have prolonged diarrhea (more than seven to ten days), they can lose a lot of nutrients in their stools. One of the important minerals lost this way is *zinc.* Zinc deficiency can also cause diarrhea.[21] Studies from India and Bangladesh indicate that zinc supplements help speed recovery from diarrhea.[22, 23] Zinc deficiency is uncommon among American children. If you believe your child has a zinc deficiency, a reasonable dosage for children six to eighteen months old is 10 milligrams of elemental zinc twice daily for one to two weeks. If your child is younger than six months old, please consult your health care professional for a proper dose.

Diarrhea is one of the side effects of too much *vitamin C.* Do *not* give your child supplemental vitamin C when she has diarrhea. Excessive *copper* can interfere with zinc absorption and increase elimination of zinc. Do *not* give your child copper supplements while she has diarrhea.[24]

The data on *vitamin A* treatment for diarrhea are conflicting. Initial reports from

Thailand and Brazil indicated that supplemental vitamin A might reduce the risks of severe diarrhea.[25] Subsequent research in India showed that it did not reduce the number of episodes, the severity, or the length of diarrhea.[26] Until research is done using vitamin A to treat American children with diarrhea, its effectiveness remains unproved.

LIFESTYLE THERAPIES: NUTRITION, EXERCISE, ENVIRONMENT, MIND-BODY

Nutrition

Nutritional therapy is the mainstay of diarrhea treatment.

Do:

- Continue to breast-feed
- Give electrolyte-balanced fluids
- Continue full-strength milk or formula unless diarrhea is severe
- Give yogurt, rice, lentils, potatoes, and other nongreasy foods

Don't:

- Give plain water alone without other fluids or foods
- Give apple or pear juice

Breast milk is the best food for an infant with diarrhea. If your infant is dehydrated, breast-feed more often and consider adding other liquids that have a balanced solution of water, salt, and sugar.

The most convenient *electrolyte-balanced liquids* to replace fluid losses from diarrhea are premixed solutions such as Pedialyte and Lytren. These solutions have been formulated with just the right amount of salt and sugar (glucose) to help your child replace the fluids she's losing with her diarrhea. Rehydration solutions are much better than half-strength Jell-O, soft drinks, or fruit juices, which have too much sugar (glucose) and not enough salt.

I asked Joe not *to replace Suzanne's fluid losses with soda or apple juice, despite his mother-in-law's advice. These fluids just don't have the proper balance of salt and sugar that a child suffering from diarrhea needs.*

You can make your own rehydration solution at home[27]:

HOMEMADE REHYDRATION SOLUTION

- 1 quart (1 liter) of clean water
- ½ teaspoon (2.5 grams) of salt
- 4–8 teaspoons (20-40 grams) of sugar

Measure the ingredients with measuring cups and spoons, and use pure water.

In many parts of the world, *rice water* is used to treat dehydration in infants with diarrhea. Several studies have shown it to be at least as effective as standard rehydration solutions, if not more effective.[28,29] In other parts of the world, other cereal powders (such as corn, millet, and sorghum) are mixed with water and salt to make the rehydration solution. An alternative recipe replaces the sugar with rice cereal. A commercial formulation, Ricelyte, is available, or you can make your own.

HOMEMADE REHYDATION SOLUTION: ALTERNATIVE

- 1 quart of water
- ½ teaspoon of salt
- 2 ounces (50–80 grams) or about 1 cup of rice cereal for babies

Joe decided that they would make their own rehydration solution at home. Because they had infant rice cereal on hand for the baby anyway, he decided to use the alternative solution. That way he could avoid giving his daughter straight sugar and save money. He wanted to know exactly how much rehydration solution he needed to give Suzanne. How much was enough?

A good rule of thumb is 2 to 4 ounces of extra fluid for each diarrhea stool. Give the fluid a little at a time. If your child is vomiting and you give her a large amount to drink at once, she could vomit it all back up. Giving a large amount at a time can also stimulate another bowel movement, making the diarrhea and dehydration worse. If your child is vomiting, try giving just a tablespoon (15 milliliters) or an ounce (30 milliliters) every fifteen to thirty minutes, increasing the amount gradually as your child tolerates it. If your child is thirsty, give fluid more frequently.

Despite well-meaning advice, you do not need to dilute milk, stop milk, or switch to a different formula. Most children recover quite nicely from their diarrhea within a few days regardless of the type of milk they drink. When I was in training to be a pediatrician, I was taught that babies who had diarrhea should be fed clear liquids, advancing to quarter-strength formula, then half-strength formula, and finally full-strength formula. Now we know that diluting milk or formula for children with diarrhea is unnecessary and may even be counterproductive.[30] Recent studies show that children who are fed full-strength milk regain weight faster than those who are fed diluted milk.[31] Diluting formula will not help your child recover from the diarrhea any faster and deprives her of needed calories.

There have been at least twenty-nine studies involving a total of over 2,000 children with diarrhea to see if feeding a lactose-free diet is helpful. Children who are mildly ill do just as well on cow's milk (or formulas based on cow's milk) as those who are taken off of cow's milk products.[32] On the other hand, some children do benefit from lactose-free milk when they have diarrhea.[33] There *are* times when it is helpful to stop milk.[34]

WHEN TO STOP MILK AND MILK PRODUCTS

IF YOUR CHILD HAS:

- severe diarrhea requiring hospital-ization
- diarrhea for more than two weeks
- doesn't tolerate lactose (milk sugar) even when she's well
- was malnourished even before she developed diarrhea[35]

Physicians used to tell parents to stop all *solids* until the child was tolerating milk and then restart solids slowly with *b*ananas, *r*ice cereal, *a*pplesauce, and *t*oast or *t*ea, the BRAT diet. While these recommendations are probably not harmful, there are no scientific studies showing they are useful. Most children do just as well by continuing their usual diet as children who are put on special diets.[36] A recent study in Pakistan showed that children with diarrhea who were fed their traditional diet of rice, lentils, and yogurt did better than children fed only rehydration fluids and soy formula.[37] Both Mexican and Peruvian studies showed that even beans can safely be included in the diet of children with diarrhea.[38, 39]

Rice and yogurt are the most easily digested foods for children recovering from acute diarrhea.[40] Rice, other cereals, potatoes, and other starchy vegetables are easy to digest and help reduce the duration of diarrhea.[41] Children with persistent diarrhea who are fed yogurt do better than those fed plain cow's milk.[42] A Finnish study showed that the

secret is the active acidophilus cultures: children who ate yogurt with active cultures recovered a day faster than children who ate yogurt with inactive cultures.[43] Homemade yogurt contains active cultures and avoids the artificial colors, flavors, and sugars contained in many commercial brands.

Extra *fiber* may make the stools look more solid, but it doesn't prevent dehydration or shorten the course of illness.[44] Some parents who are tired of dealing with the mess of sloppy diapers may want to consider fiber supplements. Fiber does *not* affect your child's illness or the risk of dehydration, but it may reduce the mess of watery stools.

Plain *water* is OK as a supplement, but it should not be the only fluid you give. When your child has diarrhea, she is losing water and salt, so both need to be replaced. The intestines actually absorb water better if it contains a little sugar. Plain water does not contain any salt or sugar, and is not absorbed as well as solutions that contain them. If a child gets too much water without replacing the salt lost because of the diarrhea, there can be blood-cell damage, seizures, and even coma.

Fruit juices and flat soda are not as helpful as the rehydration recipes described above. No one would treat diarrhea with prune juice, but many parents don't realize that as little as 5 to 8 ounces of pear juice can also cause loose stools.[45] Apple juice can also make diarrhea worse. Grape juice tends to cause fewer problems than either pear or apple juice, but purple grape juice goes right through a child with diarrhea and makes a real mess in the diaper! If you want to give fruit juice and avoid the mess, try white grape juice.[46]

Joe realized that it was time to stop giving Suzanne soda. He gave her 1/2 cup of rehydration solution to sip over fifteen minutes every time she had a diarrhea stool. He went to the store to pick up some yogurt with active cultures and made a big batch of rice as a side dish for supper. He was concerned that Suzanne was starting to get a diaper rash from all the diarrhea and wondered what he could do for that.

Environment

You can reduce the risk of diaper rash that often accompanies diarrhea by changing your child's diaper frequently and putting an ointment such as Vaseline, A&D, or Desitin on the skin with each diaper change. Diaper rashes occur when the bacteria in the stool interact with urine, forming a compound that is very irritating to babies' tender skin. If you can keep the skin clean and dry, you can reduce the risk of rash. If possible, have your baby take naps with the diaper *under* her rather than around her, exposing her bottom to air and allowing it to dry out. Some parents also use a fan or a hair dryer set at a very low setting to help dry their babies' bottoms more thoroughly. Be sure you don't burn the skin! (For more information about diaper rash, see Chapter 15.)

BIOMECHANICAL THERAPIES

There are no studies documenting the effectiveness of any biomechanical therapies in treating ordinary childhood diarrhea.

BIOENERGETIC THERAPIES: ACUPUNCTURE, HOMEOPATHY

Acupuncture

In a series of 170 infants who were treated with acupuncture for diarrhea, most children recovered in two to three days.[47] However, there was no comparison group of children who did not receive acupuncture. It is impos-sible to tell how fast the children would have improved without acupuncture or with a different treatment. Until comparative studies are done, acupuncture remains an unproved remedy for children with diarrhea.

Homeopathy

A recent randomized, controlled trial demonstrated the effectiveness of individualized homeopathic treatment for Nicaraguan children with diarrhea.[48] See Appendix B for dosing information for homeopathic remedies. Commonly recommended homeopathic remedies for diarrhea are:

Arsenicum for children who are vomiting, with tummy pain and severe, foul-smelling, burning watery diarrhea that is worse at night. *Arsenicum* is recommended for the child who is restless, exhausted, and thirsty. Children with this type of diarrhea also like to be cuddled under warm blankets. *Arsenicum* is the most commonly recommended homeopathic remedy for diarrhea due to food poisoning.

Calcium carbonate for the diarrhea that accompanies teething.

Chamomile for children whose diarrhea is related to cutting teeth, when the child is restless, whining, irritable, or clinging.

Colocynthus for children who have crampy abdominal pain.

Ipecac (the very dilute homeopathic form only) for children who have intractable vomiting along with their diarrhea.

Podophyllum for severe diarrhea when the diarrhea is worse in the morning, there isn't much vomiting, and the child is very thirsty for cold water.

Pulsatilla for diarrhea from eating excessive amounts of rich foods.

Sulfur for children whose diarrhea is worse at night or early in the morning, whose diarrhea smells like rotten eggs, or when there is redness around the child's anus.

Use only *one* remedy at a time. Do *not* combine remedies without the advice of a licensed homeopathic practitioner. If you decide to use homeopathic remedies, seek the help of a homeopathic practitioner who is experienced in treating children. Remember that the most important therapy is hydration.

WHAT I RECOMMEND FOR DIARRHEA

PREVENTING DIARRHEA

1. *Lifestyle—nutrition.* Breast-feed your child for at least the first three to four months of life.

2. *Biochemical—nutritional supplements.* After weaning, consider daily doses of yogurt with live cultures or healthy bacteria or supplements of *Bifidobacteria* or *Strep thermophilus.*

3. *Lifestyle—environment.* Use good hygiene to prevent the spread of viruses and bacteria that cause diarrhea.

- Wash your hands.

- Wash food preparation surfaces.

- Thoroughly cook all meat products.

- If your child is in day care, choose one with just a few children in uncrowded settings to prevent many infectious illnesses, including diarrhea.

- When traveling, drink bottled or filtered water. Do not drink out of streams when you are camping unless you boil, filter, or treat the water.

Take Your Child to Your Health Care Professional If She

- Looks dehydrated
- Has diarrhea for longer than a week
- Has blood in stools
- Looks sicker than you would expect with a simple virus

TREATING DIARRHEA

1. *Lifestyle—nutrition.* Give plenty of fluids. (Do *not* give apple, pear, or prune juice.)

Give one of the commercial rehydration solutions or make your own:

> 4 cups of water (1 quart)
> ½ teaspoon of salt
> 1–1½ cups (50–80 grams) of rice cereal for babies *or* 2 tablespoons of sugar

Offer 1 tablespoon to 1 ounce every fifteen to thirty minutes; increase as tolerated.

If your child is breast-feeding, continue to breast-feed. Supplement with rehydration fluids.

If your child did not have any problems with milk before, continue it or try a lactose-free soy milk or enriched rice milk. You do not need to stop milk, formula, or solids unless the diarrhea is so severe that the child is hospitalized. If any foods seem to make the diarrhea worse, stop them for a day or two, then try again.

Do not force your child to eat; offer her solids if she's hungry and not vomiting.

If your child is hungry for solids, try yogurt (with active cultures) or rice. You can flavor them with cinnamon, ginger, or mint leaves.

2. *Biochemical—medications.* Pepto-Bismol—every four hours (see label for dosing information).

3. *Biochemical—herbs.* Try herbal remedies such as ginger tea or goldenseal tinctures.

4. *Bioenergetic—homeopathy.* Homeopathic remedies must be individualized to a child's particular symptoms; consult a homeopathic physician.

17

EAR INFECTIONS

Sheryl Wu brought in her three-year-old, Nathan, because she was concerned that he might have another ear infection. He had had a cold for a few days and was more fussy and clingy than usual. He had a fever when he was put to bed at 8 p.m. and awoke at midnight, crying and holding his right ear; he was restless and irritable most of the night. He seemed better in the morning, but he'd already had three ear infections this year. Sheryl was concerned that Nathan had another ear infection, and she was frustrated that the infections kept coming back. She wanted to know why he had so many ear infections, what she could do to prevent them, and the best ways to treat them. She didn't like the idea of giving him antibiotics all the time, but she didn't want Nathan to suffer and she didn't want to jeopardize his hearing.

The number of doctor visits for middle ear infections has steadily increased over the past decade. Ear infections now account for about 25% of all doctor visits for children under five years old. The cost of treating ear infections runs about $3.5 billion a year in the United States, not counting parents' time away from work or extra day care. By the time children are three years old, about two-thirds will have had at least one ear infection,[1] and one-third of children will have

had three or more ear infections.

What we usually think of as an ear infection is actually an infection of the *middle* ear (*otitis media*). This kind of infection occurs between the eardrum and the inner ear. A middle ear infection that comes on suddenly is called *acute otitis media*. In acute otitis media, the middle ear is filled with pus. After the acute infection is over, the bacteria are gone, but some fluid persists for several weeks or months. The chronic or persistent

Inside the Human Ear

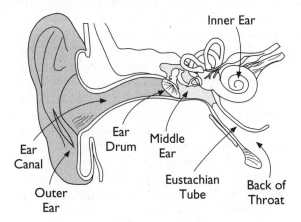

presence of fluid is called *chronic otitis media* or *serous otitis*. Colds and allergies can also cause middle ear fluid. Serous otitis is usually painless, but it can decrease hearing (which can lead to delayed speech development) and predispose a child to another bout of acute otitis media. When children suffer from repeated ear infections, it is called *recurrent otitis media*. Confusing, isn't it?

Children with acute otitis media experience a wide range of symptoms.[2]

Some children have *no symptoms* at all. These infections are usually discovered during a routine physical exam. Most children have *pain* in the infected ear, especially when they lie down. Lying down increases the blood flow to the head, resulting in more pressure in the infected ear. This is why children with ear infections are often most fussy at night. Sick children tend to be more *whiny, clingy,* or *withdrawn* regardless of why they are ill. They also tend to *behave as if they are younger than they are*; this is called *regression* and is a normal response to stress. For example, a sick child may start sucking his thumb even though he stopped sucking it six months previously. Ear infections usually are accompanied by *fever* and a *decreased appetite*. Older children may also report that they *cannot hear as well* in the infected ear or that it feels full or stuffy. If the

pressure in the middle ear builds too high, it *can rupture the eardrum*, allowing the pus to drain into the ear canal. If this happens, you might see bloody, waxy, or milky white drainage from the ear.

POSSIBLE SYMPTOMS OF MIDDLE EAR INFECTIONS

- None
- Pain in the ear, especially when the child lies down
- Pulling at ear
- Fever
- Irritability, whining, crying, sleeping less
- Clinging, withdrawn, wanting to be held
- Decreased activity, lethargy, sleeping more, decreased appetite
- Acting younger (regression)
- Decreased hearing
- Pus draining from ear
- Swollen lymph nodes in the neck

DIAGNOSIS

It is easier to diagnose an ear infection in a four-year-old who can tell you that his ear hurts than in a four-month-old who is simply feverish and irritable. Ear pain is a pretty reliable sign of an ear infection, but not always! Other causes of ear pain include sudden pressure changes (as when riding in a high-speed elevator or an airplane), headaches, infections in the sinuses, teeth, or throat, problems with the jaw joint (temperomandibular joint [TMJ]), and objects (such as crayons, pebbles, or beads) stuck in the ear. You can't depend on the color of the outer ear, because the infection is actually deep inside the ear canal behind the ear drum. The only way to be sure your child has an ear infection is to look at the eardrum.

DIAGNOSING EAR INFECTIONS

- Otoscopy
- Pneumatoscopy
- Tympanometry and acoustic reflectometry
- Tympanocentesis

A special device, an otoscope, is used to look into the ear canal and see the eardrum. Looking at the eardrum is called *otoscopy*. You can buy an otoscope to look yourself, but it is difficult to do without training and an unusually cooperative child. Medical students spend months and years learning to diagnose ear infections accurately. Exams can be tricky, especially when the child is squirming, there is wax in the canal, or the child is crying. When a child cries so hard that his face turns red, the eardrum usually turns red, too, and this redness can be mistaken for an infection. Redness doesn't predict the course of the illness.[3]

Health care professionals use several additional techniques to diagnosis ear infections. *Pneumatoscopy* is a fancy name for blowing air into the ear canal and sucking it out to see if the eardrum moves with mild air pressure. If there is pus or other fluid in the middle ear, the eardrum doesn't move very well. Accurate diagnosis depends on the combination of otoscopy and pneumatoscopy.

Before I did pneumatoscopy in Nathan's ears, I told him that I was looking for birds in his ear and that he might feel their wings softly tickling him. He sat still during the exam, absorbed in the idea of birds in his ears.

Fancier tests such as *tympanometry* and *acoustic reflectometry*, in which sound waves are bounced off the eardrum to see whether or not it moves, are also available to help confirm the diagnosis, but they aren't necessary for most children. If your child has had persistent fluid (chronic otitis) for three months or more, he should have a *hearing test* to determine whether or not the fluid is affecting his hearing. Children with persistent fluid and hearing loss may benefit from therapy with antibiotics or surgery.

The gold standard for diagnosing an ear infection is obtaining pus from behind the eardrum. This procedure, *tympanocentesis,* is done by sticking a small needle through the eardrum and withdrawing middle ear fluid into a syringe. It was routine in the preantibiotic era because it helped relieve the pressure in the middle ear by drawing off pus. Nowadays it is used in research studies but is almost never necessary for routine diagnosis. I recommend tympanocentesis only for:

- diagnosing ear infections in children less than one month old,
- children whose immune systems are weakened or suppressed,
- children whose infections have not responded to the usual antibiotics.

Blood tests are not useful in diagnosing ear infections or in distinguishing simple ear infections from other serious illnesses such as meningitis.

Ear infections are caused by the interaction of three factors.

WHAT CAUSES EAR INFECTIONS

- Blockage of the eustachian tube, which drains the middle ear
- Bacteria buildup
- The body's white blood cells' reaction to the bacteria

Under normal circumstances, the eustachian tube drains the middle ear into the back of the throat, equalizing pressure and draining bacteria and viruses out of the middle ear. Several things can block normal eustachian tube drainage.

EUSTACHIAN TUBE BLOCKERS

- Swelling (from an allergy or a cold)
- Swollen adenoids or tonsils
- An unfavorable position or weak muscles around the eustachian tube
- Bottle propping

When children have *colds or allergies*, their noses aren't the only thing that swells and feels stuffy. The lining of the eustachian tube also swells and may block drainage. Drainage from the eustachian tube can also be blocked by *swollen tonsils or adenoids* near its outlet at the back of the throat. The tonsils and adenoids are large lymph node–like tissues located near the eustachian tube opening. If they are larger than average or they swell up during an infection or allergy, they can obstruct eustachian tube drainage.

The eustachian tube is narrow in young infants and grows as the body grows. In infancy, the tube lies almost horizontally between the middle ear and the back of the throat, making it fairly easy for bacteria from the nose and throat to migrate to the ear. As children grow, the eustachian tube becomes longer and more vertical, and it is more difficult for bacteria to migrate from the back of the throat to the middle ear. This is why ear infections are much less common in older children and adults. Some children have less developed muscles around the eustachian tube, and it falls shut easily. Breast-fed babies have fewer ear infections than bottle-fed babies because breast-feeding takes a little more muscles than bottle feeding, and the eustachian tube muscles are better developed.

Propping a bottle with the baby on his back to feed him allows milk to flow back into the back of the throat, blocking the eustachian tube. Babies who are fed flat on their backs have more ear infections than infants who are held while they're fed.

The body patrols the middle ear with *immune molecules* called immunoglobulin A. It takes some experience with a form of bacteria to develop the specific kind of immunoglobin needed to manage those bacteria. As children grow older, their immune systems develop more experience and respond more quickly and efficiently.

When the eustachian tube is blocked, bacteria have no easy way out of the middle ear. They proceed to set up housekeeping, multiplying like mad. When the immune system gets wind of the situation, it rushes in to clean up the problem that should have been taken care of by an open eustachian tube. The *white blood cells* release chemicals to kill the bacteria, but these chemicals also cause swelling and irritation. With such a pitched battle going on in the tiny space of the middle ear, it's no wonder the child is in pain.

WHICH CHILDREN ARE MOST LIKELY TO GET EAR INFECTIONS?

There are two kinds of risk factors for ear infections: the kind you can do something about (modifiable) and the kind you can't do anything about (nonmodifiable).

RISK FACTORS FOR EAR INFECTIONS

NONMODIFIABLE	MODIFIABLE
Age less than two	Exposure to lots of kids
Boys more than girls	Formula feeding
Race: Caucasian, Indian, Eskimo	Feeding flat on back, or propping the bottle
Runs in families	Exposure to tobacco smoke
Season: winter and fall	No immunizations
	Pacifiers

Several *nonmodifiable factors* increase the risk of having ear infections. Because of the position of the eustachian tube and their inexperienced immune systems, younger children (under two years old) have more infections than older children. No one knows why, but boys are more likely than girls to have ear infections. Caucasian, Native American, and Eskimo children are at higher risk than are African-American or Hispanic children. Like many other characteristics, the tendency for ear infections runs in families. Ear infections are much more common during the cold and flu seasons of fall and winter.

There are also several *modifiable factors* that influence the risk of ear infections. Children who are exposed to *lots of other children* are much more likely to get ear infections than children who are spared exposure to other children's colds. Child care in large groups increases the risk of getting an ear infection by about 50% compared with keeping a child at home.[4] Nowadays it is almost impossible to avoid day care of some kind. However, if your child has been getting a lot of ear infections, you may want to look into a setting with fewer children.

Infants who are fed *formula* have more ear infections than infants who are breast-fed.[5] The risk of recurrent ear infections in a baby's first year is about 12% in infants exclusively breast-fed for the first four months of life compared with 20% among infants who are breast-fed for less than four months.[6] Breast-feeding helps protect your child because breast milk contains immune factors that help fight infections, and it spares your child exposure to potential allergens in formulas.[7] Breast milk is protective even for children at very high risk of ear infections, such as those with cleft palates.[8]

Infants who are fed while *flat on their back* are more likely to get ear infections early in life than children who are fed with their heads elevated. If you feed your child from a bottle, keep the child's head up to keep the milk from clogging the eustachian tube. Putting a child to bed at night with a bottle of milk in his mouth increases the risk of both ear infections and cavities.

Children whose *parents smoke* are far more likely to get ear infections and colds than children whose parents do not smoke.[9] *Do not smoke,* and do not allow other people to smoke around your child, especially in enclosed places such as cars.

Sheryl's mother-in-law lived with her family and was a smoker. Sheryl didn't like the fact that her children were around tobacco smoke, but she didn't feel that she could change her mother-in-law's behavior. I wrote a prescription for Nathan saying that he should not be around tobacco smoke because it increased his risk of getting ear infections, colds, and asthma. Sheryl gave this prescription to her husband, who gave it to his mother, who agreed to smoke only outside the house.

Pneumococcus bacteria are responsible for many childhood ear infections. *Immunization* with pneumococcal vaccine and daily treatment with the antibiotic sulfisoxazole (Gantrisin) results in a 90% reduction in ear infections in children with recurrent ear infections.[10] Currently the vaccine is only effective in children over two years old and is not routinely offered to all children. New vaccines on the horizon may work in younger children and provide protection against additional bacteria. If your child is over two and is still having frequent ear infections, ask your doctor about the pneumococcal vaccine.

Preliminary evidence implicates *pacifiers* as risk factors for recurrent ear infections.[11] Pacifiers may also cut down on breast-feeding. Although I used to think pacifiers were harmless, I now discourage their use. Help your baby learn to suck on his fist or fingers instead.

A note about recurrent ear infections: For children who get an ear infection within one month of a previous infection, don't blame yourself or your treatment. Most of the time (75%), recurrences are due to new bacteria altogether. They are usually due to problems in the environment, such as crowding or cigarette smoke, or problems in the child's anatomy or physiology, such as large adenoids or allergies.[12]

WHAT IS THE BEST WAY TO TREAT AN EAR INFECTION?

Even without any specific treatment, most children (70 to 80 percent) get over ear infections on their own. Then why treat? There are two main reasons: ear infections *hurt*, and they can sometimes lead to more serious problems ranging from ruptured eardrum to hearing loss to infections of the bones around the ear (mastoiditis).

About 30% of children under two years old with recurrent ear infections have some mild to moderate *hearing loss*. Hearing usually improves when the middle ear fluid finally dissipates.[13] It takes an average of one month for the fluid to clear out even with optimal treatment.[14] However, the period before two years of age is the time of major language development, and hearing loss during this period may put children behind in their language skills.

Several long-term studies have examined the impact of middle ear infections on children's language development. Doctors and psychologists in North Carolina followed a large group of children from birth until school age, checking them frequently for ear infections and monitoring their development.[15] There was *no* relationship between the number of ear infections in the first three years of life and subsequent scores on any of several IQ tests or academic achievement in kinder-

garten. There *was* an association between the number of days a child had fluid in the middle ear and subsequent teacher reports of decreased attention. Children with more ear infections tend to be less able to pay attention to their tasks and less able to work independently.[16] However, a *much* bigger factor in children's language development and school performance is parental responsiveness to the child and the creation of a stimulating home environment.[17]

If you suspect that your child has a middle ear infection, you may try home treatments for twelve to twenty-four hours before consulting a health care professional *unless*:

- your child is under twelve months old,
- the pain is severe,
- the fever is higher than 103°F,
- your child seems sicker than usual or you are concerned about his appearance or behavior.

In these cases, see your health care professional without delay. Let's tour the Therapeutic Mountain to find out what works best. If you want to skip to my bottom-line recommendations, flip to the end of the chapter.

BIOCHEMICAL THERAPIES: MEDICATIONS, HERBS, NUTRITIONAL SUPPLEMENTS

Medications

MEDICATIONS FOR EAR INFECTIONS

- Analgesics or pain medicines
- Antibiotics
- Steroids
- Antihistamines and decongestants

Pain is one of the worst symptoms for

most children suffering from ear infections. Even the most powerful antibiotics take twenty-four hours or so to improve symptoms; in the meantime, you'll want to help your child manage his pain. The most commonly used pain reliever is *acetaminophen* (the active ingredient in Tylenol, Panadol, and other nonaspirin pain relievers). Acetaminophen is an effective pain reliever and fever fighter; it is available without a prescription. It takes about forty-five minutes to start working; each dose lasts about four hours. It is very safe. Do *not* give your child aspirin. Aspirin suppresses the immune system, and it can precipitate a sometimes fatal illness called Reye's syndrome.

Anesthetic ear drops can also help reduce pain in the ear. The most commonly prescribed anesthetic ear drop is *Auralgan*. These medications do not help the ear infection go away any faster, but they can help your child feel more comfortable while he fights off the infection.

Since the dawn of the *antibiotic* era, the number of complications from ear infections has fallen dramatically. Before antibiotics, 20% of severe ear infections spread into the bones, requiring mastoidectomy (removal of the mastoid bone behind the ear). After the introduction of antibiotics, the mastoidectomy rate has dropped to less than 2%.[18]

Although this historical information is impressive, studies of the effectiveness of antibiotics have been conflicting. Some suggest that antibiotics are not helpful, but these studies were often done in older children who are less likely to have severe infections.[19] In the 1950s, antibiotics were shown to be significantly more effective than placebo in decreasing drainage from the ear,[20] resulting in fewer complications such as meningitis and mastoiditis.[21, 22] By the late 1960s, one study showed that 90 to 95 percent of children treated with antibiotics improved in one to two days, compared with 75% of those who received placebo medication.[23] A recent combined analysis of over 5,000 children with ear infections showed that the spontaneous cure rate (symptoms going away without any therapy) was 81% compared with a 92% cure rate with antibiotics. Overall, the commonly used antibiotics have similar effectiveness. That is, there is no advantage of the newer, more expensive antibiotics over plain old amoxicillin.[24] Nevertheless, the rapidly rising number of infections and parental demand have led to skyrocketing prescriptions for fancy, powerful, expensive antibiotics.[25]

The most commonly used antibiotic to treat ear infections is *amoxicillin*. Amoxicillin effectively treats most acute infections and prevents recurrent infections. It can cause upset stomach, diarrhea, allergic reactions, and diaper rashes (see Chapter 15). However, amoxicillin is still one of the safest antibiotics and is the first-line medication for children who are not allergic to it. Amoxicillin is usually prescribed to be given three times daily for ten days. However, with slightly higher doses, amoxicillin is just as effective when given twice daily.[26] Five days of treatment may be just as effective as ten days.[27] One study goes even further, suggesting that three days of antibiotic therapy may be sufficient.[28] I believe this study because I believe that most parents (even some of my medical colleagues) frequently give only three to five days of antibiotics when ten days are prescribed. Children generally recover well even though their parents don't give the whole course of therapy.

For children with allergies to amoxicillin, those whose infection does not improve with amoxicillin, or families without refrigerators (amoxicillin needs to be refrigerated), several effective alternative antibiotics are available. They include trimethoprim-sulfamethoxazole (Bactrim or Septra), clarithromycin (Biaxin), azithromycin (Zithromax), cefixime (Suprax), cefpodoxime (Vantin), cefuroxime (Ceftin), amoxicillin-clavulanate (Augmentin), erythro-mycin-sulfisoxazole (Pediazole), cefaclor (Ceclor), and others. If your child's infection does not respond to a particular antibiotic one time, he may respond to it well the next time. Don't give up on amoxicillin just because it didn't work one time. Side effects occur in 20 to 30 percent of children treated with antibiotics. If your child has a reaction to one antibiotic, remember that others are available.

For children who are vomiting or cannot take medicine by mouth for some other reason, a single shot of a new, powerful, and expensive antibiotic, *ceftriaxone*, is as effective as ten days of amoxicillin.[29] A single shot of ceftriaxone costs about four times as much as ten days worth of amoxicillin ($40 vs. $10). In emergency room surveys, parents favored the shot of ceftriaxone over the ten days of home antibiotics by four to one.

Unless your child has recurrent infections, please don't ask your doctor for a prescription for antibiotics to *prevent* ear infections. Antibiotics do *not* keep colds from turning into ear infections.[30]

Although many children get well regardless of whether or not they receive medication for their ear infections, the standard of medical care in the United States is to treat them (especially those less than two years old) with an antibiotic. This is not necessarily true in other parts of the world. In Switzerland, the Netherlands, and Britain, antibiotics are reserved for children who are not better in two to three days.[31, 32] In these countries, 92 to 96 percent of children suffering from ear infections reportedly recover within three days without antibiotic therapy.

I often recommend that parents give their child supplemental *acidophilus* or *yogurt* while they are taking antibiotics for ear infections. Antibiotics kill many of the body's normal bacteria (in addition to the bacteria causing the ear infection) and can lead to yeast

infections in the mouth (called *thrush*), the diaper area, and the vagina *(Candidiasis)*. The lactobacillus bacteria in acidophilus and yogurt help replace the body's normal bacteria and may prevent yeast infections. There are *no* studies specifically evaluating yogurt in preventing diaper rashes in children taking antibiotics, but it is harmless, and many parents report that it is helpful.

A bigger problem with the common use of antibiotics is the development of bacteria that are resistant to them. The same bacteria that cause ear infections also cause sinus infections, bronchitis, and pneumonia. As antibiotics are used more widely, the bacteria start to figure out how to work around them and eventually become totally resistant to the medication. In one suburban day care center, a strain of ear infection bacteria became resistant to four different antibiotics used in that community.[33] The development of resistance means that infections become harder and harder to treat, requiring ever newer and more powerful drugs to work.

Recurrent ear infections affect over 10% of young children. For children with recurrent infections, taking antibiotics daily is a very effective way to reduce the risk of future infections.[34] Prophylactic antibiotics cut the risk of recurrence by 40 to 80 percent,[35] but they only work as long as the antibiotic is taken. Once the child stops taking it, his risk of getting an ear infection returns to what it would have been had he never taken any. I recommend prophylactic antibiotics for children who have:

- one or more infections in the first six months of life,
- two or more infections in the first year of life,
- three or more infections in six months, regardless of age,
- four or more infections within twelve months, regardless of age.

The most commonly prescribed preventive antibiotics are amoxicillin or sulfisoxazole (Gantrisin), given once a day at bedtime.

Having had three ear infections already this year, Nathan now qualified for Gantrisin to prevent future ear infections.

When fluid stays in the middle ear for six weeks or more following an acute ear infection, it is called a *chronic* ear infection. Chronic ear infections impair hearing and predispose to repeated infections. In this situation, treatment with a combination of an antibiotic and prednisone (a steroid that decreases inflammation), followed by a second course of antibiotics may help clear up the middle ear.[36] While the antibiotic kills the bacteria, the steroid helps decrease eustachian tube swelling, thereby promoting middle ear drainage. Although steroids can have harmful effects when given over long periods of time, they have very few side effects when they are taken for less than a week.[37]

Steroid nasal sprays are more effective than placebo sprays in clearing middle ear fluid,[38] and they avoid the potential side effects of taking steroids by mouth because very little of the medicine is absorbed into the bloodstream. They reduce swelling in the adenoids and promote middle ear drainage. I recommend steroid nasal sprays for patients whose middle ear fluid has persisted for six to twelve weeks despite other treatments.

Antibiotic ear drops are *not* effective against middle ear infection, because they do not cross into the middle ear space (the eardrum is in their way). Ear drops containing neosporin and polymixin may actually damage the inner ear if they are given to a child with a punctured eardrum.[39] I do not recommend antibiotic ear drops for children unless the infection is in the ear canal (external otitis or swimmer's ear).

Antihistamines and *decongestants* (common cold medicines) are *not* effective treatments for children who have persistent fluid in their middle ear.[40] Antihistamines usually make children sleepy and dry their secretions. Paradoxically, some children react to antihistamines by becoming agitated. Decongestant nasal sprays do not reach the eustachian tube where they are needed to help drain the middle ear and are not helpful in treating ear infections.[41, 42] Decongestants taken by mouth raise blood pressure and make people feel wound up, tense, and less hungry. Many adults who take decongestants report feeling much better, but decongestants are like coffee. When you drink coffee, you may feel more awake and energetic, but you haven't really given your body any more energy. When the effect wears off, you feel exhausted and need to either rest or take more of the drug to feel better again. Obviously, this is not a cycle you want to start in a sick child. Overall, decongestants and antihistamines offer no advantage over antibiotics alone, and they demand a high price in terms of side effects.[43] I do *not* recommend them.

Herbs

Several herbal *teas* have been used for children with ear infections. These include echinacea, goldenseal, and licorice root. Other herbal teas or tinctures for children with ear infections include calendula, chamomile, elderflowers, goldenrod, ground ivy, hops, hyssop, lavender, lobelia, peppermint, passion flower, red clover, skullcap, Saint-John's-wort, and wintergreen. Chamomile, hops, and passion flower are recommended because of their powers to sedate. Herbs come in a variety of forms (dried, alcohol extracts, water extracts), and there is not much standardization in terms of dosage and frequency. Although many of these preparations have been used for many years as part of traditional herbal healing, there is *no* scientific evidence of their effectiveness in children with ear infections, and I do *not* recommend them.

Parents from many different parts of the world swear by *garlic oil ear drops* to treat their child's pain. To make garlic oil, soak four to five crushed cloves of garlic in 1/4 cup of olive oil overnight. Strain out the garlic bits. Gently warm the oil, and place one to two drops in the painful ear. Please do *not* put chunks of garlic in the ear. Garlic pieces can get stuck in the ear canal. If your child's ear hurts when you wiggle the outer ear or there is any discharge from the ear, do not place garlic oil or anything else in the ear canal without checking with a health care professional. Other herbal ear drops include mullein oil (mullein flowers, covered with olive oil overnight, then strained), Saint-John's-wort oil (Saint-John's-wort flowers, mixed with olive oil and strained), or tincture of plantain or witch hazel. Other home ear drop remedies include supersaturated solutions of sugar or epsom salts. To make a supersaturated solution, heat a cup of water and stir in sugar (or epsom salts) a teaspoon at a time until no more will dissolve. Gradually cool the solution until it is comfortable, and put a drop or two in the painful ear. If your child suffers *any* discomfort with any of these drops, flush the ear with warm water or hydrogen peroxide and discontinue their use. There are *no* studies evaluating the effectiveness of garlic or herbal ear drops.

Nutritional Supplements

Some practitioners recommend dietary supplements or foods containing high levels of vitamins A, B-complex, C, and E, zinc, and evening primrose oil to boost the immune system during an acute infection. These supplements are probably harmless, but there is *no* scientific evidence that they speed healing of ear infections.

LIFESTYLE THERAPIES: NUTRITION, EXERCISE, ENVIRONMENT, MIND-BODY

Nutrition

If your child has frequent middle ear infections, consider having him evaluated for allergies. *Food allergies* can cause swelling and inflammation of the eustachian tube and the nose. By omitting allergy-inducing foods from your child's diet, you may reduce the frequency of ear infections. Although there are many stories about children's ears dramatically improving when their parents stopped giving them milk, wheat, eggs, peanuts, soy, or other foods, there are *no* studies documenting how often such a dietary move is actually beneficial. Don't restrict your child's diet for more than a week without consulting a health care professional or he could end up with inadequate amounts of calcium, protein, or other essential nutrients.

Many parents reduce their child's intake of dairy products when he has an ear infection, because they believe that milk increases mucus production. Also, some parents restrict sugar, honey, and sources of concentrated fruit sugar when their child has an infection, based on the theory that sugar inhibits the immune system. *No* studies have documented that reducing milk or sugar during an ear infection speeds recovery.

Do make sure that your child gets plenty of *fluids*; your child will feel even worse if he gets dehydrated.

Exercise

Because one of the underlying causes of ear infections is blockage of the eustachian tube, exercises that help open the eustachian tube may be helpful. How do you exercise the eustachian tube? Think of the ways you pop your ears after a sudden change in altitude: yawning, bearing down, blowing your nose with the nostrils pinched shut, and chewing gum. Probably the easiest for children is chewing gum or blowing up balloons. Obviously it's not possible to have an infant chew gum, but most children over the age of about two and a half are delighted to practice this exercise. Sugarless gum is best. Beware: too much sugarless gum can cause diarrhea. Don't let your child go to bed with gum, or he could awaken in the morning with a gooey mess in his hair. Is there any scientific evidence as to whether chewing gum is effective? No, but it would sure be fun to find out!

Is *air travel* safe for children with ear infections? Yes. In a study of fourteen children with middle ear fluid who flew in commercial pressurized airplanes, none developed complications. Children who are on the verge of getting an ear infection or who have colds or allergies that intermittently block the eustachian tube may experience some pain, especially during landings. If your child has a cold and is prone to ear infections, let him suck on something or chew gum during takeoff and landing to help keep the eustachian tube open.

It's also helpful to prop the child's head up on a pillow to decrease pressure in the middle ear, especially when he goes to sleep. Propping the head up helps the eustachian tube drain the middle ear.[44]

Environment

Many people use *heat packs* or *ice packs* to treat the pain of ear infections. Ice packs take the heat out of inflamed tissue; heat packs increase circulation and theoretically remove toxins more quickly. I have patients who use each. Some parents apply an ice pack or a bag of frozen peas or corn to a child's ear when the child complains of ear pain. Other parents put a hot water bottle, heating pad, or warm washcloth on the painful ear while waiting for more definitive therapy. If your child doesn't respond to warm compresses, you can try ice packs, and vice versa. I don't know which of these is more effective (there are good reasons to believe in both) or if the main benefit is simply doing something for and spending time with the child. Please don't use heat packs or cold packs for more than twenty minutes at a time. Common sense precautions can prevent burns and frostbite.

Another time-honored technique is instilling *warm mineral oil* or *olive oil* in your child's ear (see section on Herbal remedies). Heat the oil as you would for a baby's bottle, and make sure it is not too hot before dropping it in your child's ear. The heat speeds circulation and comfort, but no scientific studies have evaluated its effectiveness.

Do *not* try to remove ear wax or anything else from your child's ear. Ear wax, bath water, and other things in the ear canal do not cause middle ear infections. If you see pus or any kind of drainage from your child's ear, the eardrum may have ruptured. If there is drainage from the ear, do not put *anything* in the ear until you have consulted a health care professional.

Mind-Body

Whenever a child is in pain, it is helpful to keep him calm. The best approach to keeping your child calm is to stay calm yourself. Visualize yourself as competent and able to care for and help your child; visualize your child as healthy and able to heal whatever is ailing him. Once you are in a calm frame of mind, you can distract your child from the pain by singing favorite songs, telling stories, playing quiet games, and reminding him of how much you love him.

Nathan was so distracted by the idea of having birds in his ear, he was eager for the previously dreaded ear exam!

BIOMECHANICAL THERAPIES: MASSAGE, SPINAL MANIPULATION, SURGERY

Massage

Many parents naturally massage the area affected by illness or injury. Gentle massage of the upper back, neck, and around the ears and back of the head with cocoa butter, camphorated oil, Tiger Balm, or Vicks Vaporub is soothing and relaxing. Some parents also gently massage the enlarged lymph glands in the neck. Massaging downward toward the chest may help drain the lymph glands that are swollen with white blood cells fighting the infection. Foot massage may also be relaxing and less uncomfortable if the child is very sensitive around the ears and neck. There are *no* studies evaluating the effectiveness of massage in treating children with ear infections, but I can't think of any contraindication to using massage and would love to see a study evaluating it.

Spinal Manipulation

Osteopaths claim that their treatment, particularly cranial manipulation, is effective in both preventing and treating ear infections. Osteopathic manipulation was one of the most frequent recommendations made by the American psychic Edgar Cayce for children suffering from recurrent ear infections. Although the idea of treating a fundamentally anatomic problem (eustachian tube drainage) with an anatomic therapy (spinal or cranial manipulation) is appealing, there have been *no* comparison studies evaluating the effectiveness of this kind of therapy.

Surgery

My grandfather practiced medicine in the days before antibiotics. He specialized in performing *myringotomies* on children with severe ear infections. A myringotomy involves taking a tiny scalpel and slicing a hole in the eardrum to drain the pus from the middle ear. Myringotomies help relieve the pain-causing pressure, but they can leave permanent holes or scars on the eardrum. Antibiotics are a better choice; nowadays myringotomies are rarely done—gone the way of the horse and buggy.[45]

Another one of the oldest treatments for ear infections is *tympanocentesis*, puncturing a hole in the eardrum with a needle and removing the pus. Unlike myringotomies, removing pus with a needle rarely leaves a hole in the eardrum or leads to scarring. However, as antibiotics have become more popular, fewer doctors have learned how to do tympanocentesis. It is mostly done nowadays by ear-nose-throat (or ENT) doctors, and it is rarely necessary.

Placement of *tympanostomy tubes* (ear tubes) has replaced tonsillectomy as the most common operation of childhood. A 1988 survey showed that 13 out of every 1,000 children under eighteen years of age had ear tubes.[46] This procedure involves placing a tiny plastic tube (called a grommet by the British) through the eardrum. The tube allows drainage from the middle ear to the ear canal, functioning like a backup eustachian tube. Tubes improve hearing among children who have persistent fluid (for six months or more) and hearing loss. We used to insist that children with ear tubes refrain from swimming or use ear plugs to prevent water from getting into the middle ear via the tube. Nowadays we know this is an unnecessary precaution. Two recent studies show that children with ear tubes can safely swim even without ear plugs.[47, 48]

Ear tubes only work until the tube becomes plugged up or comes out (usually within six to twelve months).[49] They also can scar the eardrum and cause other complications. Although some children experience a temporary benefit from ear tubes (while their eustachian tubes are developing to better drain the middle ear), ear tubes are overused in the United States. They are often placed before other treatments have been given a fair try.[50] Recurrent and persistent ear infections are frustrating, and ear tubes offer hope for quick relief from a chronic problem. Like many quick solutions to long-term problems, they are usually not the miracle that had been hoped for. Long-term problems usually require long-term solutions. If adequate alternative treatments have been tried for three to six months and the child has persistent middle ear fluid that interferes with hearing, families might consider surgery to prevent delayed language development. (The exception to this rule is the child who is almost certain to have frequent and severe ear infections, such as children with cleft palate. For these children, early placement of myringotomy tubes has proved helpful in maintaining hearing and developing speech.)

Because swollen adenoids can block the eustachian tubes, *adenoidectomy* (removal of the adenoid lymph tissue) is another surgical therapy for children with recurrent ear infections. Adenoidectomy done at the same time that ear tubes are placed is more effective than ear tubes alone in preventing recurrent infections.[51] This surgery should *not* be sought unless your child has had middle ear fluid for at least six months despite other therapies.

BIOENERGETIC THERAPIES: ACUPUNCTURE, THERAPEUTIC TOUCH, HOMEOPATHY

Acupuncture

Acupuncture has been recommended for treating ear infections, but there are *no* stud-

ies evaluating its effectiveness compared with antibiotics or other therapies for children with ear infections. I do *not* recommend it for this condition.

Therapeutic Touch

I use Therapeutic Touch to help me diagnose ear infections before I look in the ear. I also use Therapeutic Touch to treat children with ear infections along with other treatments. However, there are *no* studies specifically evaluating its effectiveness in treating children with ear infections.

Homeopathy

There are a variety of homeopathic remedies for children with ear infections depending on the exact symptoms. ABC is a homeopathic mixture containing minute amounts of Aconite, Belladonna, and Chamomilla; it covers all the major types of acute ear infections in children. Pulsatilla is used with almost any type of earache. There are *no* scientific studies evaluating the effectiveness of homeopathic remedies in treating ear infections. I do *not* recommend them.

If you decide to use homeopathy anyway, *if your child is not better after twenty-four hours of homeopathic treatment,* please have him examined by a health care professional. Also, if your child's earache is accompanied by a headache or stiff neck, do *not* try homeopathic remedies or any other home treatment. Go directly to a health care facility to make sure your child does not have meningitis or another serious infection that requires antibiotics.

WHAT I RECOMMEND FOR EAR INFECTIONS

PREVENTING EAR INFECTIONS

1. *Lifestyle—nutrition.* Breast-feed your infant for at least four to six months; do not feed your infant while he is lying flat on his back; do not put him to bed with a bottle of juice or milk.

2. *Lifestyle—environment.* Do not smoke, and do not allow others to smoke around your child; avoid exposure to wood smoke, other irritants, and allergens; if your child is in day care, avoid crowded settings (more than six children per room) especially during the fall and winter when cold viruses abound. Avoid using a pacifier.

3. *Biochemical—medications.* If your child is over two years old and has frequent ear infections, consider getting him immunized against pneumococcus.

Take Your Child for a Professional Evaluation If He

- Is less than twelve months old
- Has a temperature higher than 103°F
- Refuses to drink liquids
- Has severe ear pain for more than one day
- Seems sicker than usual or you are concerned about his appearance or behavior
- Has ear pain that has not improved within one or two days with home remedies

---

TREATING EAR INFECTIONS

1. *Biochemical—medications.* Consider pain medication such as acetaminophen; consider antibiotics for an acute infection; if your child has recurrent ear infections, consider a trial of three months of preventive antibiotics; after three months of persistent fluid in the middle ear, consider adding steroid nasal sprays.

2. *Biochemical—herbs or medications.* Try warm oil or garlic ear drops or anesthetic ear drops such as Auralgan.

3. *Lifestyle—mind-body.* Comfort or distract your child (rocking, holding, telling stories, etc.).

4. *Lifestyle—exercise.* Have your child exercise his eustachian tube by blowing up balloons, chewing gum, or sucking on something. Prop his head on a pillow when he goes to sleep to minimize the pressure buildup in his ear.

5. *Lifestyle—environment.* If your child has frequent colds and ear infections, have him evaluated and treated for allergies (see Chapter 4). Try putting a warm pack or an ice pack over his ear for ten minutes to reduce ear pain.

6. *Biomechanical—surgery.* If antibiotics, allergy treatments, and steroids haven't worked within six months, it's time to consider surgery.

18
ECZEMA

*Wendy Fowler brought in her ten-month-old, James, because of his recurrent
eczema. He had been seen in the clinic four months ago by another doctor
who recommended hydrocortisone cream. Although the rash initially
improved, it was back; James's itching was driving Wendy and her husband
crazy, and they were concerned that the rash on his chest was becoming
infected. James's father suffered from asthma and allergies, and James had
frequent ear infections. He was otherwise healthy. The eczema affected
about 8% of his total skin area. Wendy wondered:*

* *What caused eczema?*
* *What else could she do to rid James of this rash?*

Whether it's called eczema or atopic dermatitis, this rash is itchy and it keeps
coming back. Eczema is "the itch that
rashes." Anything that provokes itching and
scratching (such as an insect bite) can trigger
eczema. It starts out red, dry, and itchy. As it
gets worse, it contains little blisters that
break down into scabs, provoking more itching. Over time, the skin may become thickened and rough like tree bark, and the skin

color may get darker or lighter than in unaffected areas. When the rash is well managed,
the skin color improves slowly over several
months.

Eczema affects different areas of the skin
as children grow and develop. In young
infants, it usually appears on the cheeks. The
copious drooling brought on by teething often
irritates the skin around the mouth. During
toddler years, the rash tends to move to the

backs of the arms and legs. In older children and adults, the worst symptoms are on the inside of the elbows and the backs of the knees. High-top sneakers and other shoes that make the feet sweat can aggravate eczema on the feet. The backs of the hands can be real trouble spots for dishwashers and others who frequently have their hands in water.

Eczema is very common, and 85% of cases appear by five years of age. A 1994 British survey showed that about 20% of children suffered from eczema at some point.[1] People who have eczema are prone to symptoms for their whole lives, but they often improve during adolescence and early adulthood.

As if severely itchy, dry red skin wasn't enough, children with eczema frequently suffer from other problems. *Asthma* (Chapter 5) and *allergies* (Chapter 4) are much more common in eczema sufferers. Infants with eczema are also prone to getting *cradle cap* (Chapter 14). Children with eczema often put so much energy into healing their skin that there is not enough left over to grow well; thus, they may be *thin and short*. The *lymph nodes* in the neck, the armpits, and the groin can become quite *swollen* in children suffering from eczema. The neck lymph nodes swell when eczema affects the face; the armpit nodes swell when eczema affects the arms; and the groin nodes swell when eczema affects the legs. The lymph nodes usually go back to normal size when the rash improves. Probably because they are so miserable from itching, children with eczema also frequently suffer from *sleep problems*, *behavior problems,* and *difficult temperaments*. Children with eczema are also prone to developing *skin infections* and *warts*. Scratched and irritated skin is easily infected with viruses (such as Herpes) and bacteria (such as *Staphylococcus*). If your child's eczema suddenly takes a turn for the worse, especially if it becomes *painful*, take him to a health care professional to be evaluated for an infection.

It looked as if James had a typical case of hereditary eczema. He had scratched it vigorously, and a few spots were starting to look infected.

OTHER ILLNESSES THAT CAN BE MISTAKEN FOR ECZEMA

Many things besides eczema cause childhood rashes. For example, newborn *seborrhea* is frequently mistaken for eczema. Seborrhea is less itchy, and it usually appears before the infant is two months old, whereas eczema is very itchy and usually starts after three months of age. Like eczema, seborrhea tends to occur on the face and scalp, but unlike eczema, it often affects the diaper area as well. *Scabies* also causes a very itchy rash, which is very contagious; its treatment is very different from the treatment for eczema. *Skin allergies* and *contact dermatitis* also look like eczema. Children can have red, itchy skin from allergies to soap, detergent, fabric softeners, dryer sheets, and nickel jewelry. *Fungal infections* such as ringworm also look like eczema. *Rare immunological diseases* also have symptoms that look like eczema, but they have other, more serious symptoms as well. If you aren't sure what's causing your child's rash, consult your health care professional.

RISK FACTORS FOR ECZEMA

- Hereditary: sensitive immune system
- Environment: overbathing, drying soaps, allergies, irritants
- Diet: early feeding of solids, food allergies
- Mind-Body: stress

Like asthma and hay fever, eczema tends to *run in families*.[2] If one twin has eczema, chances are that the other twin has it, too. A particular configuration of chromosome 11 is associated with the sensitive immune system characteristic of eczema, asthma, and allergies. Eczema may be caused by a hereditary problem in transforming specific dietary fatty acids, such as linoleic and linolenic acids, to prostaglandin E_1.[3, 4] Prostaglandins work like local hormones, affecting the immune system and many other bodily processes. Abnormal immune function may account for the oversensitivity of children who suffer from eczema, asthma, and allergies.[5]

Paradoxically, one of the most common triggers of eczema is overzealous *bathing*. Water seems as if it should be moisturizing, but it actually dries the skin. Just as hot, soapy water helps remove grease from the dishes, it also removes the natural oils that protect the skin.[6] Soap is generally unnecessary for babies, because babies don't make the smelly sweat that older children and adults do. Babies probably don't need baths more than twice a week. Soap is only necessary for removing greasy dirt. *Soaps* and *detergents* trigger eczema in many children. In my experience, Tide detergent and Ivory soap are two of the most common culprits.

I advised Wendy to switch to Dove or another moisturizing soap if she felt she had to use soap. I also encouraged her to consider a milder laundry detergent without fragrances or softeners.

Other environmental triggers include *skin infections* (such as impetigo), *sweating*, *stress*, *irritants* (such as tobacco smoke and wool sweaters), and *allergies*. Allergies can be either from something that touches the child's skin or from something inhaled or eaten. Children who are allergic to animal fur, dust, and dust mites may have fewer eczema symptoms as well as fewer allergy symptoms when their environment is cleaned up.[7]

Early introduction of a variety of solid foods triples infants' risk of developing

severe eczema.[8] A healthy baby does not need any food other than mother's milk or formula in the first four months of life. Children can learn to like a variety of foods later in childhood; please do *not* start your baby on solids before he is four months old.

FOODS ASSOCIATED WITH ALLERGIC ECZEMA[9]

- Acidic foods, such as oranges, tomatoes, pineapple
- Proteins, such as eggs, nuts (especially peanuts), milk, soy, shellfish
- Wheat and corn
- Sweets, chocolate, soft drinks preserved with sulfur dioxide
- Artificial flavors,[10] possibly salt

Food allergies worsen symptoms in about 10 to 20 percent of children with eczema.[11] The foods that trigger eczema are the same as those that trigger other allergic symptoms such as wheezing, runny nose, sneezing, and an upset stomach.[12,13] Nursing babies whose mothers abstain from allergenic foods may have a lower subsequent risk of eczema than those whose mothers eat these foods. *Acidic foods* such as citrus and tomatoes commonly cause a rash around the mouth in sensitive children. There are a couple of case reports of reduced eczema symptoms in children who were switched to low-salt diets, but there have not been any controlled trials documenting salt's detrimental effect on eczema.[14]

Unfortunately, skin tests and blood tests are not very helpful in diagnosing food allergies. Keep a diary to record your child's symptoms and any foods that seem to make them worse. If the child's previous reactions have been mild, parents can withhold a suspected food for several days, then give it and watch for symptoms. The problem with this approach is that the parents and child know that the child is getting the suspected trigger, and negative expectations are themselves powerful triggers of adverse effects.

It is very difficult for families to test and treat their child for food allergies without professional assistance. A strong placebo effect comes into play whenever a challenging, costly treatment is recommended; this certainly applies to elimination diets in which all potentially allergic foods are avoided. It is imperative that such an effort be undertaken only under rigorous, placebo-controlled conditions.

The best test is a double-blind food challenge. In a double-blind challenge, the child avoids eating any of the suspected allergic food for a week before the test. The health care practitioner gives the child one of two different capsules—one contains the suspected allergen and the other contains an inert placebo. Neither the professional, the parents, nor the child know the contents of the capsule. Parents and professional watch the child for several hours (up to two days) to see if symptoms develop. If a child has had a previous severe reaction (including wheezing, shortness of breath, shock, or low blood pressure) to a particular food, the double-blind food challenge should only be done in a facility capable of managing pediatric emergencies. Even children who have proven severe food allergies often outgrow them within a year or two. No one knows exactly why, but you don't have to worry that a current sensitivity (or even a severe allergy) means a lifetime of restrictive diets.

How to Treat Eczema

Let's tour the Therapeutic Mountain to find out what works. If you want to skip to my bottom-line recommendations on eczema, flip to the end of the chapter.

Biochemical Therapies: Medications, Herbs, Nutritional Supplements

Medications

MEDICATIONS FOR ECZEMA

- Emollients or moisturizers
- Urea and coal tar
- Steroid creams, ointments, or pills
- Antihistamines to relieve the itch
- Antibiotics to fight infections complicating the rash
- Other

The mainstay of medical treatment is to apply *emollients* or *moisturizers* to the skin several times daily. Avoid products that contain alcohol, because alcohol can dry the skin. Effective, inexpensive emollients include Eucerin ointment, Vaseline petroleum jelly, and even plain vegetable oils. Ointments generally work better than creams or lotions because they don't wash off as easily. Hand creams containing urea are also very effective.[15] As awful as they sound, coal tar creams, such as Clinitar, are also very effective in treating chronic eczema when the skin has become thick and rough like tree bark[16]; newer formulations don't smell as bad as older preparations.

The second medical therapy for eczema is *steroid cream or ointment*. Steroid preparations come in many varieties and strengths. The mildest, 0.5% and 1.0% hydrocortisone cream, are available without a prescription. Most physicians recommend applying steroid ointments after a bath when the skin is warm and the pores are open to absorb the medicine. After applying the steroid, cover it with an emollient to seal it in. Stronger, prescription steroids can cause side effects such as weakening and thinning of the skin and even high blood pressure.[17] They should be used only under professional supervision and only as long as necessary to treat severe symptoms. When symptoms are under control, return to milder preparations. Your health care professional will help you determine the best regimen for your child.

Steroids often improve symptoms dramatically, but they do not "cure" eczema. When treatment stops, symptoms recur. On the other hand, there is *no* evidence that treating eczema with steroid creams (or any other treatment) "drives" the problem deeper into the body or that eczema treatment "causes" asthma or other problems.

Antihistamines, such as Benadryl (a non-prescription brand of diphenhydramine), reduce itching and scratching.[18] Your doctor can prescribe stronger antihistamines to help your child sleep when the itching is particularly fierce.[19] Daytime antihistamine use is for those children who can't stop itching and who are willing to be a little sleepy. *Note*: A few children have just the opposite reaction to antihistamines; they get hyper. Kids who react one way to one of these medicines won't necessarily react the same way to all of them. If you don't like the side effects with one antihistamine, be reassured that there are several other options. Although antihistamines don't cure the underlying cause of eczema, they can help interrupt the itch-scratch-itch-scratch cycle and help improve symptoms.

Prescription *antibiotics* are useful for treating the skin infections that frequently complicate eczema. Usually a five- to ten-day course of an oral antibiotic that kills staph bacteria is sufficient to get the infection under control. Antibiotic ointments are useful if the infected area is small; they cause fewer side effects than antibiotics that are taken by mouth.[20] Occasionally, eczema is complicated by yeast or a fungal infection. In this situation, the combination of a steroid and an antiyeast antifungal medication may be helpful.[21]

When they can't find anything else to put on eczema, some parents have resorted to *Calamine* lotion. Though it may provide temporary relief, Calamine's drying effect makes it a poor choice for long-term use.

Herbs

Two randomized, controlled trials of Chinese herbal tea showed a significant improvement in children's eczema symptoms.[22, 23] Traditional Chinese medical herbal teas contain ten or more ingredients, and the potency of different ingredients can vary as much as fivefold between different batches; it is not clear which of the herbs is responsible for the beneficial effect. There are several reports of patients who developed liver toxicity while taking Chinese herbal remedies for eczema; the liver toxicity markedly improved once patients stopped taking the tea but returned when the tea was resumed.[24, 25] Many of these teas taste bad, and children cannot easily be persuaded to drink them. Still, if your child has severe eczema that is not responding to simple treatments, consider consulting an herbalist who is trained in traditional Chinese medicine *and* having your child's liver function tested periodically to avoid harmful side effects.

Licorice root's active ingredient, glycyrrhetinic acid, has anti-inflammatory properties similar to those of steroids.[26] Several case reports in the 1950s British dermatology literature claimed benefits from ointments containing glycyrrhetinic acid.[27, 28] Unfortunately, other studies failed to reproduce these promising results, possibly because of the natural variation in the potency of licorice extracts.[29] Consequently, licorice root never caught on as an eczema remedy.

Other herbs recommended for treatment of eczema are aloe vera, calendula, chamomile, lemon balm, coleus root (recommended for asthma and allergies as well), gotu kola, and Saint-John's-wort oil (used for skin wounds and infections), yellow dock root, Oregon grape, and echinacea. Old-fashioned blood-purifying teas thought to be helpful in treating eczema are sarsaparilla root and dandelion green. Sage, nettle, and burdock tea added to the bath are said to be helpful for weepy, blistery eczema. Poultices made from plantain, strawberry leaves, goldenseal, and violet are traditional cures for eczema. Whatever the cause of the itch, oatmeal compresses or oatmeal baths are soothing. Despite years of anecdotal experience, all of these herbs remain *unproved* scientifically as treatments for childhood eczema.

Beware of tea tree oil, *Melaleuca alternifolia.* Although it is a proved antiseptic, it can actually *cause* allergic, eczema-like rashes.[30]

Nutritional Supplements

HELPFUL SUPPLEMENTS FOR ECZEMA

- Essential fatty acids: evening primrose oil
- Vitamin C

Because of the presumed defect in metabolizing *essential fatty acids* in children with eczema, supplemental essential fatty acids may be helpful.[31] Evening primrose oil (EPO Efamol) contains high amounts of one of these essential fatty acids, gamma linolenic acid. A randomized, controlled crossover trial in Italian children showed a significant improvement in eczema symptoms when the children received 3 grams daily of EPO compared with children who received placebo olive oil.[32] A 1989 study summarized nine controlled trials and concluded that EPO improves eczema symptoms.[33] Recent studies have both refuted and confirmed these results.[34, 35, 36] EPO is very safe.[37] You might

want to try EPO supplements if your child has severe, recurrent eczema. Be persistent. It takes four to twelve weeks for EPO to achieve maximal benefits.

Other sources of essential fatty acids can be found in both the plant and animal kingdoms. Blackcurrant oil and borage oil also contain the essential fatty acids found in evening primrose oil. Herring, mackerel, and salmon contain other essential fatty acids, which offer intriguing possibilities for eczema treatment.[38] Still, there are not enough studies to recommend their routine use.

In a recent double-blind, placebo-controlled crossover trial, supplemental *vitamin C* (50 to 75 milligrams per day—or the amount in one tall glass of orange juice) significantly improved eczema in children.[39] At these doses, it is safe and may be worth a try.

I suggested that Wendy start giving James evening primrose oil and 100 milligrams of vitamin C mixed in applesauce.

Despite initially hopeful case reports, subsequent studies have shown that vitamin E and selenium are *not* helpful for most people with eczema.[40] Vitamin A supplements have also been shown *not* to be helpful.[41] Zinc supplementation was *not* helpful for children with eczema in a British randomized, controlled double-blind trial.[42] If anything, the children taking extra zinc had a little worse itching. I do not recommend vitamin A, vitamin E, or zinc supplements for children with eczema.

LIFESTYLE THERAPIES: NUTRITION, EXERCISE, ENVIRONMENT, MIND-BODY

Nutrition

Altogether food allergies trigger symptoms in about 20% of children who have eczema. Allergies to milk protein are among the most common, but they trigger symptoms in fewer than 10% of children with eczema.

Still, some food-sensitive children notice big improvements if they totally eliminate food triggers.[43, 44] (See Chapter 4, Allergies.) Complete elimination of all possible food allergies (as in hospital programs relying on artificial food substitutes) can result in marked improvements in skin symptoms.[45]

Of course, eliminating dietary staples runs the risk of starvation, or at least severe nutritional imbalance.[46] Up to 75% of children on cow's milk elimination diets receive insufficient calcium.[47] Despite the occasionally impressive short-term benefits of elimination diets, ongoing studies have shown that a year after starting them, even children who initially improved with the diet were no better off than children who maintained their usual diet.[48] The emotional and financial costs to the family of a child following a strict elimination diet are high. Even highly motivated families of children who have well-defined food allergies frequently find it impossible to maintain elimination diets.[49] Only try the food elimination diets if your child has severe, extensive (more than 20% of the skin affected) eczema that is not controlled by other regimens *and* you seek the help of a nutritionist or dietitian.

Many children outgrow their sensitivity to foods. Even if your child's eczema is clearly worse with a certain food, it doesn't mean she can never have it again. You may carefully reintroduce it in six to twelve months. If there is still a reaction, wait another few months and try again.

We decided not to pursue possible food allergies at our initial visit and to wait to see how well James responded to other therapies.

Environment

In general, heat makes all itching worse. Sweating washes the protective, lubricating natural oils off the skin. Cold relieves itch. I advise many of my patients with a small itchy area to rub an ice cube on it. Avoid overdressing your child, and avoid giving him baths in very hot water.

Make sure your child's fingernails are cut short and kept clean to reduce the risk of infection from constant scratching. You may want to put a pair of gloves or socks over your child's hands at night to keep him from scratching himself in his sleep.

Too much bathing dries the skin and makes eczema worse.

BATH-TIME HINTS FOR CHILDREN WITH ECZEMA

- Give your child fewer baths.
- Use tepid (not hot) water.
- Avoid vigorous scrubbing and rough loofah sponges.
- Avoid soaps or use only moisturizing types such as Dove.
- Soap only the armpits, groin, feet, diaper area, and greasy, dirty areas.
- Put a tablespoon of vegetable oil in the bathwater to soothe the skin; *or* put 2 cups of oatmeal in an old stocking or pillowcase, tie the end in a knot, and throw it in the bathwater for a soothing soak; *or* add a cupful of baking soda to the bathwater.
- After the bath, pat, rather than rub, the skin dry.
- Apply an emollient, such as Eucerin or Vaseline, immediately after bathing.

Avoid bubble baths because they can dry the skin and may cause an allergic reaction.

Many children with eczema have worse symptoms in the winter, when indoor air is dry. You might keep a *humidifier* going in the child's bedroom to add moisture to the air.

A recent study showed that some children with eczema had markedly improved symptoms when careful attention was paid to cleaning their environment.[50] The culprit here isn't dirt itself, but a microscopic critter called the *dust mite*. This bug also aggravates asthma and allergies in sensitive children (see Chapters 4 and 5).

Avoid using detergents, soaps, fabric softeners, and dryer sheets that contain *perfume*. Nearly 4% of eczema patients are allergic to perfumes.[51] Interestingly, those who react to the perfumes in dishwashing detergent seem to be most sensitive when the dishwater is very hot; washing in more tepid water causes less of an allergic reaction.[52]

Sunlight, especially the ultraviolet end of the spectrum, has been reported to help reduce eczema symptoms. Although sunlight therapy has been used for years, there are *no* comparison trials assessing its effectiveness. Sweating can definitely aggravate eczema, and excessive sunlight increases the risk of developing skin cancer later on. Definitely avoid the most intense rays between 10 a.m. and 2 p.m.; use a sunscreen.

The most effective environmental therapies involve a *combination* of all the above *plus* avoiding smoking around your child *plus* the Nutrition and Biochemical therapies described above.[53]

Wendy decided to decrease James's bathing from daily to twice a week, stop using soap, and use a milder detergent. She decided to add a cup of oatmeal to James's bathwater and to apply Eucerin and steroid cream immediately after the bath. She also went on a cleanup campaign to destroy dust-mite strongholds in James's room.

Mind-Body

Hypnosis can effectively alter skin sensations such as itch and pain. Hypnosis has proven very effective in reducing pain in adults with eczema.[54] Any treatment that reduces itching could be useful for children with eczema. Hypnosis may also help children learn to manage the stressors that make their symptoms worse. (See Appendix A for additional resources for hypnotherapy.)

Biofeedback aimed at relaxation and hand warming has also proved effective in a study of five patients with severe eczema.[55] Any other mind-body technique such as visualization or deep breathing that helps children relax and manage stress is also helpful. Such techniques may eventually be shown to affect the oversensitive immune system itself—the source of eczema symptoms.

BIOMECHANICAL THERAPIES: MASSAGE

Massage is a natural way to apply emollients and other skin treatments for eczema. Vegetable oil, evening primrose oil, jojoba oil, and even plain old Vaseline and Eucerin have all been recommended as excellent emollients. Some herbalists recommend adding a drop or two of chamomile or yarrow oil to 1 teaspoon of vegetable oil to enhance its healing effects. There are *no* studies showing that massage itself actually heals eczema.

BIOENERGETIC THERAPIES: ACUPUNCTURE, THERAPEUTIC TOUCH, HOMEOPATHY

Acupuncture

Although one case report indicated that transcutaneous electrical nerve stimulation (TENS) was helpful in treating an adult with eczema,[56] there are no scientific trials evaluating acupuncture's effectiveness in treating childhood eczema. I do *not* recommend it.

Therapeutic Touch

Therapeutic Touch has been shown to reduce pain, to improve wound healing, and to be calming. I use Therapeutic Touch when I see patients with eczema in the office, although it remains scientifically untested as a specific eczema remedy.

Homeopathy

The most commonly recommended homeopathic remedies for eczema are *Carcinosin,* *Housedust, Medorrhinum, Oleander, Pulsatilla, Sulfur,* and *Tub bov.* Homeopathy was reportedly helpful in a series of ninety children treated with these and other remedies.[57] Unfortunately, there was no comparison group of children who did not receive homeopathic remedies. This makes it impossible to tell if symptoms improved because of patients' expectations, by chance, or as the natural course of the illness over time. Although homeopathic remedies may be safe, they remain unproved until better studies are performed. I do *not* recommend them.

WHAT I RECOMMEND FOR ECZEMA

PREVENTING ECZEMA

1. *Lifestyle—nutrition.* Do *not* introduce any solids in the first four months of life; after four months, introduce no more than one new food per week.

2. *Lifestyle—environment.* Do not smoke, and do not allow others to smoke around your child. Minimize your child's exposure to allergens such as dust, dust mites, furry pets, and pollens. Do not use drying soaps on your baby or bathe him too frequently. Use tepid water in her baths.

Take Your Child to a Health Care Professional If

- You are concerned that the rash could be caused by something else
- The eczema takes a turn for the worse, becomes painful, or looks infected
- There is no improvement after four weeks of home therapy

TREATING ECZEMA

1. *Lifestyle—environment.* Bathe your child less often. Avoid drying or perfumed soaps. If you do use soap, try a moisturizing type. Avoid strong, scented detergents. Make sure that all clothing has been rinsed well to remove soap residues before drying. Try putting 2 cups of dry oatmeal in an old stocking and drop it in your child's bathwater. Let your youngster "scratch" with an ice cube.

2. *Biochemical—medications.* Use Eucerin, Vaseline, or vegetable oil as a moisturizer or emollient after baths and before bed. Avoid "moisturizers" that contain alcohol. Talk with your health care provider about treatment with a steroid ointment. Follow recommendations exactly. Consider using an antihistamine at night to reduce nighttime scratching. If the rash looks infected, try an antibiotic ointment or see your doctor.

3. *Biochemical—nutritional supplements.* Supplement your child's diet with at least 50 to 75 milligrams per day of vitamin C. Consider supplementation with 3 grams daily of evening primrose oil.

4. *Biochemical—herbs.* Consider consulting a practitioner of Traditional Chinese Medicine to discuss herbal tea.

5. *Lifestyle—mind-body.* Consider taking your child for hypnotherapy or biofeedback to help him learn to desensitize his skin and to learn to deal with stressful triggers.

6. *Lifestyle—nutrition.* If your child has severe, extensive eczema, talk with a nutritionist about trying an elimination diet.

19

FEVER

Greg Edgecomb called me one Sunday evening because his three-week-old daughter, Nicole, had developed a fever of 102°F (39°C) and was not interested in breast-feeding. She was also sleepier than usual. I asked Greg to bring Nicole to the emergency room, so we could make sure she did not have a serious infection.

Sarah Klein called before work to ask if she should bring in Jacob, her two-year-old son, for an evaluation of his fever of 103°F (39.4°C). Jacob had had a cold for several days but had been drinking, playing, and sleeping normally until this morning when he awoke with a fever and rapid breathing. Sarah had given Tylenol and sponged Jacob, but his temperature was still 101°F (38.4°C). Sarah was concerned that Jacob might have pneumonia, and I agreed to see him as the first patient that day. On the way into the clinic, Jacob had a seizure. Sarah wanted to know if a seizure could be caused by a fever alone or if it meant that Jacob had meningitis.

Frank LittleBear brought in his eighteen-month-old, Tara, for a checkup and immunizations. The nurse noticed that Tara felt warm and checked her temperature: 101.5°F (38.7°C). Frank said that Tara had a cold but had been behaving completely normally. He wondered if Tara could still get her scheduled immunizations or if they would have to make another visit.

Although they are frightening for many parents, fevers are a natural defense against infections. Even cold-blooded animals such as fish and reptiles seek warmer surroundings to boost their temperatures when they are fighting infections. Those that are allowed to raise their temperatures have higher survival rates than those that are kept cool.[1]

Fevers are a leading cause of children's doctor visits. Winter is the peak fever season. Fever is not a disease itself, but it is a symptom of many common childhood illnesses. Most children who have fevers can be safely managed at home. Knowing a few basic facts about fevers may save you a trip to the doctor's office.[2]

WHAT IS A FEVER?

Temperatures normally vary up to one full degree over the course of a day, with lower readings in the morning and higher ones in the afternoon. Children tend to run slightly higher temperatures than adults. Normal temperatures range from 97.1°F (36.2°C) to 99.5°F (37.5°C) when measured in the mouth or ear. Temperatures vary depending on where they are measured. Rectal measurements are generally higher than oral, underarm, or ear measurements.

TEMPERATURES CONSIDERED FEVERS

- *In the mouth or the ear*: above 99.5°F(37.5°C)
- *Under the arm (axillary)*: above 98.6°F(37°C)
- *Rectally*: above 100.4°F (38°C)

- *Low-grade fevers*: less than 102°F (38.9°C), measured rectally
- *Moderate-grade fevers*: between 102°F (38.9°C) and 104°F (40°C), rectally
- *High fevers*: greater than 104°F (40°C) measured rectally

Even among children with temperatures higher than 105°F (40.5°C), only about one-third have a serious bacterial illness. It is not until temperatures exceed 106°F (41C) that the majority of children have a serious illness such as pneumonia.[3] Infections rarely cause a fever of 106°F and *never* cause a fever over 107°F. Only heatstrokes or rare medical conditions cause temperatures higher than 107°F.

WHAT CAUSES FEVER?

Infections such as colds, flu, ear infections, and sore throats are the most common causes of fever. Rheumatoid arthritis and cancer are uncommon childhood illnesses, but they can cause fevers. Teething does not raise the temperature above 101°F (38.4C).[4] Overbundling can cause fevers in babies. The temperature in a closed car in summer sunshine can easily exceed 110°F (43.2°C) and cause heat illness in a child left inside while the parent makes a "quick stop" at the store.

Our temperature is normally controlled by a "thermostat" in the hypothalamus, a small area in the middle of the brain close to the pituitary gland. When a child has an infection, the white blood cells fighting the infection send chemical messengers called interleukins to the hypothalamus. The thermostat, normally set at 98.6°F (37°C), is raised to help the white blood cells fight the infection.[5] The hypothalamus sends orders to the rest of the body to raise the temperature. The body responds by seeking a warm room, putting on more clothes, and shivering. When the new set-point is reached, the child relaxes and stops shivering. When the set-point returns to normal, new orders go out; the body reduces the temperature by sweating, throwing off covers, and drinking cool water.

This explains the "chills and fever" when a fever builds and the sweating when a fever "breaks." When our body temperature is lower than the brain's thermostat, we feel chilled and try to warm up. Shivering is one of the most effective ways to warm up quickly. This is what happens when someone has the "shaking chills." When the set-point returns to normal and our temperature remains high, we feel hot and start to sweat. Sweating is a sign that the set-point has been lowered and the fever has broken.

When a child is overbundled, the temperature may rise even though the thermostat remains set at 98.6°F (37°C).[6] Babies can't easily remove their own clothes, move to a cooler place, or sweat enough to cool off, so they can get overheated and have a higher temperature just from being overdressed or in a hot environment.

Fever raises the heart rate and breathing rate and increases the loss of fluids.[7] Blood levels of zinc and iron fall, while copper levels rise. Levels of the stress hormone cortisol double.[8]

DO FEVERS CAUSE BRAIN DAMAGE?

There is *no* risk of brain damage unless the temperature rises above 107°F (41.7°C) and stays there. Fevers even from serious illnesses such as pneumonia and kidney infections do not cause temperatures high enough to cause brain damage. The only thing that causes that kind of temperature is *heatstroke*. Heatstroke occurs when someone is overexercised or overdressed in a hot environment and cannot cool off. During heatstroke, the internal thermostat remains set at 98.6°F (37°C), but the body can't dissipate the heat from exercise and the environment. Eventually it gives up.

I saw heatstroke knock down a North Carolina teenager who was playing basketball indoors in August and who didn't stop to rest or get a drink of water until he passed out with a temperature of 107.6°F (42°C). He was fine once we got some fluids into him and cooled him off.

Many parents worry that fevers less than 102°F can cause brain damage.[9] This fear has created an epidemic of overtreatment even when the child has a low-grade fever, which may be helping him fight an infection.[10] Many physicians and pharmacists have perpetuated fever phobia by fixating on the child's temperature when inquiring about symptoms.[11] Fever phobia contributes to a lot of unnecessary medication for children with low-grade fevers.[12, 13]

DO FEVERS CAUSE SEIZURES?

Sometimes. Between the ages of three months and five years, about 3 to 5 percent of children have seizures when they have a fever. This is *not* the same as epilepsy. Seizures triggered by fevers last less than 15 minutes and typically involve jerking movements of the whole body, not just one side or one part.

Sarah's son, Jacob, fit this picture.

Seizures triggered by fevers run in families, are more common in children who have seizures even when they don't have fevers, and are more common among children who attend day-care.[14] Why are they more common in day care attendees? Probably because children in day-care get more infections and more fevers. In children who are otherwise healthy and developing normally, a typical fever-triggered seizure does *not* damage IQ or cause later school problems or epilepsy.[15]

Seizures look very scary. Most parents who see their child have a seizure are afraid the child is going to die, even though the typical seizure stops within a few minutes and does not cause any long-term harm.[16] If your child has a seizure with a fever, remain calm, check your watch to see how long the seizure actually lasts (even though it seems like hours, it probably will be less than five minutes), make sure he is lying on his side on the floor or bed in a safe place away from sharp objects. Do not try to put anything in his mouth. Old-fashioned beliefs that seizures make people swallow their tongues are just plain wrong. If the seizure lasts longer than four minutes, call 911 or take him immediately to the nearest emergency room. If it lasts less than four minutes, take him to your regular health care provider or the emergency room.

When I examined Jacob fifteen minutes after his seizure, he was sleepy and had pneumonia. Sarah was scared by the seizure, which had lasted about two and a half minutes. She said she finally understood what her mother had gone through when Sarah had fever-triggered seizures as a child. We treated Jacob with an injection of antibiotics for his pneumonia. He was better by the next day. As with most children who suffer a fever-triggered seizure, Jacob has never had another one. Note: Giving your child Tylenol at the first sign of illness will not necessarily prevent seizures.[17]

Fevers are uncommon in children under three months old. It's hard to tell just by looking at them whether or not young babies are ill; special blood tests, urine tests, spinal taps, and X rays are needed. If your child is under three months old and gets a fever, have her evaluated by a health care professional. Do *not* try to treat a fever in an infant yourself without having her professionally evaluated. Feverish children under one month of age may need to be hospitalized while the cause of the fever is being sorted out.[18]

Nicole's tests showed that she had a kidney infection. She was hospitalized and received antibiotics by vein. Later tests showed that the infection had been caught in time and there was no permanent kidney damage. Her parents were relieved that their quick response to Nicole's fever spared her problems she might have developed if they had delayed care.

Fevers can be signs of serious illness.

SEEK PROFESSIONAL HELP FOR FEVER IF THE CHILD

- Is less than three months old
- Is lethargic, refuses to drink fluids, is not interested in play
- Has a seizure, stiff neck, limb or abdominal pain
- Has trouble breathing or swallowing her own saliva
- Has pain when she urinates, is vomiting or not keeping down liquids
- Looks sicker than you'd expect from a viral illness

DO FEVERS DO ANY GOOD?

Yes. Fevers kill many germs. *Strep pneumonia*, the bacteria responsible for many ear infections and pneumonia, is killed at temperatures over 104°F. In the preantibiotic era, practitioners often *caused* fevers in patients (e.g.,with steam baths) to cure disease. I do *not* recommend that you give your child a fever on purpose, but you don't need to worry about the fever either. Instead, try to figure out why your child's body may be creating one. Treat the child, *not* the thermometer.

CAN CHILDREN WITH FEVERS RECEIVE THEIR REGULAR IMMUNIZATIONS?

Yes. Children with fevers and minor illnesses such as colds and ear infections can receive immunizations safely.[19]

Frank's daughter, Tara, could receive her scheduled immunizations even though she had a fever.

WHAT'S THE BEST WAY TO TAKE A CHILD'S TEMPERATURE?

The new *digital thermometers* work quickly (in less than thirty seconds) and are accurate and easy to read. Check *Consumer Reports* for the best values. Many doctors' offices now use electronic thermometers that measure the temperature in the ear. Even if your child has an ear infection, the reading in that ear will be less than half a degree higher than the child's real (core) temperature. Ear wax doesn't affect the accuracy of temperatures measured by ear thermometers.[20] *Glass thermometers* can be difficult to read and take several minutes to reach core temperature.

The new temperature *strips* and *temperature-sensitive pacifiers* are easy to use, but they tend to underestimate the true temperature. I do *not* recommend them. Our hands are also not very accurate in judging fevers. Most parents and health care professionals tend to overestimate a child's temperature when feeling the forehead.[21,22] However, I still feel foreheads on my patients because I often get a sense of the child by touching him and most children feel soothed when someone who cares about them strokes their forehead.

Measuring the temperature *under the armpit* is the safest and easiest for most parents. The temperature under the armpit usually is a little lower than the temperature inside the body. Electronic thermometers are not accurate for measuring armpit temperatures. You must use a glass mercury thermometer and hold it in place for several minutes to obtain an accurate reading. Do *not* leave your child alone with the thermometer under the arm. It can slide out, resulting in an inaccurately low reading.

Temperatures measured *rectally* are the most accurate, especially in children under five years old, but taking a rectal temperature can be tricky. Please ask your health care provider to show you how. Be sure to clean the thermometer carefully with rubbing alcohol and wash it in cool water before and after measuring a rectal temperature. Use a lubricant such as petroleum jelly on the thermometer before trying to insert it. The tip of the thermometer should be about 1 inch inside the rectum for the most accurate temperature; don't force it in. You will need to hold your child still with his "cheeks" (buttocks) together to hold the thermometer in place. Do *not* leave your child alone, even for a minute, with a rectal thermometer in place. The thermometer can slide in too deep or slide out completely. Glass thermometers can break if your child moves suddenly.

Temperatures can be measured in the *mouth* (*orally*) with the thermometer under the tongue in older children. It is difficult to get an accurate reading in children whose noses are so stuffy that they have to breathe through their mouths. In these cases, an armpit (axillary) temperature may be better. For the most accurate reading with an oral thermometer, don't start to measure until several minutes after your child has eaten or drunk anything cold or hot. Be sure to clean the thermometer with rubbing alcohol and rinse it in cool water before and after using it. Let it dry thoroughly before putting it in the mouth. Place the tip of the thermometer under the tongue and have the child close her mouth, holding the thermometer in place with her hand, *not* her teeth. Glass thermometers need to stay in place for at least three minutes to be accurate. You can read an electronic thermometer as soon as it beeps (usually in thirty seconds or less).

Do *not* leave a child alone with an oral thermometer in place. Sick children may be distracted easily and forget to keep the thermometer under their tongue, resulting in an inaccurately low reading. Older children may have learned that they can create a "fever" (and thereby avoid an unwanted activity such as school) by holding the thermometer near a light bulb, rubbing it between their hands, or running it under hot water. Don't tempt your child to use one of these common tricks by leaving her alone with the thermometer.

WHAT'S THE BEST WAY TO TREAT A FEVER?

Most parents can tell when their child is sick because the child doesn't eat, sleep, or play as she normally does. The child may whine, cling, and regress to more babylike behavior or become quiet and withdrawn. If your child isn't acting sick, there's no reason to take or treat her temperature. The only reason to treat the child's fever is to help her feel more comfortable. Let's tour the Therapeutic Mountain to learn what works safely; if you want to skip to my bottom-line recommendations, flip to the end of the chapter.

BIOCHEMICAL THERAPIES: MEDICATIONS, HERBS, NUTRITIONAL SUPPLEMENTS

Medications

PROVED SAFE AND EFFECTIVE

- Acetaminophen (Panadol, Tylenol, Tempra)
- Ibuprofen (Pediaprofen, Children's Advil)

How does *acetaminophen* (the active ingredient in Tylenol, Panadol, Tempra, and other nonaspirin fever medications) work? It resets the brain's temperature thermostat. Acetaminophen also helps the child feel more comfortable with her other symptoms. It does *not* make the illness go away any faster. You can't tell how sick your child is (that is,

whether you are dealing with a cold or pneumonia) by how much the temperature goes down when taking Tylenol.[23, 24] A child with a high fever is unlikely to achieve a completely normal temperature from Tylenol, but she may well feel more comfortable. *Don't watch the temperature, watch the child.*

If you decide to use acetaminophen, read the package instructions carefully for the correct dosage for your child. Do not give it more often than every four hours. Overdoses can cause liver damage. There is no benefit to dividing doses every two hours. Keep medicine out of your child's reach (in a childproof or locked cabinet) between doses. It takes about forty-five minutes to an hour for acetaminophen to start working. The effects wear off in four to six hours, so if your child is uncomfortable again in that time you can repeat the dose. Please do *not* wake up your child to give her acetaminophen. If she's sleeping, the medicine is much less important than the rest she needs to fight the infection.

Acetaminophen is very safe when taken in recommended doses. I've never seen a child experience side effects from it when it was taken as recommended. Acetaminophen does not prolong most illnesses or other symptoms.[25] Generic or store brands are just as effective and safe as name brand acetaminophen.

Do *not* use *aspirin* without talking to your child's doctor. Giving aspirin when a child has influenza or chicken pox is associated with a sometimes fatal condition called Reye's syndrome. Other side effects of aspirin include upset stomach, prolonged bleeding, and allergic reactions, especially in asthmatic children.[26, 27] It is not worth the risks when good alternatives are available.

Ibuprofen (Children's Motrin or Advil) works a bit longer (six to eight hours instead of four hours for acetaminophen) and may reduce fever a bit more than acetaminophen (by about one degree Fahrenheit).[28] However, ibuprofen is more likely than acetaminophen to cause an upset stomach.[29]

What about alternating acetaminophen and ibuprofen? Before we realized that fevers can be helpful, we often treated them aggressively with two medications. There is no evidence that this is helpful, and it doubles the risks of side effects. If your child's discomfort is not better with either acetaminophen or ibuprofen, it's time to call the doctor and get some help figuring out what's making the child so uncomfortable. Don't experiment by combining medicines on your own.

Herbs

A number of herbs used in other parts of the world have proved effective as fever fighters in animal studies. These include the East Indian plant known as Akra (*Calotropis procera*),[30] the African and Chinese fever remedy rhinoceros horn,[31] and the herb *Euphorbia hirta*.[32] A German combination containing ash tree, poplar, and goldenrod, known as STW 1, was shown in animal studies to be as effective as aspirin in reducing fever.[33, 34] Despite their effectiveness in animal studies, I do *not* recommend any of these herbal remedies for treating feverish children until additional studies have evaluated their safety and effectiveness in humans.

White willow bark is the original source of common aspirin. It has been used since ancient times around the world to treat fever and the aches and pains of a variety of illnesses. Willow bark tea does not taste very good. Because the active ingredient in willow bark is metabolized in the body to salicylic acid (aspirin), it is likely to have the same risks as aspirin (upset stomach, suppressed immune system, possible allergies, and possible Reye's syndrome).

Other traditional remedies have not been evaluated in comparison studies, although they have been used for centuries. Bitters, such as Angostura bitters or gentian, have long been recommended to reduce fever, especially in illnesses characterized by upset stomach and diarrhea. Boneset tea was used by Native Americans to break the bone-breaking fevers and chills of influenza. It is bitter and may cause nausea and vomiting. Catnip tea is used in treating low-grade fevers to help a child relax and induce sweating. Echinacea attacks some bacteria directly, helps bolster the immune system, and is used to treat infectious illnesses characterized by fever. Elder flower tea is sometimes used in combination with catnip or peppermint and yarrow to treat fevers. Licorice root has some antibacterial and anti-inflammatory properties and is used to treat fevers accompanying inflammation. Bitter-tasting yarrow flowers were said to have been used by the Greek hero Achilles to stanch the flow of blood from his battle wounds. Modern herbalists recommend a tea from its flowers to reduce fever and as a general tonic. There are *no* scientific studies evaluating the effectiveness of any of these herbal remedies in treating fever in children.

Herbal remedies are not necessarily safe just because they are natural. A traditional Asian remedy for fever, star anise (*Illicium verum*), proved an effective fever fighter in rodents but also caused seizures.[35] Feverfew is used primarily as a painkiller for headaches and arthritis, but it can cause allergic reactions.[36] Beware of possible contamination in herbal products. Most have been used for many years and generally are considered safe if given in small doses over a few days. If a child does not respond within a day or two to home remedies, her temperature exceeds 103.9°F, or she is lethargic, having trouble breathing, or acts very ill, take her to be evaluated by a health care professional.

Nutritional Supplements

NUTRITIONAL SUPPLEMENTS AND FEVER

- Vitamin A: no
- Vitamin C: maybe
- Zinc: maybe
- Ginger, bee products, garlic, beet juice: maybe

Chronic *vitamin A* overdoses can actually *cause* fevers.[37]

Blood levels of *vitamin C* decline during fever. High doses (1 gram or more in adult volunteers) of vitamin C temporarily *raise* the temperature by almost one degree.[38] In animal studies, giving vitamin C supplements along with acetaminophen (Tylenol) boosts Tylenol's antifever effects and decreases its potentially toxic effects on the liver.[39] It has not yet been studied as a fever fighter in humans.

Children with Down's syndrome have weak immune systems and tend to get a lot of fevers. Among children with Down's syndrome, daily *zinc* supplements of 25 to 50 milligrams significantly reduced episodes of cough and fever compared with similar children given placebos.[40] Zinc supplements have not been studied as preventive therapy in healthy children.

In animal studies, *ginger* has proven to have fever-fighting properties.[41] There are *no* studies evaluating ginger's effectiveness in treating fevers in children. *Bee products* such as propolis have also gained popularity recently for treating a variety of illnesses, but animal studies have *not* demonstrated any antifever effects of propolis and there are *no* studies evaluating its effectiveness in feverish children. *Garlic* has been used to treat infectious illnesses since ancient times by Egyptians, Greeks, and Romans and is known as Russian penicillin. *Beet juice*, sometimes combined with carrot juice, is a British folk remedy for fever. There are *no* studies on the effectiveness of garlic or beets for reducing fever in children.

LIFESTYLE THERAPIES: NUTRITION, EXERCISE, ENVIRONMENT, MIND-BODY

Nutrition

Feed a cold and starve a fever? Most children with fevers are not hungry. Neither force-feed nor withhold food from a feverish child. Let appetite be the guide. Offer her foods that are easy to digest (such as rice, crackers, yogurt, and broths) several times a day, but let her appetite guide what and when she eats.

Do give your child *extra fluids* while she has a fever. Higher body heat causes extra sweating, and this fluid needs to be replaced. Fresh fruit juices are excellent. Carrot and beet juices are good choices as vegetable juices for feverish children. Some children like to suck on ice cubes or fruit juice popsicles when they have a fever.

Exercise

Having a fever takes a lot of energy. Let your feverish child *rest*. Athletes also should take rest breaks and drink plenty of fluids to avoid becoming overheated on hot days. Gentle exercises, such as swimming, yoga, and tai chi, may be good exercise alternatives in August.

Environment

When a child has a fever, the body's thermostat is set higher temporarily and the body will try to maintain the new higher temperature. Children maintain a higher temperature by shivering, moving to a warm room, or asking for extra blankets or to be held close. Removing all the child's clothes or giving sponge baths will make her uncomfortable and more likely to shiver because it does *not* reset the internal thermostat. Sponging does *not* affect the underlying cause of the fever. By artificially lowering body temperature without resetting the internal thermostat, sponging may make things worse. It is not more effective than Tylenol.[42] If your child is sweating because her fever set-point has been reduced (the fever has "broken"), sponging away the sweat with tepid water may help her feel more comfortable.

Do *not* sponge your child with rubbing alcohol. Rubbing alcohol can be absorbed through the skin, causing low blood sugar, seizures, and even coma.

Mind-Body

Remain calm yourself. Keep your child company. Read her stories while she is awake. Cuddle her and let her know she is loved. Remind her that she will be feeling better soon and that while she is sick it is OK for her to rest. The behavior of many children regresses when they are sick to that associated with younger ages. Your child may want to cuddle an old favorite teddy bear or prefer stories that were outgrown months previously. This is normal; your child will be back to her usual self soon. You may want to play soothing music or children's books on tape. You can play videos that you have approved as appropriate for your child. Do not give in to the temptation to let the TV be your sick child's baby-sitter.

BIOMECHANICAL THERAPIES

Massage feels wonderful and can be very soothing for a sick child, but there are *no* scientific studies evaluating its effectiveness in treating fevers.

There is *no* role for surgery in the treatment of simple fevers, but it may be needed if the underlying problem is appendicitis!

BIOENERGETIC THERAPIES: ACUPUNCTURE, HOMEOPATHY

Acupuncture

Acupuncture treatment effectively reduces fever in arthritis-like disorders in animals.[43] Until such studies have been performed on human children, I do *not* recommend acupuncture as a primary treatment for typical fevers.

Homeopathy

Several remedies are traditionally used by homeopathic practitioners in extremely dilute doses (more concentrated doses can be poisonous) for treating various kinds of fever: *Aconitum, Arsenicum, Belladonna, Bryonia, Ferrum phos, Gelsemium, Nux vomica, Pulsatilla,* and *Sulfur.* In higher (nonhomeopathic doses) *Pulsatilla* effectively reduced fever in experimental rats.[44] The primary Bach flower remedy for fever is Rescue Remedy. There are *no* scientific studies evaluating the effectiveness of homeopathic remedies in treating children with fever. I do *not* recommend them.

WHAT I RECOMMEND FOR FEVERISH CHILDREN

Seek Immediate Professional Help If Your Child

- Is under three months old and has any degree of fever
- Is any age and the temperature is over 104°F
- Looks very sick
- Is more difficult than usual to awaken
- Won't stop crying with your usual loving care
- Is confused or delirious
- Loses consciousness or has a seizure
- Has a stiff neck
- Has painful or very frequent urination
- Is unable to keep down clear fluids
- Has trouble breathing or can't swallow her own saliva
- Cries when you touch or move her
- Has a rash with deep red or purple spots that don't fade or blanch when you press on the skin

WHAT TO AVOID WHEN YOUR CHILD HAS A FEVER

1. *Lifestyle—environment. Don't* sponge your child with alcohol or ice water. Sponge only when the fever is breaking, use tepid (not ice) water, and sponge only as long as it helps her feel comfortable. Neither overdress nor completely undress your child. Her body will find its own proper temperature if you dress her as usual and offer a light blanket or two.

2. *Biochemical—medications. Avoid* aspirin. Do *not* awaken your child to give antifever medicines.

When to Call or Visit Your Health Care Provider

- If your child is less than two years old and the temperature is above 102°F
- If your child is urinating less often than usual (fewer than four wet diapers a day). This may be a sign that your child is becoming dehydrated. Offer additional fluids.
- If the fever lasts more than a day or two, especially if it's not clearly associated with a simple cold or flu.

TREATING A FEVER AT HOME

Remember, treat the child, not the thermometer reading.

1. *Lifestyle—nutrition.* Give your child plenty of extra fluids to drink. Juices and broths are excellent and easily digested.

2. *Biochemical—medications.* Try acetaminophen or ibuprofen to reduce your child's discomfort. Do not exceed the doses recommended on the package label.

3. *Lifestyle—environment.* You may give a tepid water sponge bath if your child is sweating (the fever has "broken").

4. *Lifestyle—exercise.* Encourage your child to rest.

5. *Lifestyle—mind-body.* Stay with your child, offering love, support, and encouragement. Remember that most fevers resolve in two to three days on their own.

20

HEADACHE

Mike Fahnestock called me shortly after he and his wife moved to town. Their eleven-year-old daughter, Kim, had started having headaches a few weeks before they moved. She was now having them almost twice a month. She had told Mike that she knew when she was getting a headache because she saw flashing lights. Shortly afterward, she complained of terrible pain, usually on the left side of her head. She had tried aspirin, but that didn't help very much. She felt better after a long nap. Mike initially attributed the headaches to the stress of the move, and then he thought Kim might be getting migraines like her mother and grandmother. He called me to see if there were any new treatments for migraine and to make sure Kim didn't have something more serious, like a brain tumor or meningitis.

Headaches are very common. Americans spend over $300 million a year on nonprescription headache remedies alone, plus the cost of doctor visits, prescription medications, and time off from school or work. Children with migraines miss more than twice as many school days each year as children without recurrent headaches.[1] In a 1989 survey of teenagers and young adults, over 50% of boys and 75% of girls had had a headache in the previous month; migraine headaches were reported by 3% of boys and 7% of girls.

Many parents worry when their child has recurrent headaches that there is a brain tumor, but tumors are incredibly rare. Other causes are far more common. About half of all headaches in children are due to muscle tension. About 25% are due to migraine, and the rest are due to fever, head injuries, sinus infections, dental problems, jaw joint problems, uncorrected vision problems, and ear infections. Less common causes of headache include very high blood pressure, meningitis, lead poisoning, carbon monoxide poisoning, eating very cold foods, altitude sickness, and vitamin overdoses.

Tension headaches are caused by clenched muscles in the face, jaw, scalp, neck, or shoulders. Chronically contracted muscles squeeze off their own blood flow, limiting the supply of oxygen, allowing toxic waste products to build up, triggering inflammation.

TENSION HEADACHE TRIGGERS

- Emotional stress
- Physical stress, lack of sleep, fatigue, heat, noise
- Poor posture
- Pain, pinched nerves
- Eyestrain, poor lighting
- Other illnesses, colds, flu

Muscular tension headaches can be caused by emotional stress, anger, and depression. They can also be caused by physical stress (e.g., fatigue, cold, heat, irregular meals, noisy environment), poor posture, pain, pinched nerves, grinding teeth, eyestrain, poor circulation, and illnesses elsewhere in the body.[2] Whew! Given this long list, it's surprising that not *all* kids get tension headaches. Tension headaches are usually most painful in the forehead or the back of the head. They feel like a band tightening around the head or a steady pressure.

Migraine headaches can provoke pain, clenched muscles, and thus tension headaches. Often the two go together. Although migraine headaches and tension headaches can occur simultaneously, migraines have their own painfully unique characteristics.

Migraine headaches actually occur in two phases:

1. the preheadache phase, in which the blood vessels in the scalp and head squeeze down, followed by

2. the actual headache phase, in which there is dilation, pounding pain, and inflammation of the blood vessels in the scalp and head.

CHARACTERISTICS OF MIGRAINE HEADACHES

- Run in families
- Recurrent headaches; pain-free between episodes
- Symptoms preceding the headache: aura
- Typically last two to seventy-two hours
- Pounding or throbbing on one side of head; can hurt all over
- Often very sensitive to light or sound
- Often have upset stomach, nausea, or vomiting
- Prefer to remain lying down in quiet, dark room
- Improved with sleeping

Mike was really on the ball in putting together his daughter's symptoms with his wife's history of headaches. Migraine headaches run in families. Migraines are also more common in women, adding more weight to the possibility that Kim was having migraines.

Like Kim, some people with migraines experience symptoms such as flashing lights or other images *just before* the headache starts. These symptoms are known as the headache's *aura*. Less often, people with migraines have other symptoms such as temporary blindness, tingling, or severe weakness in the arms or legs on one side of the body. Usually these symptoms go away when the actual headache begins. Some people are so troubled by the aura symptoms that they actually look forward to the headache itself. This is the case with one of my colleagues. His aura symptoms include temporary blindness; when the headache starts, he can finally see again.

A migraine headache is typically a throbbing or pounding headache on one side of the head. However, many children experience migraine headaches as a kind of vague pain all over the head. Most migraines are accompanied by nausea or a stomachache, making the sufferers truly miserable. When struck with a headache, most prefer to lie in a very quiet, dark room. Migraines typically last several hours, but they can last up to three days. Even after the headache is over, many sufferers feel wiped out and achy for a day or so.

Like tension headaches, migraines can be triggered by many different things.

MIGRAINE HEADACHE TRIGGERS

- Stress, tension, or anxiety
- Being overtired, late nights
- Diet: chocolate, cheese, aspartame, nitrites, MSG, caffeine
- Menstrual period
- Bright light, flashing lights

Children who suffer from migraines do not necessarily experience any more *stress* than other children, but they seem to respond differently to stress, often feeling more anxious about life's challenges than other children.[3] Many children get their migraines after the tension has eased (e.g., after the exam is over) rather than while they are worried about it. *Anxious* children tend to get more frequent and more severe migraines than children who are not anxious. This provides the rationale for mind-body

therapies such as self-hypnosis, biofeedback, and meditation.

About 25% of families identify *fatigue* as a trigger for migraines.

Missing meals or *eating certain foods* (such as chocolate, cheese, aspartame, nitrites, MSG, caffeine, and red wine) have also been blamed for migraines.[4] Although some children and adults are certainly sensitive to certain foods, foods have taken an unfair rap in many cases. *Chocolate* may indeed be a trigger for some migraine sufferers,[5] but in a randomized, double-blind crossover trial only *two* out of twenty-five adults who initially attributed their symptoms to chocolate had consistently negative reactions.[6] If your child gets headaches after eating chocolate, try going three months without any chocolate and keep track of whether or not she has fewer headaches. Children do not *need* chocolate as part of a healthy diet, but they may not need to live a life of total deprivation either.

The amino acid tyramine, found in *cheese*, especially aged cheeses, has also been blamed for migraines. However, the vast majority of people can eat cheese safely. Several studies in children have shown that tyramine does *not* trigger migraines.[7,8]

Despite suggestions that the artificial sweetener *aspartame* (Nutrasweet) triggers some adult migraines,[9,10,11] there are no studies linking it to headaches in children. Controlled studies show that aspartame does *not* trigger migraines in adults, even among those who had thought they were highly sensitive to it before the studies.[12,13] As with chocolate, if your child has frequent migraines, try omitting aspartame for three months and keep track of her headaches. Careful monitoring may uncover other triggers, too.

Nitrites and nitrates are used to cure and preserve many meats such as hot dogs, bacon, salami, and dried meat sticks. Nitrites and nitrates trigger migraines in some people.[14] Again, try going several months without these products and monitor your child's headaches carefully.

MSG is the key ingredient held responsible for the "Chinese restaurant syndrome": headache, dizziness, flushing, sweating, and abdominal cramps. When you eat out, be sure and ask to have your child's food prepared without MSG; most restaurants accommodate this request without a fuss. Because many people now steer clear of MSG, manufacturers have started calling it by other names: hydrolyzed vegetable protein (HVP), hydrolyzed plant protein (HPP), and natural flavor enhancers.[15] Read labels carefully. Sensitive children who consume small amounts of MSG in ordinary foods every day may end up with chronic headaches.[16]

Caffeine, found in coffee, tea, cola, and chocolate, is addictive. Quitting coffee cold turkey not only results in more yawns, but in more headaches, irritability, and depression.[17] Children who drink two to three cans a day of caffeine-containing sodas are just as susceptible to withdrawal headaches as adult coffee drinkers who try to quit suddenly, who oversleep on the weekend and miss their morning dose, or those who are forced to abstain because of hospitalization or surgery.[18, 19, 20, 21] If your child is a regular cola drinker, gradually reduce her intake over two weeks to avoid withdrawal headaches.

Paradoxically, caffeine is a potent pain reliever that effectively combats headache pain. It is so effective, it is included in many headache remedies including Anacin and Excedrin. People who start taking these medications every day for mild aches and pains may end up addicted to caffeine and suffer severe headaches when they try to quit.

Menstrual periods are a common trigger for migraines in teenage girls and adult women. *Bright* or *flashing lights* trigger symptoms for some sufferers. Although some factors seem to trigger migraine headaches

directly, others seem to work in combination. A teenager who usually tolerates nitrates without any problem could develop a raging headache if she has a bacon cheeseburger the day after a sleepless slumber party, especially if it's the wrong time of the month.

Migraine sufferers who keep careful track of their headaches using a *headache diary* often find that their headaches occur more often at certain times of the day. In a study of fifteen meticulous migraine sufferers, the headaches occurred most often between 6 a.m. and 10 a.m. and were less likely between 8 p.m. and 4 a.m.[22] This is the same timing as adult heart attacks. It is also the rhythm of the rising and falling of several stress hormones, suggesting a complex interaction between hormones, blood vessels, inflammation, and pain.

Have you ever had an *ice cream headache*? Many people have. The problem is not the ice cream per se but the temperature.[23] The headache occurs when cold food hits the nerves on the roof of the mouth, triggering a pain sensation that feels as if it comes from the forehead or behind the eyes. This type of headache may have a strikingly sudden onset, but it usually resolves within a minute. Your child can still eat ice cream and popsicles, but she may have to go slowly, allowing the ice cream to melt on her tongue before letting it hit the roof of her mouth.

DIAGNOSIS

There are no blood tests or X rays that differentiate between tension headaches and migraines. X rays may help make the diagnosis of a sinus headache. Expensive tests such as CT scans and EEGs are rarely necessary.[24, 25] The most helpful information is a complete picture of the child's symptoms. If your child has frequent headaches, keep a diary or calendar noting the headaches, when they start, what seems to trigger them, how long they last, what seems to relieve them, and any other symptoms. This kind of record is more useful than a hundred CT scans or MRIs, and it doesn't cost you a penny.

What Is the Best Way to Treat Headaches?

The two most important aspects of any headache treatment are:
- recognize and address the underlying cause of the headache,
- prevent it or treat it early rather than wait it out.

The treatment for a sinus headache involves treating the sinus infection, while the treatment for a stress headache involves relieving the stress. A headache signifying meningitis requires different therapy than a headache from a head injury. No matter what causes the pain, it's better to treat it early rather than wait until the body starts screaming even more loudly with worse symptoms.

This chapter does *not* cover the specific treatments for all causes of headaches. It focuses on treatments for tension headaches and migraine headaches.

SEE YOUR HEALTH CARE PROFESSIONAL IF YOUR CHILD HAS

- A very severe headache
- Headache accompanied by fever or stiff neck (possible meningitis)
- Headache and vomiting following a blow to the head (possible brain injury)
- Headache with seizures, dizziness, trouble seeing or hearing

---

Also seek professional care if you suspect that your child might have a sinus infection, a dental problem or jaw problem, lead poisoning, high blood pressure, or some other serious problem underlying her headaches.

Let's tour the Therapeutic Mountain to find out what works for tension and migraine headaches. If you want to skip to my bottom-line recommendations, flip to the end of the chapter.

Biochemical Therapies: Medications, Herbs, Nutritional Supplements

Medications

For regular everyday *tension headaches,* all your child may need is a nonprescription pain reliever and a nap in a dark, quiet room.

NONPRESCRIPTION PAIN RELIEVERS

- Aspirin
- Acetaminophen (Tylenol, Panadol, and other brands)
- Ibuprofen (Advil, Motrin, and others)
- Naproxen (Aleve. Prescription names: Anaprox or Naprosyn)

Aspirin is inexpensive and widely available. It has even proved effective in treating migraine headaches.[26] Aspirin should *not* be taken when your child has influenza or chicken pox because of the risk of developing Reye's syndrome, a potentially deadly disorder of the liver and brain. Because of this risk, many physicians now steer clear of aspirin. It can also cause an upset stomach and even bleeding of the stomach lining.

Acetaminophen (Tylenol and other brands) is the most widely used nonprescription pain reliever. Generic brands are just as effective as name brands. Acetaminophen is inexpensive and is very safe if taken in recommended doses. Acetaminophen starts to work in thirty to forty-five minutes; benefits last for about four hours.

Ibuprofen (Advil, Motrin, and other brands) is at least as effective as acetaminophen[27] and lasts about two hours longer. However, it is somewhat more expensive. Ibuprofen can cause upset stomach. If used as recommended, it is safe, and many kids prefer its flavor to acetaminophen's.

Naproxen (Aleve) recently made the transition from a prescription to a nonprescription medication. In the process, the price dropped about 75%. Naproxen is a powerful pain reliever that lasts up to twelve hours. It can cause stomach upset and may only be tolerable if taken with food. It is very useful for migraines but is probably overkill for simple tension headaches. Since it became a nonprescription medication, I have begun recommending that migraine sufferers keep some on hand because it is so effective in treating severe headaches.[28] It is even more effective than the old standard of ergotamine.[29]

For *migraine headaches,* additional medications have proved effective in prevention and treatment. If your child has migraines more than once a month, talk with your health care professional about preventive medications.

PREVENTIVE PRESCRIPTION MEDICATIONS FOR MIGRAINES

- Beta-blocker medications: Propranolol (Inderal) and others
- Antidepressant medication: amitryptiline (Elavil)
- Methysergide (Sansert)
- Antihistamines: cyproheptadine (Periactin)
- Seizure medications: phenobarbital, phenytoin (Dilantin), carbamazepine (Tegretol)

Beta-blocker medications such as propranolol (Inderal) have been the treatment of choice for preventing migraine headaches for over twenty years. In adults, propranolol reduces migraine headaches an average of 43%—about the same reduction achieved with biofeedback training.[30] Propranolol also prevents pediatric migraines.[31, 32] Because of its success, new related drugs appear every year. Promising candidates for preventing childhood migraine include nadolol, timolol, atenolol, and metoprolol.[33] Propranolol should *not* be used in children suffering from asthma, heart failure, or depression, because it can worsen the symptoms of these disorders.

Certain *antidepressant* drugs (amitryptiline) have been successfully used to prevent migraines in adults (even those who were not depressed!),[34] but they have not been tested with controlled trials in children.

Sansert is an effective migraine preventer, but because of its severe side effects it is not much used in the United States.[35] *Periactin,* a widely used prescription antihistamine, also prevents migraines[36]; its side effects include drowsiness and increased appetite. Periactin has not yet been compared to other treatments. I do *not* recommend it.

In the past, the seizure medications *phenobarbital* and *Dilantin* were used to prevent migraines, but they have substantial side effects and have not been rigorously tested as migraine treatments in children. *Tegretol* is effective in preventing migraines in older children and adults,[37] but it is rarely used unless the migraine sufferer also suffers from seizures.

Until recently, *ergotamine* had long been the standard treatment for migraine headaches. Ergotamine was originally derived from ergot, a fungus that grows on wheat. It has proved effective in adults.[38] The injectable form, dihydroergotamine, used in emergency rooms, is especially useful in treating children who are nauseated with their migraines. Ergotamine is better absorbed and more effective when *caffeine* is added.[39] If it is taken as soon as the child feels the headache coming on, Cafergot (caffeine and ergotamine) is frequently successful in minimizing subsequent symptoms. Cafergot has significant side effects including cold hands and feet from blood vessel spasms. Nowadays more potent medications with fewer side effects are available.

TREATMENT MEDICATIONS FOR MIGRAINE (PRESCRIPTION ONLY)

- Ergotamine (available for oral use, as a suppository, and as injection)
- Sumatriptan: Imitrex (injection only)
- Antinausea medications: metoclopromide (Reglan), prochlorperazine, (Compazine), and chlorpromazine (Thorazine)
- Sedatives and narcotics (butalbital, Valium, Demerol, morphine)
- Combinations: Midrin and Fiorinal

Sumatriptan is the newest wonder drug for the quick relief of migraine headaches.[40] Its biggest drawbacks are that it has to be taken as an injection (at least until the oral form is approved in the United States) and it is expensive. However, I know several migraine sufferers who have happily learned to give themselves injections (just as diabetics learn to inject insulin) because of the rapid relief afforded by sumatriptan. It starts to work in ten minutes, relieving the pain, the oversensitivity to lights and sounds, and the nausea and vomiting of migraine headaches.[41] It works best when given at the beginning of headache symptoms; it is *not* a preventive medication. Sumatriptan causes a brief rise in blood pressure, which is safe for most adolescents but may be hazardous in those with severe heart disease. Pain, tingling, and red-

ness at the injection site are common but short-lived and not serious in the long run.[42] Other side effects include flushing, tingling all over the body, warmth, and light-headedness.

Nausea and vomiting are among the most troublesome migraine symptoms. *Antinausea medications*, such as metoclopromide, not only treat this symptom, but by promoting normal intestinal movement, they aid the absorption of other pain medicine. Recent studies have shown that two other powerful prescription antinausea medications (prochlorperazine and chlorpromazine) effectively relieve migraine headaches on their own.[43,44] They are generally only used in emergency rooms, where they are given by injection to migraine sufferers who have not found relief with typical home treatments.[45] These medications may cause drowsiness, dizziness, and a drop in blood pressure.

Many of the *sedative* medications used to treat migraine work by promoting sleep, which is the way people throughout history have dealt with migraines. Sedatives such as butalbital and Valium work solely by putting the patient to sleep; they do not address the underlying cause of the headache, and I do *not* recommend them. *Narcotic* pain relievers (such as Demerol, morphine, and codeine) are widely used in emergency rooms as migraine treatments, but they carry the risk of addiction. None of these medications actually addresses the cause of headaches, but they have been used for many years when no other effective medication was available.

Midrin is the brand name of a combination medication: acetaminophen, isometheptene, and dichloralphenazone. Midrin has proved effective in several studies in adults but has *not* been evaluated in children. *Fiorinal* is the combination of aspirin, caffeine, and butalbital (a sedative). Midrin and Fiorinal can be addicting and are not any more effective than other headache medications. I do *not* recommend them.

Herbs

Herbal remedies traditionally used to treat headaches include angelica, balm mint, chamomile, cowslip flowers, ginseng, feverfew, hawthorn, lavender, peppermint, rosemary, skullcap, valerian, violet flowers, and white willow bark. Migraine sufferers who eat as little as two to three feverfew leaves a day report a dramatic decrease in the frequency and severity of their headaches.[46, 47] Feverfew is a member of the *Chrysanthemum* family of plants and is easily grown in the home garden. A recent double-blind study showed that 25 milligrams twice daily of freeze-dried feverfew leaves effectively prevented migraines in adults.[48] Feverfew must be taken daily for weeks or months before the benefits are noticeable; you cannot wait until your child has a headache and then expect feverfew to relieve it. Although feverfew is widely used in Great Britain, there are *no* studies of its safety or effectiveness in treating children suffering from headaches. Biochemical analysis has shown great variability in the strength, potency, and purity of commercially available feverfew preparations.[49]

Valerian and skullcap have traditionally been used to treat headaches because of their sedative effects, but recent reports raise the possibility that chronic use of valerian can cause liver trouble. Lavender, chamomile, and mint are used in many stress-related conditions because they are so calming. Unfortunately, there are *no* studies evaluating their effectiveness in treating adults or children suffering from headaches.

White willow bark is the original source of acetylsalicylic acid, aspirin's active ingredient. It is an effective pain remedy, but the amount of pain reliever in willow bark is fairly small and varies from batch to batch as all herbal products do.

An herbal bath may be soothing for the headache sufferer. Herbs traditionally added to the headache sufferer's bath include balm mint, chamomile, hops, Saint-John's-wort, lavender, rosemary, peppermint, and rose. Put the dried herbs in an old pillowcase or a stocking to make cleanup easier. Alternatively, you can add a few drops of the essential oils of these herbs to the bathwater. There are no scientific studies evaluating the effectiveness of herbal baths as headache treatments; you will have to experiment to find out what works best for your child.

Headaches can be a *side effect* of herbs. Gingko causes headache and upset stomach even at normal doses. Hops (even in the innocuous sleep pillow, see Chapter 24) have also been accused of causing headaches and nausea. Ephedra, commonly used to treat congestion and colds, can cause high blood pressure, rapid heart rate, and headache.

Nutritional Supplements

NUTRITIONAL SUPPLEMENTS FOR HEADACHES

No: vitamin A, vitamin D, zinc, niacin

Maybe: magnesium, capsaicin (hot peppers), ginger

It is much better for your child to get her vitamins and minerals from foods rather than from pills. Excessive *vitamin A* causes a buildup of pressure inside the brain that produces such severe symptoms it has been mistaken for a brain tumor.[50] Overdoses of *vitamin D* can also cause headaches. Excessive *zinc* can cause headaches as well as stomachaches, nausea, vomiting, and decreased appetite.[51] *Niacin* injections were used in the 1940s to treat headache pain, but later studies showed that they were no better than a placebo for curing headache pain.[52] I do *not* recommend them.

Magnesium functions in balance with calcium. High blood pressure medications that slow the flow of calcium in and out of cells have proved effective in preventing migraine headaches and reducing blood pressure. Magnesium levels are lower among children who suffer from migraines than among healthy children, with even lower magnesium levels during headaches.[53] So far, the only studies of magnesium supplements have been done in women whose migraines are part of the premenstrual syndrome. In a comparison study, magnesium supplements (360 milligrams taken three times daily) were significantly more effective than placebo pills in reducing premenstrual symptoms including migraine.[54] These results are very promising, but we are a long way from completely understanding all of the risks and benefits of supplements with a single mineral and how megadoses might affect the balance of other minerals and functions elsewhere in the body. I recommend that your child eat plenty of magnesium-rich foods such as figs, nuts, seeds, citrus fruits, corn, apples, and dark green vegetables rather than relying on magnesium supplements.

Capsaicin is the spicy ingredient in hot peppers. It appears to decrease the nerve transmitters responsible for pain. Hot peppers have long been a folk remedy for painful conditions. In an experimental trial, capsaicin nasal spray successfully reduced pain in adults suffering from cluster headaches (a type of adult headache related to migraine).[55] Capsaicin has *not* been studied as a treatment of childhood headaches. It can certainly sting and cause severe irritation if it gets in the eyes. Do not spray pepper up your child's nose. If you want to try it, use it in food.

Ginger is a traditional remedy for headaches and upset stomachs. It is widely used in East Africa and in Ayurvedic medicine as a headache cure. Certain compounds in ginger appear to work the same way as aspirin does, blocking inflammation and pain. There are several case reports that taking raw ginger or ginger powder daily helped prevent migraines in adults.[56] There are *no* studies evaluating its effectiveness in preventing or treating children's headaches. Nevertheless, ginger is safe, inexpensive, and widely available. If you want to give it a try for your headache-prone child, keep careful track of her headaches for a month before and for at least three months after boosting her ginger intake.

LIFESTYLE THERAPIES: NUTRITION, EXERCISE, ENVIRONMENT, MIND-BODY

Nutrition

Food allergies and food sensitivities are commonly blamed for migraine headaches. A British study showed that 93% of children suffering from weekly migraines and other allergy symptoms (e.g., skin rashes, diarrhea, wheezing) markedly improved when they consumed a low-allergen diet.[57] This diet (only one type of meat, one fruit, one vegetable, one carbohydrate, water, and vitamins allowed) for three to four weeks is gradually supplemented with one new food each week.[58] Any foods provoking headaches are withdrawn. The foods that provoke symptoms most often are cow's milk, egg, chocolate, orange, wheat, corn, cheese, tomato, cane sugar, benzoic acid, and the yellow dye tartrazine.[59] Several other studies have confirmed these findings in adult migraine sufferers.[60, 61] In another study, however, even children with frequent migraines that were thought to be triggered by foods did not have symptoms when given them under double-blind study conditions.[62]

Avoiding allergenic foods is rarely successful because it is very difficult to change family eating habits. In a study of adults with chronic headache, 75% identified one or more foods as headache triggers. However, most of them did not act on this knowledge. They ate just like people who didn't suffer from chronic headaches, except they drank a little less red wine.[63] This may be one reason physicians rarely pursue food sensitivities in the treatment of headache; even when extensive tests are done, families rarely follow through on the rigorous diets required.

There are no reliable tests that can tell you in advance which foods will cause problems for a particular child, so if you want to find out whether your child has a true sensitivity, you need to start with the bare bones and gradually add things. An alternative approach is to eliminate those foods most commonly associated with headaches in other children: chocolate, caffeine, cow's milk, cheese, processed meats (nitrites and nitrates), citrus fruits, wheat, tomatoes, aspartame, and MSG. For children with severe, frequent migraines, this approach might be worth a try. Many children who are sensitive to particular foods do eventually "outgrow" their sensitivity and tolerate these foods later without any symptoms. Besides being extremely difficult to institute, these diets run the risk of nutritional deficiencies unless supervised by a pediatric nutrition expert. *See your health care professional before starting any special diet.*

Exercise

Being overly tired is a setup for developing a headache. Make sure your child gets *plenty of rest*, especially during periods of increased stress. Going to bed in a quiet, dark place is useful even after one feels the aura for a migraine starting. For many people,

going to bed is the main treatment for migraines. Usually by the time the sufferer awakens, the headache is gone. Rest is also helpful for many of the illnesses (such as influenza, intestinal flu, strep throats, and sinus infections) that cause headaches.

Vigorous *exercise during the day* (when the child is not having a headache) is one of the best remedies for stress. Aerobic exercise seems to be a natural antidepressant. Exercise programs can be very useful in preventing migraine headaches as well as relieving the stress that triggers tension headaches.[64]

Environment

Being in a *quiet, dark environment* is soothing for many headache sufferers. Often the stress that precipitates a headache is due to loud noises (e.g., construction noises right outside), bright lights, or overstimulation. Relaxing in bed in a quiet, dark room helps reduce the environmental stress level.

Ice packs to the back of the neck or forehead are commonly used and effective headache remedies.[65] Ice packs are most helpful if they are applied to the back of the neck when the headache starts. Other home remedies include a ten- to fifteen-minute *hot foot bath or soak*. The heat dilates the blood vessels of the feet and promotes general relaxation.

Exposure to *toxic chemicals, fumes, and carbon monoxide* is a hidden cause of many headaches. When I was studying hypnosis, we learned of a girl with severe recurrent headaches who had been evaluated for several serious illnesses. Her headaches responded briefly to hypnotherapy but then recurred. Finally her parents looked for an environmental cause. They found it in their own garage (which was next to the girl's bedroom); a faulty furnace was spewing carbon monoxide into the air and poisoning their daughter. When the furnace problem was corrected, their daughter's headaches disappeared. Carbon monoxide poisoning can occur wherever there is incomplete combustion such as from a leaky car exhaust pipe, smog, and fumes from charcoal being burned indoors during a power outage.

Mind-Body

If your child suffers from recurrent headaches, keep a diary or log of her symptoms. You can use a regular calendar or make your own. Write down the date and time of the headache (was it a school day? a weekend? first thing in the morning? after school? just before or during a menstrual period?), the events, food, or other factors that seemed to trigger it, what you did to treat it, how long it lasted, and if anything seemed to make it worse or better. By keeping careful track of your child's symptoms, you will be well on the way to determining their cause and the best ways to prevent and treat them.

Children do especially well with mind-body therapies such as *biofeedback, hypnosis*, and *progressive relaxation*.[66] None of these methods is 100% effective for all children, and when the child does get a migraine, it may be just as bad as before—just not as often. On the other hand, some comparison studies have found that the combination of *deep breathing, autogenic training,* and *progressive muscle relaxation* can reduce the headache's severity and length, leading to less pain medication and less time out of regular activities. Mind-body therapies can help 50 to 75 percent of headache sufferers.[67] These techniques require training and regular practice. Most adults require about two months of practice before they notice fewer symptoms. (See Appendices A and B for additional information.)

EFFECTIVE MIND-BODY THERAPIES FOR PREVENTING MIGRAINES

- Hypnosis
- Autogenic training
- Biofeedback: thermal and EMG
- Progressive relaxation

Several studies have demonstrated that the most effective preventive therapy for migraines in children is *relaxation,* whether through self-hypnosis, the relaxation response (meditation), autogenic training, biofeedback, or progressive muscle relaxation.[68, 69, 70, 71] As with other therapies, one type may work better for your child than another. A review of many studies found that relaxation therapy alone improved symptoms for 38% of adults with migraine headaches and 45% of those with tension headaches. Unlike the benefits of medication, which tend to wear off soon after the medication is stopped, the benefits of relaxation training last for several *years* beyond the initial training.[72] Some of these therapies can be learned and practiced at home after a few training sessions with a professional—all of which leads to lower cost than continuous treatment with prescription medications.[73]

Self-hypnosis is even more effective than the most commonly prescribed medication, propanolol, in preventing migraines in children.[74] Children as young as six years old can learn hypnosis to help them prevent headaches. Hypnosis is simply being in a very relaxed state of mind in which the child's attention is focused on pleasant, healing images.

You can help your child relax through *deep breathing exercises* (in which the child watches her belly rise and fall with each breath), *progressive muscle relaxation,* or repeating a favorite phrase, affirmation, or prayer. Relaxing, pain-reducing images for your child might include the following:

1. Imagine that the pain is like a bunch of bubbles. Take a deep breath in. Each time you breathe out, blow the bubbles out of your head and watch them disappear as they float up into a soft blue sky.

2. Imagine yourself in your favorite place. It may be home in bed with your parent reading you a story. It may be at the beach or in the woods. Imagine yourself there feeling very safe and happy.

3. Imagine the sun warming your hands and feet.

4. Imagine the pain as a point on a dial inside your head. Reach over and gradually turn the dial down until it is at zero.

5. Imagine the pain as a thermometer reading. Watch the thermometer go down and down as the headache disappears. Imagine putting an ice cube at the bottom of the thermometer so it goes down even faster.

I'm sure you and your child can imagine even more ways of blowing away or turning down the pain. (See Appendix A for more information about Hypnotherapy resources.)

Autogenic training is a kind of self-hypnosis in which the person tells herself several relaxing statements over and over. Autogenic training is an effective treatment for chronic headaches.[75, 76] (See Appendix B for more information on autogenic training.)

Biofeedback is any technique in which one receives amplified feedback about a normal body function. For example, when a temperature sensor is applied to a fingertip and connected to a machine that uses lights or sounds to indicate higher and lower temperatures, this *thermal biofeedback* can be used to begin to consciously control the temperature

of the fingers. *Electromyographic (EMG) biofeedback* provides information about muscle tension to help one learn to relax specific muscles.

Preventing and treating headaches is an area in which biofeedback therapy really shines.[77,78] By relaxing tense muscles, EMG biofeedback has been especially helpful for those with chronic tension headaches.[79,80] Controlled studies document the effectiveness of EMG biofeedback training in reducing the pain and frequency of muscle tension headaches in children as young as six years old.[81] Thermal biofeedback has proved especially helpful for migraine sufferers. Benefits have persisted for at least six years in adults who participated in just eight to ten weeks of biofeedback training.[82] (See Appendix A for more information on how to find a biofeedback therapist in your area.)

Progressive relaxation exercise combined with *diaphragmatic breathing* can help reduce the frequency and intensity of headaches for many children. As preventive therapy for headaches, they can be as effective as biofeedback training and less costly.[83] Relaxation exercises increase the child's sense of mastery, decrease her sense of distress, decrease her muscle tension, and distract her from pain. The benefits of progressive relaxation exercises, self-hypnosis, and autogenic training can persist for years in children with both tension headaches and migraine headaches. (See Appendix B for information on how to do progressive relaxation and diaphragmatic breathing.)

Mind-body techniques are most effective if practiced regularly.[84] Children benefit from home practice and the encouragement of supportive parents.[85] Most successful programs combine biofeedback training with imagery, breathing, or relaxation techniques.[86, 87] I recommend professional relaxation, hypnosis, or biofeedback training for children whose headaches have not responded to home therapies. (See Appendix A to find resources on Mind-Body therapies.)

BIOMECHANICAL THERAPIES: MASSAGE, SPINAL MANIPULATION, SURGERY

Massage

Massage is one of the most widely used headache remedies. It is a perfectly natural response to headache pain, and it has proven effectiveness.[88]

Recipe for a Heavenly Headache Massage

1. Start by massaging your child's forehead. Put your thumbs together at the center and top of her forehead and slowly stroke away from the center. Repeat this movement, moving gradually down toward the eyebrows with each repetition.

2. Next, massage her temples slowly using tiny circular motions.

3. Move to the back of the skull at the place where the skull meets the spine. Rub from the center away toward the ears and make slow, gentle circles in all the tender spots.

4. Then massage the back of the neck, moving from the back of the skull downward toward the shoulders.

5. Before doing the shoulders themselves, try a brisk scalp rub. Use your fingertips or knuckles to lightly "scrub" your child's scalp as if you were giving her a shampoo, first one side, then the other.

6. Gently knead the muscles of the shoulders and upper back. Experiment with what feels best for your child.

7. Finish the head and neck massage by massaging your child's face. In general, it feels best if you use your thumbs, moving from the center toward the sides of the face. Slide along the bones that form the rim of the eye socket. Rub from the bridge of the nose down to the tip. Be sure to massage the jaw from the chin up toward the ears. Gently tug and wiggle her earlobes.

Be very gentle. There are often sore spots where the muscles have been tightly tensed. It is better to massage these spots lightly, focusing on the less painful areas and coming back to the tight spots, gradually increasing pressure as your child tolerates it. If your child's head or neck is very tender, you may want to give her a foot massage first to help her relax. You might try adding one or two drops of peppermint or eucalyptus oil to 1 teaspoon of plain vegetable oil as a special headache massage lotion because they are relaxing and may decrease pain sensitivity.[89] If your child's headaches are particularly severe or recurrent and you want professional assistance, see a massage therapist or physical therapist to learn how to help.[90]

Spinal Manipulation

Although cranial and spinal manipulation are widely used to treat headaches and neck aches, there are no comparison studies evaluating their effectiveness in treating childhood headaches.

Surgery

There is no need for surgery to treat most childhood headaches. However, surgery can be lifesaving when severe head trauma results in brain injuries.

Bioenergetic Therapies: Acupuncture, Therapeutic Touch, Homeopathy

Acupuncture

Several articles report that acupuncture effectively prevents many *migraine headaches*.[91, 92, 93, 94] Unfortunately, most of these studies did not include a group of migraine sufferers who were *not* treated with acupuncture. Because migraines come and go, it is difficult to tell how helpful a treatment is without a comparison group. Two small studies found that adult migraine sufferers improved as they monitored their headaches over time *regardless* of whether they received real therapy or placebo therapy.[95,96] (Keeping track of your child's headaches can be therapeutic in itself!) On the other hand, at least two studies show that true acupuncture *is* more effective than sham treatment in reducing migraine frequency and pain as well as the need for pain medications in adults.[97, 98] Another study in adults showed that acupuncture was as effective in preventing migraines as a standard beta-blocker medication.[99] Studies on acupuncture for children suffering from migraines have not yet been reported. If your child's migraines have not responded to other treatments, you may want to consider acupuncture therapy.

Acupuncture has also been recommended for *muscle tension headaches*.[100] A Swedish study compared acupuncture to physical therapy (massage, ice massage, progressive relaxation, biofeedback, transcutaneous electrical nerve stimulation, and general relaxation) for adults with chronic tension headache; both treatments improved symptoms, but the combination of physical therapies was better than acupuncture.[101] It is not surprising that a multifaceted approach worked better than a single therapy. In a controlled study, true acupuncture was more effective than sham acupuncture in preventing adults' chronic tension headaches.[102] More studies are needed to examine the role of acupuncture in the treatment of tension headaches in children. So far, it looks very promising. If your child's headaches have not responded to other remedies, acupuncture therapy is worth trying.

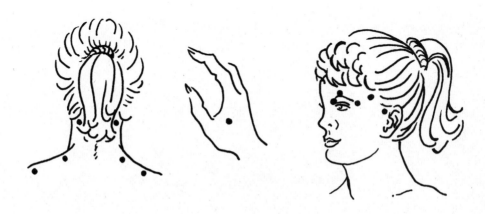

Therapeutic Touch

Therapeutic Touch successfully treats tension headaches in adults. In a comparison trial, Therapeutic Touch effectively relieved tension headaches in 90% of recipients, and relief was sustained for over four hours.[103] Therapeutic Touch is safe, and I often use it in my practice for both patients and colleagues who have headaches. (See Appendices A and B for more information on Therapeutic Touch.)

Homeopathy

The most commonly recommended homeopathic headache remedies are *Belladonna*, *Bryonia*, *Gelsemium*, and *Nux Vomica*. There are no studies evaluating their effectiveness. I do *not* recommend them.

WHAT I RECOMMEND FOR HEADACHES

PREVENTING HEADACHES

If your child has frequent headaches, *keep a diary or log of the headaches, headache triggers, and remedies.*

1. *Lifestyle—exercise.* Make sure your child gets plenty of regular sleep at night and vigorous aerobic exercise during the day.

2. *Lifestyle—nutrition.* If your child suffers from other allergy symptoms (runny nose, diarrhea, skin rashes) as well as frequent headaches, see your health care professional or a nutritionist to discuss the possibility of a low-allergenic diet. Try avoiding nitrates, nitrites, aspartame, MSG, chocolate, and aged cheeses and monitor your child's headaches. Avoid sudden changes in caffeine consumption. Give your child magnesium-rich foods. Also consider including ginger and hot peppers as part of her diet.

3. *Lifestyle—environment.* Avoid known allergens and toxins such as carbon monoxide and lead.

4. *Lifestyle—mind-body.* Have your child practice relaxation exercises or meditation regularly to help minimize stress and build a sense of mastery. Consider professional mind-body therapies such as self-hypnosis, guided imagery, or biofeedback training.

5. *Biochemical—medications.* See your physician about preventive prescription medications such as beta-blockers.

6. *Bioenergetic—acupuncture.* If other preventive therapies have not helped, consider acupuncture therapy.

See Your Health Care Professional If Your Child Has a Headache and

- You are concerned about possible meningitis (fever, stiff neck, spotted rash) or your child is lethargic or irritable
- Your child has recently suffered a head injury *and* vomits more than three times, vomits more than one hour after the injury, has difficulty hearing or seeing properly, has clear or bloody fluid coming out of the nose or ears, has a seizure, or becomes more clumsy, off-balance, or dizzy
- The headache is severe and won't go away with simple home remedies
- You are concerned about a possible sinus or tooth infection: facial pain, runny nose or thick mucus from the nose, fever, or pain in the jaw, teeth, ears, or eyes
- You are concerned that your child has an underlying serious illness: frequent recurring headaches despite home remedies, the child seems unwell, tired, has a poor appetite, is not growing well, has a change in personality, or becomes clumsier

---

TREATING HEADACHES

1. *Biochemical—medications.* Try a nonprescription pain reliever such as acetaminophen (Tylenol), ibuprofen (Advil or Motrin), or naproxen (Aleve). For a severe migraine, see your physician about an injection of sumatriptan or a prescription for ergotamine to have on hand to treat the headache in its early stages.

2. *Lifestyle—environment.* Have your child lie quietly for a few minutes in a dark room; try an ice pack on the back of her neck. Alternatively, try a hot foot bath or warm towels around her feet.

3. *Biomechanical—massage.* Try a head, neck, and shoulder massage. If she is too sore, try a foot massage instead. Consider adding oil of peppermint or eucalyptus to the massage oil. Consider seeking professional help from a licensed massage therapist or physical therapist.

RESOURCES

National Headache Foundation
5252 N. Western Avenue
Chicago, IL 60625
1(800)843–2256

American Council for Headache Education
875 Kings Highway, Suite 200
West Deptford, NJ 08096
1(800)255-ACHE

To find a biofeedback therapist in your area, contact:
Biofeedback Certification Institute of America
10200 West 44th Avenue, Suite 304
Wheatridge, CO 80033
1(303)420–2902

Books

Lipton, Richard, Newman, Lawrence, MacLean, Helene. *Migraine: Beating the Odds: The Doctor's Guide to Reducing Your Risk.* Addison Wesley, 1992.

Soloman, Seymour. *The Headache Book.* Consumer Reports Books, 1991.

Saper, Joel R., Magge, Kenneth. *Freedom from Headaches.* Fireside Books, 1986.

Sinclair, Marybetts. *Massage for Healthier Children.* Wingbow Press, 1992.

Thomas, Sara. *Massage for Common Ailments.* Fireside Books, 1988

21

HYPERACTIVITY
(ATTENTION DEFICIT DISORDER)

Sandra Vincent called me shortly after the beginning of the school year about her first-grader, Brian. She had always known Brian was an active boy, but his teacher had called her in to discuss the possibility that Brian was hyperactive. The teacher noted that Brian had a hard time sitting still in class and was usually out of his chair even before she'd finished calling attendance. He frequently shouted out answers impulsively, even if another child had been called on. Sandra wanted to bring him in for an evaluation and discuss the possibility of medication. She didn't like the idea of Brian having to take medicine every day just to be able to go to school, but she didn't know if there were any other options.

Hyperactivity is shorthand for the diagnosis of attention deficit disorder with hyperactivity (ADDH). Attention deficit can also occur without hyperactivity (simple ADD), but it is much less troublesome. With or without the H, ADD is the most commonly diagnosed behavioral or psychiatric disorder of childhood.

Between 3 and 10 percent of school-age children suffer from hyperactivity. A 1987 survey found that 6% of elementary school children were prescribed medications for hyperactivity. As of 1993, nearly 1% of Baltimore County high school students were taking medications for hyperactivity.[1] Prescriptions for hyperactivity medications doubled every four to seven years between 1971 and the late 1980s.[2] Boys are ten times as likely as girls to be diagnosed with ADDH, but diagnosis and treatment rates have recently risen in girls, too.

Before 1900 hyperactivity was not described as a medical condition, leading to speculation that it simply reflects a poor fit between children's temperaments and current cultural expectations.[3] Rather than being confined to crowded classrooms year after year, children used to stay at home and learn from their parents by active example. Although most children seem to have adapted to the demands of modern society, some simply don't have the disposition to sit still, pay attention, and wait their turn without one-to-one supervision. It doesn't take long before these children are labeled as troublemakers; the label often becomes a self-fulfilling prophecy.

Even during its brief history, ADDH has undergone numerous name changes. Prior to the 1960s, hyperactivity, minor neurological problems, and a variety of learning disabilities were lumped under the label of *Minimal Brain Dysfunction (MBD)*. In 1968 hyperactivity and learning disabilities were divided into separate diagnoses. In the 1970s, hyperactivity became known as *hyperkinetic syndrome* or the *hyperactive child syndrome*. In the 1980s the American Psychiatric Association defined specific criteria for *attention deficit disorder* (with or without hyperactivity). The psychiatric criteria continue to be modified every few years. These changing definitions make diagnosis difficult and have led to widely ranging estimates about its prevalence.

To some degree, impulsiveness, short attention span, and high activity levels are normal. Normal toddlers are messy, impatient, distractible, and seem to be always on the go. Things that are normal for two-year-olds are not necessarily normal for ten-year-olds. Before diagnosing ADDH, one has to be sure that the child is not simply acting his age.

SYMPTOMS OF ADDH

- Severe impulsiveness
  - Often acts before thinking
  - Has difficulty organizing work
  - Often blurts out answers, interrupts others' activities
  - Has difficulty waiting his turn in group games or activities
  - Shifts excessively from one activity to another
  - Needs a lot of supervision
  - Often engages in physically dangerous activities (e.g., runs into the street without looking)
- Shorter than average attention span; distractibility
  - Often fails to finish things he starts
  - Has difficulty sustaining attention to tasks or activities
  - Has difficulty following through on instructions
  - Is easily distracted
  - Does not seem to listen to what is being said to him
- Hyperactivity
  - Runs about or climbs things excessively
  - Difficulty sitting still, fidgets with hands or squirms in seat
  - Has difficulty staying seated
  - Moves about excessively during sleep
  - Is always on the go or acts as if "driven by a motor"
- Other symptoms
  - Is often messy or sloppy
  - Often loses things necessary for homework or activities

Symptoms of ADDH appear before the child is seven years old, but often the diagnosis is not made until the child's behavior starts causing problems in the classroom. Children don't have to have all of the above symptoms to be diagnosed as having ADDH, but they do need to exhibit at least several of these characteristics more than is normal for their age *for at least six months*. Other causes of disruptive behavior (such as a stressful situation, schizophrenia, depression, mental retardation, or petit mal seizures) must also be accounted for. Certain illnesses can also make children irritable, distracted, and squirmy. These conditions must be addressed before diagnosing hyperactivity.

After hearing this brief history of hyperactivity, Sandra was curious about what causes it—is it a health problem? too much sugar? bad parenting? or what?

POSSIBLE CAUSES OF
HYPERACTIVE BEHAVIOR

- Other medical problems
- Genetic factors or congenital problems
- Learning problems and other mental health issues
- Dietary problems
- Problems of arousal and low self-esteem

Physical problems such as impaired hearing and vision can cause problem behavior that is easily mistaken for hyperactivity. If your child can't hear the teacher, he can't very well pay attention to what she says. If your child can't see the blackboard, he's likely to pay more attention to what's on his neighbor's desk. Hyperactive children also have a higher than normal risk of having thyroid problems,[4] which can be evaluated with simple blood tests.

Another physical problem that can cause

daytime hyperactivity is poor sleeping at night. Among the many causes of sleep problems, one of the biggest culprits is partially blocked breathing.[5] Breathing can be temporarily blocked during a cold or sinus infection. In these cases, breathing, sleep, and behavior return to normal when the infection clears. Chronic blockages are usually due to large adenoids or tonsils. Nighttime breathing blockages result in loud snoring and frequent stops and starts in breathing, daytime sleepiness, and poor growth. These obstructions can be easily corrected with surgery, which often results in dramatic improvements in behavior and growth.

Brain damage due to lead poisoning has long-term effects on language and concentration skills.[6] Lead levels are often elevated in hyperactive children.[7] The higher the lead level, the more hyperactive symptoms.[8] Chelation therapy (which removes lead from the system) may improve hyperactive behavior in children with elevated lead levels.[9]

Cigarette smoke adversely affects many aspects of a child's health, including behavior.[10] Maternal *smoking during pregnancy* increases later problem behaviors such as hyperactivity.[11] Maternal smoking subtly limits the developing infant's oxygen supply, impairing brain development. In studies of children whose mothers used moderate amounts of alcohol, marijuana, and cigarettes during pregnancy, cigarettes had even more impact on intelligence and behavior than alcohol or drugs.[12] Maternal *smoking after pregnancy* also affects children's behavior: the more she smokes, the worse the child's behavior, including hyperactivity.[13] Being exposed to smoke at home is a bigger risk factor for school failure than recurrent ear infections are.[14] Maternal use of alcohol or drugs during pregnancy can lead to lower IQ, decreased attention, and increased distractibility in the child years later.[15, 16, 17] Children of *alcoholic fathers* are also at increased risk of behavioral problems such as hyperactivity.[18]

Brain damage from any cause can result in problems in thinking, memory, and attention. Even minor damage from head injury can cause learning and behavior problems.

Pinworms are a common childhood infection. The worms live in the large intestine and crawl out of the anus at night to lay their eggs on the skin. This infection leads to several symptoms in the child: an itchy bottom at night and irritability and distractibility throughout the day. Pinworms can be easily eradicated with medication, dramatically improving a child's disposition and behavior.

The diagnosis of ADDH or hyperactivity is based on your child's symptoms. There are no blood tests, urine tests, X rays, or other laboratory tests for ADDH. Parents and teachers may be asked to complete questionnaires or daily diaries of the child's behavior to help confirm the diagnosis. The most widely used daily behavior diaries are the *Conners Parent Rating Scale* and *the Conners Teacher Rating Scale*. Other questionnaires include the *Child Behavior Checklist*, the *Yale Children's Inventory*, the *Behavior Rating Profile*, and the *ADD-H Comprehensive Teacher Rating Scale* (ACTeRS).[19] If your child's symptoms and tests are not suggestive of any other physical, emotional, or learning problems and *are* consistent with ADDH, the diagnosis is made.

I gave Sandra copies of the Conners Parent *and* Teacher Rating Scales *for her and the teacher to fill out over the next two weeks.*

Hyperactivity does *run in families*. Many parents whose children are diagnosed with hyperactivity report that they, too, had problems paying attention in school. Between 50 and 70 percent of children who meet the criteria for ADDH *also* have learning disabilities, language problems, or slow learning. *Learning problems* such as dyslexia can also lead to distractibility. Language problems can be addressed by proper school evaluations. It's hard to pay attention if you can't understand what's being said or can't understand directions. Improved language skills can dramatically improve academic and social performance.

Brian's physical exam didn't indicate that any of these physical ailments were contributing to his behavioral problems at school. Sandra said that Brian's father had also had problems in school and wanted to make sure that Brian didn't have a specific learning disability. She scheduled an appointment for him to be tested by the school psychologist.

Children who are *grieving* for a significant loss, such as the loss of a parent through death or divorce, are often inattentive to their school environment, may act out their sadness through aggression, or act impulsively in dangerous situations out of despair and hopelessness. *Anxiety* and *depression* can also mimic attention deficit disorder. Before a child is diagnosed with attention deficit disorder, consider whether the child has a long-term behavioral disorder or a reaction to an upsetting situation.

Brian didn't seem to be suffering from any particular stresses this year and didn't appear to be anxious or depressed except about his school performance. While she was filling out the Conners scale and waiting for the results of the school psychologist's tests, Sandra wanted to do something to help Brian. She wondered if his problems weren't just caused by his grandparents' frequent indulgence of Brian's sweet tooth.

The anti-*sugar* mania of the 1970s and 1980s was highlighted by the famous Twinkie defense. In 1978, a gunman named Dan White shot San Francisco's mayor and city supervisor. In his defense, White pleaded that his criminal behavior was due to his steady diet of Twinkies! Excellent double-blind studies since then have proven that hyperactive children, even those whose parents swore the problem was sugar before the studies, were *not* made hyperactive by eating large amounts of sugar.[20, 21] Sugar is not the culprit; sugar does not make kids or adults crazy, criminal, delinquent, or aggressive.[22, 23] This is fortunate because almost all healthy fresh and dried fruits, starches, and grains are broken down into sugar during digestion.

On the contrary, sugar and other carbohydrates may exert a calming effect.[24] Have you ever indulged in "comfort foods"? Rice pudding, oatmeal, ice cream, and other high-carbohydrate foods actually seem to calm the brain, reducing aggressive behavior.[25] Sucrose (plain table sugar) given before painful procedures such as blood drawing or circumcision helps calm infants and reduces pain.[26] Hyperactive children may unconsciously be trying to treat their symptoms by eating sweets.

After sugar was off the hyperactivity hook, another dietary villain was sought. Despite much concern about artificial sweeteners, *aspartame* has been exonerated from blame for hyperactivity.[27] Even in amounts ten times higher than that consumed by the average child, aspartame has *no* adverse effects on the behavior of hyperactive children.[28]

The same thing may be true of *caffeine*. More than 75% of all children regularly consume caffeine, usually from soft drinks and chocolate.[29] On a weight basis, children typically consume more caffeine than adults. For example, a 25-pound toddler who drinks a can of cola consumes about twice as much caffeine (for his size) as a 120-pound woman who drinks one strong cup of coffee a day. Caffeine improves attention in normal children and adults.[30] Hyperactive children tend to drink more caffeine-containing sodas than their unaffected peers. Again, hyperactive kids may be unconsciously treating their symptoms with caffeine.

Dr. Ben Feingold, a San Francisco allergist, developed his theory about hyperactivity from the observation that hyperactivity has increased as Americans have increased their intake of *artificial colorings and flavorings*. He was also alarmed at the increasing use of children's aspirin in the 1960s and 1970s, knowing that its active ingredient, salicylate, can trigger asthma symptoms in some patients. He became convinced that subtle allergic symptoms to artificial colorings and salicylate were the basis for about 50% of cases of hyperactivity.

Based on this belief, he began treating hundreds of children with the Feingold diet.[31] Although he did not perform any controlled scientific studies, enthusiasm for his approach infected millions of frustrated families with hope that radically restricting their child's diet would improve intolerable behavior.

FEINGOLD DIET AVOIDS

- Artificial colors and flavors, especially yellow dyes (tartrazine)
- Medicinal salicylate compounds such as aspirin, Pepto-Bismol, and oil of wintergreen
- Foods containing natural salicylates such as almonds, apples, apricots, berries, cherries, citrus, cloves, cucumbers, currants, grapes, raisins, nectarines, peaches, plums, prunes, strawberries, tea, and tomatoes

There has been a great deal of confusion about what items are actually excluded from this diet. For example, artificial preservatives, stabilizers, and other chemical ingredients shunned by many parents were not excluded from Feingold's original diet.

The best study of the Feingold diet was performed at the University of Wisconsin in the mid–1970s. Three dozen hyperactive children and their families were placed on experimental diets for up to two months.[32] The participating families were told only that the study was evaluating the effect of different foods on behavior. For this reason, every week during the study, all of the food in the study households was removed and replaced with free food, prepared and delivered by study personnel. The families did not know when they were on the Feingold diet and when they were on a similar diet that contained hidden artificial colors and natural salicylates. The children's behavior was closely monitored at home, at school, and in behavior/learning laboratories by parents, teachers, and trained observers, none of whom knew which diet the children were eating during any given week. Among school-age children, the Feingold diet did *not* improve attention, hyperactivity, or disruptive behavior. Among the preschool children, parents reported modest improvements during the Feingold diet weeks, but these improvements were not discernible in the lab by objective observers. The researchers concluded that there may be some preschool children whose behavior is improved by the Feingold diet, but there was no benefit for school-age children.[33]

In a somewhat similar study in Pittsburgh, a nutritionist gave families advice about two different diets, each of which was to be followed for a month: the Feingold diet (though it was not named as such) and a comparison diet. The families in the study bought and prepared their own food based on the nutritionist's recommendations.[34] The children's teachers noted somewhat improved behavior on the Feingold diet, but parents did not.

In three later studies, children were knowingly placed on the Feingold diet. Those who seemed to improve were kept on the diet and later tested the forbidden foods. Those who seemed to react to the foods were instructed to adhere strictly to the diet. Later, they were tested in double-blind studies comparing capsules or foods containing artificial colors vs. placebos. Their behavior was closely monitored by parents and others who did not know when the child was given the real test substance and when the placebo was given. Under these conditions (in which parents had been strongly convinced of the efficacy of the Feingold diet before the study),[35] fewer than 5% of children had consistently negative reactions to the artificial substances.[36] The negative reactions included irritability, restless sleep, and other allergic symptoms, not just hyperactivity.[37] Similarly, double-blind challenges of yellow dye vs. placebo in children whose parents had believed they were very sensitive to artificial colors demonstrated that the majority were *not* affected by it.[38]

Numerous studies have also evaluated the possibility that hyperactivity is due to *food allergies*.[39, 40, 41] For the most part, these studies are not convincing that food allergies play a significant role in hyperactive behavior in most children. When allergies *do* play a part, the child often has other symptoms, such as eczema or hay fever, that make him uncomfortable and irritated.

The bottom line about food sensitivities is that the vast majority of hyperactivity is *not* due to food sensitivity of any kind. The main benefit of restrictive diets seems to be in the powerful placebo effect of making an entire family change its eating habits.[42] There are rare children who experience behavioral as well as physical changes because of food allergies (see Chapter 4).[43] If you suspect that your child has a food allergy, please have him evaluated by a health care professional who is experienced in pediatric nutrition.

"If it's not sugar or food additives, then what is it? And is there any possibility that this is just a phase he's going through and that he'll outgrow it?" Sandra wanted to know.

The real situation underlying ADDH seems to be a *problem with arousal*.[44] Arousal or vigilance is the state of being watchful, awake, and alert. Hyperactive children actually seem to be less aroused (sleepier) than other children. Have you ever noticed that when you are very tired it is difficult to concentrate and that the only way to stay awake (if you must stay awake) is to move about or fidget? In addition to fidgeting, you might daydream, complain of being bored, or fall asleep. Medications that increase arousal allow children to stop fidgeting and to pay attention more easily.[45]

Without help, hyperactive children frequently become disruptive in a regular classroom and are soon labeled as the "bad kids." Children whose behavior frequently meets with disapproval often end up with poor self-images. This is certainly true of hyperactive children, who frequently suffer from *low self-esteem*. Low self-esteem exacerbates feelings of hopelessness and aggressiveness. This is the basis for the mind-body therapies that form the backbone of treatment for hyperactivity.

Some children do outgrow their hyperactive behavior, but the tendency for short attention span, easy distractibility, and impulsiveness remains at least throughout adolescence and young adulthood.[46] Some learn to compensate for their disability as they grow older, developing different strategies for staying focused and attentive. About two-thirds of children improve during early adolescence, but a third continue to suffer the full spectrum of symptoms. Even those without hyperactivity continue to have problems with distractibility and impulsiveness, impaired school work, and social interactions. Children who suffer from hyperactivity during early school years remain more accident-prone and have higher rates of car crashes than other teenagers and young adults as they begin to drive.[47] Untreated, they are also at much higher risk of developing substance abuse problems and antisocial behavior, resulting in rates of unemployment and imprisonment that are five to ten times higher than in the general population.[48]

WHAT IS THE BEST WAY TO TREAT HYPERACTIVITY?

Now that we know that hyperactivity is common, how it is officially defined, what other things can look like it, what causes symptoms, and what tests your doctor and psychologist may do to diagnose it, let's talk about what you really want to know: how to treat it. We'll tour the Therapeutic Mountain to find out what works. If you want to skip to my bottom-line recommendations, flip to the end of the chapter.

BIOCHEMICAL THERAPIES: MEDICATIONS, HERBS, NUTRITIONAL SUPPLEMENTS

Medications

Stimulant medications have been the mainstay of medical treatment for hyperactive children for over twenty years. These medications have proven effectiveness in helping children improve classroom behavior and academic performance.[49, 50] Although stimulant medications are effective, the American Academy of Pediatrics recommends that they *never* be used as the *only* treatment for hyperactivity. Lifestyle, especially mind-body, therapies are integral to the success of a comprehensive treatment program.[51] Medications help with symptoms of impulsiveness, distractibility, and hyperactivity, but they do *not* correct the underlying disorder or correct learning disabilities such as dyslexia.

PRESCRIPTION MEDICATIONS TO TREAT HYPERACTIVITY

- Methylphenidate: Ritalin
- Dextroamphetamine: Dexedrine
- Pemoline: Cylert
- Others such as clonidine and desipramine

It may seem paradoxical that the medications that are most effective in treating hyperactivity are stimulants, but it is true. This is probably because ADDH is primarily a problem of low arousal. By increasing arousal, stimulants decrease symptoms. Tranquilizers and sedatives are *not* helpful for hyperactive children.[52]

Ritalin is the most widely prescribed medication used to treat hyperactivity, accounting for 93% of all stimulant medications prescribed for children. Ritalin benefits attention, impulsiveness, and activity, but it has little effect on aggressive behaviors or poor social skills.[53] Ritalin is helpful for adolescents suffering from attention deficits and impulsiveness as well as younger children who are hyperactive.[54]

The best way to tell if your child will benefit from Ritalin is the double-blind, placebo-controlled crossover trial.[55] This means that you, your child, and your health care provider agree to participate in a brief (three-week) study to determine whether or not Ritalin actually helps your child. The physician will talk with a pharmacist, who will make up three different preparations: a dummy or placebo pill, a low dose of Ritalin, and a higher dose of Ritalin. Your child will take each of the medicines for one week. Neither you nor your child nor your child's physician will know the order of the medications. During each week, you and the child's teacher or day care provider will keep careful track of your child's symptoms in a symptom diary (such as the Conners parent or teacher questionnaire).

At the end of the three weeks, you return to your doctor with the symptom diaries for each of the three treatment periods and your best guess about when your child was taking the real medication. After reviewing the records, the physician will contact the pharmacist to find out when the child was taking the placebo, low dose, and higher dose of Ritalin. This may sound like a complicated process, but it is the easiest and most objective way to determine if your child will really benefit from taking Ritalin. Most parents would rather go through a three-week trial and know for sure than have their child on months and years of medication without really knowing if that's what he needs. I do not prescribe Ritalin to any of my patients until we have gone through this process. Not all pharmacies are geared up to do this kind of study. Your physician may need to contact a pharmacy at the closest university or children's hospital to prepare the trial medications; it's definitely worth the effort.

Children can continue taking Ritalin for years and still receive the same benefits without increasing the dose.[56] Side effects include decreased appetite, stunted growth, insomnia, dizziness, stomachaches, tics, and headaches.[57, 58] On the other hand, Ritalin results in less daydreaming, staring, irritability, and nailbiting.[59] Despite older warnings against epileptic children using Ritalin, recent studies show that it does *not* provoke seizures.[60] The regular form must be given at least twice daily (at breakfast and lunch time) in order for effects to last throughout the school day. A sustained-release preparation is available, which may be more convenient for those who have difficulty taking the second dose at school.[61]

Dexedrine is chemically related to Ritalin. It has been used for over fifty years to treat school children with behavior problems. It is an effective stimulant medication that starts acting within an hour.[62] Dexedrine is as effective as Ritalin, and sustained-release forms are also available. It is less commonly prescribed because there is more concern about its side effects, which are similar to but perhaps more intense than with Ritalin.

Several studies have shown *Cylert* to be as effective as Ritalin and Dexedrine in improving attention and learning.[63, 64] It is long-acting and can be given just once a day, but your child may need to take it for several days before improvements become apparent. Cylert may cause liver problems. If your child takes Cylert, he needs regular tests to monitor liver function.

Other medications used to treat hyperactive children include antidepressants and the blood pressure medicine *clonidine*. Clonidine can worsen depression. Antidepressant medications such as *desipramine* are effective[65] but can result in serious side effects. Five children have died as a result of cardiac side effects while taking antidepressant medication for hyperactivity. All of these prescription medications should be taken *only* under the close supervision of a qualified health care professional.

Herbs

Traditional herbal medicine has remarkably little to say about hyperactivity, probably because it is largely a twentieth-century diagnosis. Sedative herbs, such as valerian, are recommended by some German herbalists, but sedatives are *not* helpful for hyperactive children. In fact, sedatives may make them drowsy, confused, and even more likely to be erratic and impulsive.

Because heavy metals (such as lead poisoning) have been blamed for problem behavior in some children, a few herbalists recommend detoxifying teas such as red clover lemon grass, and milk thistle. There are *no* scientific studies showing that these herbs help alleviate symptoms.

Nutritional Supplements

Caffeine has been evaluated in numerous studies as an alternative treatment that is fairly safe, inexpensive, and readily available.[66] However, caffeine is not nearly as effective as the prescription stimulant medications.[67, 68, 69] Low doses of caffeine may benefit children who are already taking Ritalin, boosting the benefits without substantially increasing side effects.[70] Caffeine's own well-known side effects include feeling jittery, nervous, anxious, and eventually feeling tired when the effects wear off.

Deficiencies of vitamin C and zinc have been suspected of causing hyperactivity in some children. One study showed that hyperactive children who had low zinc levels were less likely to respond to stimulant medications than children with normal zinc levels.[71] On the other hand, a New Zealand study showed no association between children's zinc levels and their behavior as rated by parents and teachers.[72] A double-blind controlled study of hyperactive children given megadoses of vitamin C, B-vitamins, and calcium (vs. placebo) showed no behavioral improvements with the supplement. If anything, children tended to have *worse* behavior, and some developed signs of liver toxicity.[73] I do *not* recommend them for this condition.

LIFESTYLE THERAPIES: NUTRITION, EXERCISE, ENVIRONMENT, MIND-BODY

Nutrition

Just because there is compelling evidence *against* the "sugar causes hyperactivity" hypothesis does *not* mean your child should subsist on cookies, cola, and candy bars. Sugar is bad for your child's developing teeth, and it replaces many more healthy foods your child needs for a balanced diet. If you are convinced that sugar makes your child's symptoms worse, temporarily eliminate all sweets from his diet (without telling anyone else), and then ask his teachers or other adults how they think he's doing. Check it yourself several times. If you remain convinced that sugar is the culprit, your child can live without cakes, cookies, and candy, but don't expect it to be easy![74]

Avoiding artificial dyes may be helpful in a very small minority of hyperactive children.[75] Rare children do have reproducible reactions (including irritability, restlessness, and sleep disturbances) to the yellow dye tartrazine.[76]

Despite vivid testimonials to the contrary, there have been numerous studies demonstrating the ineffectiveness of the Feingold diet.[77, 78, 79] The diet is so restrictive, it's quite possible that children who adhere to it will end up with more nutritional deficiencies than those who eat a normal diet. On the basis of all existing evidence to date, I do *not* recommend the Feingold diet.

Others suggest that hyperactive children might benefit from a "few foods diet."[80] This diet includes only lamb and turkey, rice and potato, bananas and pears, root vegetables, green vegetables, sunflower oil, milk-free margarine, and bottled water. If children improve after two weeks on this diet, one new food per week is gradually added. A few allergic children improve on this regimen (see Chapter 4, Allergies).[81] The provocative foods most commonly implicated are well-known allergens such as chocolate, cow's milk and cheese, oranges, wheat, tomato, and egg. This restrictive diet is extremely difficult for most families to maintain.

Most studies do not show any benefit for most children from restrictive diets. Avoiding food allergens and food sensitivity probably helps only a small minority of children. I do *not* suggest that you pursue restrictive diets unless all other measures have failed to help or your child has other allergic symptoms. If you decide to pursue dietary therapy, make sure you seek the help of a trained nutritionist so your child does not develop any preventable nutritional deficiencies.

Exercise

Exercise is great for hyperactive kids. Kids with ADDH are often a bit clumsy, struggling with eye-hand coordination. Go for large muscle exercises such as running, soccer, and swimming. If your child is involved in team sports, let the coach know that extra directions may be needed. Keep the child close to the coach or team leader so his attention is less likely to wander. Teams and activities with close adult supervision (such as Scouting) are better bets than unorganized after-school pickup games.

Martial arts training in small groups may be helpful in promoting discipline, coordination, and self-esteem. Relaxing exercise such as yoga may have special benefits for the hyperactive child. A comparison study showed that hyperactive children who were taught simple yogic breathing exercises, slowly moving stretches, and relaxing postures had improved self-esteem.[82] Teaching a child how to relax through movement is a perfect therapy for hyperactive children, who are on the move and need to develop relaxation skills.

Because hyperactive kids tend to have a lot of injuries, they often end up in the emergency room for stitches and casts. Make sure your youngster wears proper protective gear whenever he goes out to rollerblade, ride a bike, or engage in contact sports.

Environment

ENVIRONMENTAL STRATEGIES

- Reduce lead exposure
- Organize home environment
- Music

Help prevent your child from developing *lead poisoning* by keeping your home free of paint chips and dust. Dry dusting and sweeping just stir up the dust, so use a wet mop and a damp duster. High-phosphate cleaners are especially effective at removing lead dust. Wet-mop hard floors at least twice a month, vacuum and damp dust window ledges weekly, and have toddlers wash their hands several times daily (at least before all meals and bedtime).[83] Do not store your child's juice in glazed pottery or pewter containers, because both may contain lead that can leach into your child's juice. Keep lead-containing objects, such as watch batteries, fishing weights, and old soldered toy soldiers away from toddlers. If you or your spouse work in a high-lead occupation (e.g., foundries, firing ranges), change your clothes as soon as you get home so you don't spread lead dust from your clothes to your house. Removal of lead-based paint should always be done by professionals who are trained and have the proper equipment to get rid of the lead without astronomically increasing airborne lead levels.

Your health care practitioner can test your child for lead poisoning. Most pediatricians test at least once during infancy and toddlerhood if lead poisoning is a problem in your area. If levels are high, medical treatment can help your child excrete the lead.[84] Lead screening and treatment is best done by the time a child is two or three years old, long before hyperactivity becomes an issue.

Help your child create an *organized environment* at home. Minimize clutter to minimize distractions. Calm colors and simple

lines help reduce overstimulation.

Can *music* therapy help? An interesting Israeli study compared normal and hyperactive boys' work performance while they listened to different kinds of music: fast-paced vs. slower tempo vs. no music.[85] As expected, the hyperactive boys tended to make more mistakes than the normal boys. Their performance plunged even more while listening to fast-paced music. While listening to calmer, slow-tempo music, however, they did nearly as well as the normal boys. These intriguing results bear repetition in a variety of classroom settings. Pending such studies, it makes sense to keep all environmental cues (musical and otherwise) as calm as possible to help hyperactive children maintain a steady pace.

Mind-Body

Mind-body therapies are the cornerstone of treatment for hyperactive children. Parents must learn to express disapproval of a child's unwanted behavior while still expressing love for the child himself. Take every opportunity to praise your child whenever he behaves as you would like, even if it is only for a few minutes. Over the long term of months and years, appropriate treatment can eventually rebuild self-esteem,[86] but it is far easier to maintain and improve self-esteem from the time your child is young rather than waiting until it is already severely impaired.

MIND-BODY THERAPIES

- Structured schedule
- Step-by-step instructions
- Positive reward for desired behavior
- Tutoring
- Biofeedback and relaxation training
- Professional counseling

First, review your child's *daily schedule*. Make sure there *is* a schedule. Everything should be as routine and predictable as possible—meal times, nap time and bed time, exercise time, story time, day care or school time, bath time, cleanup time, relaxing time, chore time, and so on. It may help for you and your child to sit down and make a poster or chart together, listing all the day's activities and the times and places they occur. Try to stick as much as possible to the schedule, even on weekends and vacation time. Organization and structure are very important for hyperactive children.

Break every activity down into smaller steps. Hyperactive children need specific, detailed, step-by-step instructions. You can't just say, "Get ready for dinner." You have to tell them to first wrap up the game, then put it away, then go wash their hands and face, and finally, come to the table and sit down. You may have to go through this exact same routine a thousand times before they get it. If you vary it, your child may not get it right, even though he's done it many times before.

Reward your child for getting it right. He should get at least four compliments for every correction! Many families find a chart and sticker system very helpful. Put all your child's daily activities on a chart hung on his bedroom door. He gets a regular star (or ordinary sticker) for doing each activity when you remind him and a gold star (or special sticker) for doing each activity *without* needing to be reminded. Some parents use vouchers instead of stickers. When he has earned a certain number of vouchers, he can trade them in for a special reward.

Tutoring can be extremely helpful. It provides one-to-one attention and more easily addresses a child's other learning disabilities than can a single teacher in a crowded classroom. Tutoring also provides an opportunity for immediate feedback. Private tutoring can be expensive, but volunteer tutors are often available through community centers and literacy programs. Also, call your school to arrange an Individual Educational Assessment and Plan so your child gets all the school services to which he is entitled by law.

Biofeedback that focuses on reducing muscle tension in the forehead (EMG biofeedback) not only reduces muscle tension but seems to result in more relaxed behavior and improved attention.[87] EMG biofeedback also seems to improve language skills and helps children feel more in control of their behavior.[88] A comparison study showed that EMG biofeedback produces behavioral improvements that are comparable to Ritalin.[89] Biofeedback is especially helpful when used along with other behavioral therapies such as structured scheduling and rewards for relaxed behavior.[90] Don't expect results overnight. Biofeedback training takes at least six to eight weeks and possibly as long as six months with regular practice at home to achieve maximal effectiveness.

Relaxation training can be very helpful in teaching hyperactive children how to relax.[91] It can be done in groups or with an individual therapist. There are several types of relaxation training: progressive muscle relaxation, deep breathing, autogenic training (similar to self-hypnosis), and even yoga exercises. Relaxation training of any sort works best if the parents are involved and the child continues to practice regularly at home. Learning the relaxation skills can help improve the hyperactive child's self-esteem as well. (See Appendix B for relaxation techniques.)

Professional counseling by a psychologist or psychiatrist can be very helpful for a number of reasons. First, a mental health professional can help ensure an accurate diagnosis and can reassure you that your child is not suffering from another problem such as depression or anxiety, both of which are difficult to diagnose in young children. Second, a professional can provide more in-depth education about attention deficit disorder. Professionals can also provide additional behavioral, communication, and problem-solving strategies for dealing with the child's hyperactivity and self-esteem.[92] They can also help families deal with the stresses inherent in having a child labeled difficult, different, bad, or handicapped.

Last, but not least, seek the support of other parents and families with hyperactive children. You are not alone and you don't need to feel alone. National support groups, local support groups, and even Internet support groups are available.

Neurophysiological retraining therapies, which have *not* been proved effective in comparison studies, include patterning, visual retraining, and vestibular stimulation.

BIOMECHANICAL THERAPIES: MASSAGE

Although it makes sense that massage would help children learn to relax, it has not been evaluated for hyperactivity; I cannot recommend it on the basis of existing evidence.

BIOENERGETIC THERAPIES: ACUPUNCTURE

Although acupuncture has been tried for hyperactivity, it has not been evaluated in comparison studies. I cannot recommend acupuncture for this condition until more studies have been done.

WHAT I RECOMMEND FOR HYPERACTIVITY

PREVENTING HYPERACTIVITY

1. *Lifestyle—environment.* Do not smoke, drink, or use recreational drugs during pregnancy. Do not smoke around your child even after birth.

Keep your child's environment free of lead. Get professional help in removing lead paint. Keep your dust levels down with weekly damp-mopping and dusting.

2. *Lifestyle—exercise.* Protect your child from damaging head injuries by insisting he use proper protective equipment while bicycling, rollerblading, and engaging in contact sports. Always use seatbelts and child restraint devices when riding in a car.

Take your child to your health care provider to be evaluated for:

- hearing problems, vision problems, thyroid problems, breathing obstructions during sleep, lead poisoning, pinworms, allergies, eczema, and other health problems that may interfere with his learning and behavior.

Take your child to a clinical psychologist or educational specialist for:

- intelligence testing and testing for special learning problems, additional testing for emotional problems or stresses that may trigger problem behavior, additional advice about behavioral management, additional information about hyperactivity, and support.

Do fill out formal behavior rating scales such as the Conners parent and teacher scales. These will help you determine objectively how serious your child's symptoms are and how much he improves with various treatments.

TREATING HYPERACTIVITY

1. *Lifestyle—mind-body.* Accept your child as he is. Avoid blaming him or yourself. Be patient and persistent in reminding him of your expectations about his behavior.

Give your child clear structure. Make his routine consistent, orderly, low-key, and predictable. A wall chart of his daily activities may be very helpful. Have consistent meal time, bed time, chore time, study time, play time, etc. Also be consistent in terms of your expectations.

Break down tasks into smaller steps and make sure they're clear to him.

Reward him regularly for desired behavior. Lavishly praise positive behavior; he should get at least four compliments for every correction. Give feedback immediately. Use time out rather than physical punishment for discipline. Focus on building self-esteem.

Consider having him tutored in his most challenging subjects.

Teach your child relaxation skills. These can be breathing exercises, progressive muscle relaxation, yoga, or other methods. Reward your child for his efforts to practice relaxation skills.

Consider taking your child to a professional counselor for training in relaxation exercises or biofeedback. Support and encourage your child's practice at home.

Recognize that having a child with ADDH is stressful for most parents. Recognize your own needs for time out and breaks. Seek support. Regularly talk with your child's teachers and other parents whose children are hyperactive.

2. *Lifestyle—exercise.* Regular vigorous exercise and stretching relaxing exercise such as yoga or tai chi may be very helpful. Focus on sports with close interaction between child and coach (such as martial arts training or small teams).

3. *Lifestyle—environment.* Reduce excessive stimulation in your child's environment. Consider playing slow-tempo rather than fast-paced background music.

4. *Biochemical—medications.* In conjunction with your health care provider and your child's teacher, do a double-blind crossover trial of stimulant medication (such as Ritalin) vs. placebo to determine whether or not your child will benefit from medical treatment. If he does, make sure he gets it regularly and recheck his need for the same dose every year. Do *not* rely on sedative medications.

5. *Biochemical—nutritional supplements.* If you are interested in milder, natural stimulants, consider giving your child extra caffeine in the form of coffee, tea, or cola beverages. Remember that even natural stimulants can have side effects such as decreased appetite, feeling jittery, and insomnia.

RESOURCES

Books

Gordon, Michael. *Jumpin' Johnny Get Back to Work!*. GSI Publications, 1991.

Grant, Martin. *The Hyperactive Child*. Victor Books, 1992.

Kennedy, P., Terdal, L., Fusetti, L. *The Hyperactive Child Book*. St. Martin's Press, 1994.

Kurcinka, Mary. *Raising Your Spirited Child: A Guide for Parents Whose Child Is More Intense, Sensitive, Perceptive, Persistent, Energetic*. HarperCollins, 1992.

Moss, Robert A. *Why Johnnie Can't Concentrate: Coping with Attention Deficit Problems*. Bantam Books, 1990.

Silver, L.B. *The Misunderstood Child: A Guide for Parents of Learning Disabled Children*. 2nd ed. McGraw-Hill, 1992.

Support Groups

CHADD: Children and Adults with Attention Deficit Disorder
National Headquarters of CHADD
499 NW 70th Avenue, Suite 109
Plantation, FL 33317
1(800)233–4050 or 1(305)587–3700

Attention Deficit Disorder Association
Child and Family Center–Suite C14
801 Encino Place
Albuquerque, NM 87102
1(800)413–3902

National Attention Deficit Disorder Association
1(800)487–2282

Learning Disabilities Association
4156 Library Road
Pittsburgh, PA 15234

ERIC Clearinghouse on Disabilities and Gifted Education
Council for Exceptional Children
1920 Association Drive
Reston, VA 22091–1589
1(800)328–0272

Internet Newsgroups

alt.support.attn-deficit is supported by champion@well.sf.ca.us

FAQ (frequently asked questions) about ADDH is maintained by Frankk@canada.sun.com

For a parents' support group, send e-mail to: add-parents-request@mv.mv.com
In the body of the message, type: add-parents YOUR-NAME

22

JAUNDICE

Steven Chen called me just as the office opened one morning about his newborn daughter, Maggie. Steven's mother, Rose, was in town helping with the new baby and had noticed that Maggie was becoming jaundiced. Maggie had been a little yellow in the face the previous evening, but now the jaundice was noticeable on her chest as well. Rose had told Steven that when he was a baby, he also had jaundice and underwent many blood tests. She had been told to stop nursing him and he had had to stay three extra days in the hospital under special lights. Rose had continued to be extra cautious with his health throughout his infancy. She wanted him to make sure that his bad luck wasn't starting in his daughter.

Steven's wife, Bonnie, was much less concerned. Her pregnancy and delivery had been completely normal. Maggie had weighed 7 pounds, 6 ounces at birth and had gone home twenty hours after her delivery. After a day or so, Bonnie's milk supply had come in, and now she was nursing six or seven times a day. A public health nurse was coming to visit them later that afternoon for a routine checkup following the early discharge, but Rose was urging him to come in right away to get Maggie started on therapy. He felt trapped between his mother's concern and his wife's confidence, and he wanted some professional advice about what to do.

Jaundice is a yellow color of the skin and the whites of the eyes. It is caused by a buildup of the yellow pigment *bilirubin* in the blood. Bilirubin is a normal breakdown product of red blood cells. Every day about 1% of our red blood cells die and are replaced with new cells. Rather than waste the precious iron carried by the dead red blood cells, our body recycles it. Iron's carrier, hemoglobin, is easily replaced, so while the iron is saved, the old hemoglobin is broken down and metabolized in the liver.

The first by-product of hemoglobin breakdown is biliverdin, which is a green pigment. Biliverdin is transformed into bilirubin, which is yellow (see Figure 1). This is why bruises change color over several days from reddish-purple (fresh blood) to green (biliverdin) to yellow (bilirubin). The liver further metabolizes bilirubin to prepare it for excretion. If the liver gets backlogged, some of the bilirubin spills over into the bloodstream, turning the skin and the whites of the eyes yellow. Once the liver has finished with the bilirubin, it passes it on to the gallbladder (which functions as a kind of holding tank), which in turn passes it on to the intestines for excretion. Before it passes out of the body, it faces another hurdle. An enzyme in the intestines can free the bilirubin to be reabsorbed into the blood. The longer it takes for the intestinal contents to be excreted, the more chance there is for bilirubin to be reabsorbed into the blood. It then has to return to the liver to be reprocessed and resecreted into the gallbladder and intestines.

Where Bilirubin Comes from and Where it Goes

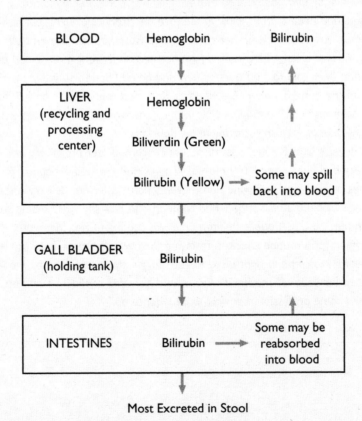

Most Excreted in Stool

Jaundice is not an illness; it is simply a sign that bilirubin has built up in the blood. Now that you know where bilirubin comes from, you can easily see the different reasons it can build up.

WHY BABIES HAVE HIGH
BILIRUBIN LEVELS

- Higher turnover of red blood cells
  — Fewer red blood cells needed after birth
  — Bruising during birth (forceps or vacuum-assisted deliveries)
  — Diseases such as Rh, ABO, genetically fragile blood cells
- Slower liver metabolism or excretion
  — Babies are slower than adults; genetic differences in metabolism
  — Diseases slow down liver metabolism
  — Diseases block secretion from the liver to the gallbladder
- Slower movement through the intestines, allowing time for reabsorption

First, babies have more red blood cells for their size than adults. They need more red blood cells to help carry oxygen before they are born. Once they are breathing on their own, babies do not need so many red blood cells. The extra blood is broken down, recycled, and metabolized to supply future needs. The extra work of breaking down blood cells creates a backlog for the liver, and some bilirubin tends to spill over into the blood. To compensate for thinner air (less oxygen), babies born at high altitudes have higher hemoglobin levels than their sea-level counterparts; babies born at high altitudes are also more likely to be jaundiced than babies born at sea level.[1] Babies who get bruises on their head from pushing during delivery (or from the forceps or vacuum extractors used to assist delivery) are also more likely to become jaundiced because of the extra work for the liver in breaking down the blood in the bruises.

Certain diseases can also cause a higher turnover of red blood cells. In the bad old days, the most feared cause of jaundice was *Rh disease*. Rh disease occurs when the mother has Rh-negative blood and the baby has Rh-positive blood. Rh-negative mothers make antibodies to the Rh factor in their baby's blood cells, causing them to break down rapidly, leading to anemia (a shortage of red blood cells), very high bilirubin levels, and sometimes death or permanent disability, called *kernicterus*. Fortunately, scientists found a way to block this reaction: Rhogam. Rhogam derails the destructive reaction against babies' blood so Rh-negative mothers can have normal, healthy Rh-positive babies without breaking down their red blood cells.

Rh disease was terrible and frightening. High bilirubin levels meant the possibility of kernicterus, which was to be avoided at all costs. The memory of kernicterus has been linked to jaundice in the minds of older parents and physicians alike. The fear of kernicterus is why many people fear jaundice. This is the main reason for the persistence of aggressive diagnostic studies and treatments. Kernicterus has virtually disappeared in full-term babies with the advent of Rhogam, so younger parents and physicians are less likely to panic at the first tinges of yellow skin.[2]

Other blood group differences (such as A, B, O, AB blood types) between mother and baby can also lead to breakdown of the baby's red blood cells. These differences are rarely as severe as Rh disease.[3] Mothers with type O blood are the most likely to have an immune reaction to their babies' blood. A mother who has O-positive blood makes antibodies to blood types A, B, and AB. If the mother has blood type O and the baby has one of the other types, it is called an *ABO setup* or *ABO incompatibility*. This is why physicians check mothers' blood types during pregnancy. If the mother is type O, her baby's blood type is checked soon after delivery. Careful monitoring and early treatment can prevent damage from ABO incompatibility.

Some *genetic diseases* cause fragile blood cells, which are easily destroyed. These diseases have long names such as glucose–6–phosphate dehydrogenase (G6PD) deficiency and hereditary spherocytosis. G6PD is common among Sephardic Jews, Greeks, and Nigerians and is rare in most other peoples.[4] Genetic diseases causing fragile blood cells are unusual in the United States and can be diagnosed with simple blood tests.

Even under normal circumstances, the newborn's liver has a lot of work to do metabolizing broken-down blood cells. However, babies' livers, like the rest of them, are not as speedy or developed as adults'. They just aren't as quick at the hemoglobin recycling program. Bilirubin builds up as it waits for the liver to metabolize and excrete it. Excessive bilirubin spills into the bloodstream and appears as yellow in the skin and eyes. Low-birth-weight and premature babies are more likely to become jaundiced because their livers are even less fully developed and ready to metabolize bilirubin than full-term babies.

The rate at which the liver gets up to full speed varies slightly from baby to baby and in different ethnic groups. Asian babies have a higher rate of jaundice than other races. Hispanic babies are more prone to jaundice than Caucasians, and African-American babies are least likely to be jaundiced.[5, 6] These differences are not just because it's easier to see jaundice in certain racial groups; the bilirubin levels really differ in different races. The differences are probably due to differences in liver metabolism in different racial groups. For unknown reasons, boys are more likely to become jaundiced than girls are.

If there are *liver diseases* such as hepatitis or other illness that slow down the liver, a backlog of bilirubin accumulates, spills into the blood, and causes jaundice. Any major illness, such as sepsis or meningitis, can also slow liver metabolism. Hypothyroidism slows metabolism throughout the body, including the liver. Blockages in the pathway from the liver to the intestines by way of the gallbladder can also lead to bilirubin buildup.

Once bilirubin has made it to the *intestines*, you'd think the way would be clear to excretion in the stool, but there is another hurdle before bilirubin's final exit. The longer the bilirubin stays in the intestines, the more chance it will be reabsorbed into the blood. From there it has to go back to the liver to be remetabolized and reexcreted. This process is known as the *entero* (intestinal) *hepatic* (liver) *circulation*.

Anything that slows down the intestines can slow the excretion of bilirubin and increase its enterohepatic circulation.[7] Everyone who has changed a newborn baby's diaper knows that newborn stool is thick and sticky. This thick, sticky stool, known as *meconium*, builds up before the baby is born. It needs to be cleared out before normal stool can pass. Every time a baby drinks milk (mom's or formula), the intestines contract, moving the meconium and stool along on their way out. The less often the intestines contract, the more slowly meconium is excreted. Babies who are constipated or who don't pass a stool within the first day of life are more likely to develop jaundice than those who pass a stool in the first twenty-four hours.[8]

The most common cause of slowed excretion is not consuming calories frequently. Formula-fed babies get a full complement of calories at every meal from day one. Breast-fed babies initially have smaller meals until their mother's milk supply comes in. The less frequently breast-fed babies nurse (for example, if the baby is fed only every four hours or if water is substituted for a feeding), the less the intestines are stimulated and the more slowly the mom's milk supply comes in. For reasons no one quite understands, there is an enzyme in some women's breast milk that enhances bilirubin's reabsorption from the intestines.[9] For these reasons, breast-fed babies are about twice as likely to be jaundiced as formula-fed babies.[10, 11] In the first few days of life, they tend to take in fewer calories,[12] have less stimulation to move their bowels, may have an extra enzyme that enhances bilirubin's reabsorption, and have fewer bowel movements. All of this increases the chances for intestinal bilirubin to be reabsorbed into the bloodstream.

In light of all the factors that can cause increased bilirubin, it's not surprising that so many babies become jaundiced. Jaundice is very common even among perfectly normal, healthy babies with perfectly normal deliveries. About 35% of babies have visible jaundice (bilirubin levels of 7.0 or higher), but only about 1 to 2 percent have bilirubin levels above 15 (the old treatment level),[13] and only 0.17% (about 2 per 1,000) reach bilirubin levels of 18 or more, the current treatment level for most full-term babies.

Jaundice typically becomes noticeable around the third day of life as the unneeded red blood cells break down and the liver falls behind on metabolizing them. Bilirubin levels are highest on the fourth or fifth day of life. They gradually decline over the next several days as the liver gets into gear and the mother's milk supply comes in. However, breast-fed babies can be jaundiced for several weeks.

Maggie had typical newborn jaundice. Because she was breast-feeding, Asian, and jaundice ran in her family, she was at higher risk than the average baby of being visibly jaundiced, but she was not necessarily in any danger.

TAKE YOUR CHILD TO A HEALTH CARE PROFESSIONAL FOR AN EVALUATION IF

- The mother is Rh-negative or blood type O
- Abnormal or fragile blood types or severe jaundice run in your family
- Jaundice is apparent within the first forty-eight hours of life
- The jaundice lasts longer than ten days
- The jaundice extends all the way down the chest to the belly button
- The baby is more than three weeks premature
- The baby develops dark urine or pale stools
- The baby acts sick, is very sleepy, or is not interested in nursing
- The baby has trouble breathing or is breathing very fast
- The baby vomits frequently
- You are concerned about the baby in any way

These could be signs that your baby has a serious problem or needs additional treatment.

Maggie first became visibly jaundiced when she was three days old. She had no signs of serious illness.

DOES JAUNDICE CAUSE BRAIN DAMAGE?

In the days when Rh disease caused devastating red blood cell destruction, anemia, and even death, autopsies showed bilirubin deposits (or staining) in the brain. This brain stain accompanied by either death or disability was attributed to bilirubin toxicity.[14] Many studies have looked at whether bilirubin causes brain damage in babies who are *not* affected by Rh disease.

In the short term, bilirubin does affect *hearing*. However, highly sensitive and complex tests show that these hearing deficits resolve as soon as the bilirubin levels drop to normal.[15] Many babies also become *sleepier* when they are jaundiced, but when the jaundice resolves, their sleepiness disappears.[16] Long-term follow-up studies of thousands of otherwise healthy, full-term babies have failed to demonstrate any long-term adverse effects of jaundice on IQ, development, or behavior.[17, 18] These studies do not necessarily apply to very premature babies or babies whose jaundice is due to other serious problems such as hypothyroidism. Sick babies tend to have persistent problems following high bilirubin levels, but among healthy premature babies, the long-term effects are not serious if the jaundice is monitored and treated.[19] Some researchers have even suggested that bilirubin itself is not toxic to the brain; in fact, it may be a protective antioxidant, which simply marks injured areas.[20] For the vast majority of babies, jaundice is not dangerous, not brain-damaging, and not life-threatening. On the other hand, for a few, it can be a sign of a serious problem that requires prompt medical attention. So how do you know whether or not to be worried?

DIAGNOSIS

Talking to parents about family history of jaundice, liver disease, blood problems, and how the baby is currently doing (feeding, sleeping, voiding, and stooling) can uncover other clues to the diagnosis. A physical examination can point the way to other conditions contributing to jaundice. The bilirubin level in the blood can be determined easily by a blood test. Along with a bilirubin level, your health care professional will also check the baby's and mother's blood type and may test the blood cells themselves. Depending on the results of the initial discussions, examination, and blood tests, other laboratory studies may be helpful.[21]

I reassured Steven that based on what I had observed while they were in the hospital, Maggie was probably fine, but I'd have the public health nurse check her and draw a blood sample that afternoon to measure her bilirubin level.

WHAT IS THE BEST WAY TO PREVENT AND TREAT JAUNDICE?

The best way to *prevent* jaundice is to feed your baby early and often—at least eight to ten times daily during the first week of life. Also, make sure your baby is exposed to some sunlight every day. Let's tour the Therapeutic Mountain to find out what works in treating jaundice; if you want to skip to my bottom-line recommendations, flip to the end of the chapter.

BIOCHEMICAL THERAPIES: MEDICATIONS, HERBS, NUTRITIONAL SUPPLEMENTS

Medications

Although a number of medications have been tested over the years, none has caught on as the primary treatment for newborn jaundice.

MEDICATIONS TO PREVENT OR TREAT JAUNDICE

- Activated charcoal (no longer used)
- Agar (rarely used as an adjunctive treatment)
- Phenobarbital (effective but has side effects)
- Protoporphyrin (experimental; high-risk groups only)

Activated charcoal binds bilirubin. It is not absorbed into the bloodstream but simply passes through the intestines, absorbing bilirubin and preventing its reabsorption. A Minneapolis study from the 1960s showed that feeding babies activated charcoal from the time they were four hours old decreased their bilirubin levels.[22] However, the charcoal was not very helpful if it was started later when the babies were actually jaundiced. Because it didn't have a big impact on eventual bilirubin levels, had to be given before anyone knew if a baby would be jaundiced or not, and was very messy, activated charcoal never really caught on.

Agar, an extract of seaweed, also absorbs bilirubin in the intestines and helps prevent its reabsorption. Different kinds of agar have varying abilities to absorb bilirubin. Most absorb far too little to affect newborn jaundice. Even the highest medical-grade agar is not very potent. In our 1988 study at Yale, we found that the most absorbent agar does lower bilirubin levels by a couple of points, but it probably has little long-term benefit for most babies.[23] High-grade agar is used in some medical centers as an adjunctive treatment to light therapy (see Lifestyle-Environment).

Phenobarbital, the well-known seizure medication, lowers bilirubin levels by revving up liver metabolism. Because of its sedative effects, it is rarely used nowadays to treat typical newborn jaundice.

Protoporphyrins are chemicals that look enough like hemoglobin to fool the enzymes that usually break it down, thereby blocking bilirubin breakdown. Giving an injection of protoporphyrin on the first day of life lowers bilirubin levels throughout the first weeks of life (when they are typically highest).[24] The trouble is that you have to know in advance which babies are going to have jaundice or a lot of babies end up being treated unnecessarily. Protoporphyrins also have side effects

such as skin irritation. They have not caught on as primary therapy for jaundice except in countries where there are many babies with fragile blood cells and very high rates of jaundice, but you may see them used more often in the United States in coming years.[25]

Several medications increase bilirubin levels. They are *contraindicated in newborns* because of the risk of shifting jaundice from a benign condition to a worrisome problem. For this reason, medications such as sulfa drugs and ceftriaxone are not used in babies less than two weeks old.

Herbs

No herbs have proven safe and effective in treating newborn jaundice. Herbal remedies traditionally used for adults with liver disease or jaundice (such as aloe vera gel, cascara bark, dandelion root, parsley, and milk thistle) have not been evaluated in babies. Several herbal remedies can actually *cause* liver damage and jaundice. For example, the Chinese herbs *Yin-Chen* and *Chuen-Lin,* which are traditionally used to treat jaundice, do lower bilirubin levels, but they do so by displacing bilirubin from the blood to other tissues such as the brain![26, 27] Other herbs, such as chaparral and *Jin Bu Huan* (Lycopodium serratum) actually cause liver toxicity and jaundice.[28, 29] Do *not* resort to herbal remedies to treat newborn jaundice.

Nutritional Supplements

Fearing that the baby might be dehydrated, many mothers give water supplements. Jaundice is not caused by dehydration. Water supplements have *no* benefit for bilirubin levels or the course of jaundice.[30]

Megadoses of niacin can actually cause jaundice in older children. *No* vitamins or mineral supplements have proved helpful in treating newborn jaundice.

LIFESTYLE THERAPIES: NUTRITION, ENVIRONMENT

Nutrition

Feeding Frequency

As they used to say about Chicago voting, do it early and often. Frequent feeding, especially for breast-fed babies, results in lower bilirubin levels and less jaundice.[31] Nursing mothers should breast-feed their newborn babies *at least eight to ten times daily*. Jaundiced babies may be a little sleepy, but make them nurse every two to three hours. Frequent nursing in the first week of life helps mothers produce more milk more quickly, stimulates the babies' intestines to move things along, and helps babies eliminate bilirubin.[32]

Formula Supplements

In the 1980s there was a raging controversy about whether or not to temporarily interrupt breast-feeding in jaundiced babies, feeding them formula instead. Supplementing a nursing baby's diet with formula in the first few days of life before mother's milk comes in can reduce bilirubin levels. However, supplementing with formula seriously sabotages the eventual success of breast-feeding.[33] Because jaundice is generally so benign and breast-feeding is so beneficial, most pediatricians no longer recommend formula supplements for jaundiced breast-fed babies. Rather than stopping or interrupting breast-feeding, I recommend that you nurse your baby more often, at least eight times daily. If your baby is very jaundiced and seems to be hungry even after she nurses, please discuss the situation with your health care professional or a lactation (breast-feeding) specialist.

Environment

Light therapy (phototherapy) is the mainstay of jaundice therapy. Phototherapy was discovered years ago by a nurse and physician in England who observed that infants whose cribs were near the window were much less likely to be jaundiced than babies whose cribs were far from the window. Astute pediatricians since then have noted that jaundice occurs more commonly during the fall and winter months when babies are exposed to less sunlight.[34]

In the presence of sunlight, our skin changes bilirubin to another form that is much more easily excreted by the kidneys. This change allows bilirubin to bypass the liver and intestines to be excreted directly without the possibility for reabsorption.

Phototherapy is recommended at different bilirubin levels depending on the baby's age.[35] These levels are a few points higher than in the 1970s and 1980s, which means that fewer babies need to be treated.[36] The changes were based on evidence that most jaundice is not harmful and many treatments are costly and distressing.[37] The changes mean that many parents can be spared the costs and concerns of repeated tests and hospitalization.[38]

BILIRUBIN LEVELS LEADING TO PHOTOTHERAPY AT DIFFERENT AGES

BABY'S AGE	BILIRUBIN LEVEL FOR PHOTOTHERAPY
Less than 24 hours old	Any jaundice
25–48 hours old	12–15 or higher
49–72 hours old	15–18 or higher
73 or more hours old	17–20 or higher

Maggie's bilirubin level was 15 at four days of age, and both she and her mother had type A

(Rh-positive) blood. The nurse encouraged more frequent breast-feeding and two outdoor strolls per day to help bring down the bilirubin. However, it was overcast and rainy, and Maggie never made it outside. When the nurse returned the following day, Maggie's bilirubin had climbed to 18 so she was started on home phototherapy.

Phototherapy can be provided by standard fluorescent lights, special blue-green spectrum fluorescent lights, halogen lights, or special blankets containing fiber-optic lights ("bili blankets"). These phototherapy devices are available only by prescription. The most potent type of light therapy is the combination of placing a baby on top of a bili blanket while shining standard fluorescent lights a few inches above the baby.[39, 40] Sandwiching the baby between lights is called double phototherapy. Single phototherapy, such as the bili blanket alone, is also effective, particularly with the newer high-intensity devices.[41] Bili blankets have two main advantages over conventional light therapy: (1) the baby's eyes do not need to be covered, and (2) the baby can be snuggled by the parents rather than being confined to an incubator.

Phototherapy has few side effects. Because of the light intensity with overhead light therapy, the baby's eyes need to be protected to prevent eye damage. The room temperature may need to be turned up if the baby is lying naked on top of a bili blanket. The baby may also need some extra milk to compensate for the increased water evaporation from the skin during phototherapy. Long-term follow-up studies have not indicated any increased risk of skin cancer or other skin diseases in children who received phototherapy as infants.

By the time Maggie was a week old, her bilirubin level was down to 13; she was nursing well, and her mother's milk was in. She had had a total of three blood tests, four nurse visits, five calls to the physician (me), two days of home phototherapy, and had avoided extra trips to the office and an expensive hospital stay. Her grandmother, Rose, was very impressed at the changes in health care in the twenty-three years since Steven was born. Bonnie was confident that Maggie was basically a healthy baby and was glad not to have had to make repeated trips to the clinic in the first week after her delivery.

BIOMECHANICAL THERAPIES: SURGERY

If a baby's bilirubin level climbs to potentially dangerous levels despite changes in feeding and despite light therapy (phototherapy), *blood transfusions* can be helpful. This is called an exchange transfusion because some of the baby's blood (containing high bilirubin levels) is removed and exchanged for low-bilirubin blood. This procedure must be done in the hospital by physicians who are very experienced in the care of newborn infants. It can rapidly reduce the blood levels of bilirubin,[42] but the potential for side effects is great: problems with circulation and with the balance of salt and water in the blood. Because of the risks of this potentially lifesaving procedure, most physicians use it as a last resort, relying on *frequent feeding* and *phototherapy* as the mainstays of treatment.

BIOENERGETIC THERAPIES: THERAPEUTIC TOUCH, PRAYER, HOMEOPATHY

Therapeutic Touch, Prayer

Prayer-healing has been shown to prevent red blood cells from breaking down in test tubes.[43, 44] Other studies have shown that prayer-healing and Therapeutic Touch can increase hemoglobin levels in healthy adults.[45] There are *no* studies specifically evaluating the effectiveness of prayer or Therapeutic Touch in treating jaundiced newborns, but because both therapies are safe, I encourage you to try them along with other therapies if they are consistent with your family's beliefs. (See Appendix B for more information on how to use Therapeutic Touch.)

Homeopathy

Traditional homeopathic remedies for adult jaundice include *Chelidonium* (celandine), *China officianalis* (or Chinchona officianalis), *Natrum Sulfuricum* (sodium sulfate). There is *no* scientific evidence that homeopathy is useful in treating newborn jaundice. I do *not* recommend it.

WHAT I RECOMMEND TO TREAT NEWBORN JAUNDICE

Take Your Child to a Health Care Professional for an Evaluation If

- The mother is Rh-negative or blood type O
- Abnormal or fragile blood types or severe jaundice run in your family
- Jaundice is apparent within the first forty-eight hours of life
- The jaundice lasts longer than ten days
- The jaundice extends all the way down to the chest or the belly button
- The baby is more than three weeks premature
- The baby develops dark urine or pale stools
- The baby acts sick, is very sleepy, or is not interested in nursing
- The baby has trouble breathing or is breathing very fast
- The baby is vomiting frequently
- You are concerned about the baby in any way

---

1. *Lifestyle—nutrition.* Feed your baby at least eight to ten times daily.

2. *Lifestyle—environment.* Take your baby outside to get some sunlight every day. Avoid the high-intensity hours between 10 a.m. and 2 p.m. If your baby develops higher bilirubin levels, use professional phototherapy.

3. *Biochemical—medications.* If you are Rh-negative, see your doctor about receiving Rhogam to prevent hemolytic disease in your baby. If your baby develops high bilirubin levels, consider prescription protoporphyrins or supplementary medical-grade agar.

4. *Bioenergetic—prayer, Therapeutic Touch.* If they are consistent with your family beliefs, try prayer and Therapeutic Touch to help stabilize hemoglobin and reduce bilirubin levels.

5. *Biomechanical—surgery.* If your baby develops very high bilirubin levels despite other therapies, she may need an exchange transfusion, exchanging her high-bilirubin blood for lower bilirubin blood.

23

RINGWORM AND OTHER FUNGAL INFECTIONS

Marie Washington brought in her sons, Irving and Michael, to be treated for ringworm and athlete's foot, which they'd picked up at school. Eight-year-old Irving had silver-dollar-size scaly patches on his arms and legs. Michael, the sixteen-year-old star of his basketball team, was complaining of itching and burning on his feet. He had cracked, peeling skin around his toes. Marie wanted to know:

- *if ringworm was really caused by worms,*
- *if only athletes could get athlete's foot,*
- *what was the best way to treat both boys?*

Despite its name, ringworm is caused by a fungus, not worms. Ringworm (*tinea corporis*) is the most common fungal infection in children over a year old. The same types of fungus that cause ringworm also cause infections on the feet (athlete's foot, or *tinea pedis*), in the groin (jock itch, or *tinea cruris*), and in the scalp (*tinea capitis*). *Tinea* simply means fungal infection. The second part of each medical name refers to the body part affected (*capitis* = head, *corporis* = body, *pedis* = feet). Several types of fungus cause infections in humans. They have long, poetic names such as *Trichophyton*, *Microsporum*, and *Epidermophyton*.

Tinea capitis (ringworm of the scalp) is usually caused by *Trichophyton tonsurans* and less commonly by *Microsporum canis*. Although most fungal infections are passed from person to person, these two can be caught from dogs or cats. These fungi can cause big pimplelike swellings, mushy areas, and crusting on the scalp, called a *kerion*. Kerions can look so serious they have fooled experienced doctors into thinking that something other than a simple fungal infection was responsible, leading to costly treatment errors and even hospitalization.[1] Alternatively, the fungi can simply cause the scalp hairs to break off, resulting in bald patches with dots of broken hairs, called *black dot ringworm*.

Athlete's foot is incredibly common. In one study of marathon runners, about 11% had symptoms, though twice as many carried the ringworm fungus.[2] This finding points out the need for careful hygiene in the locker room. Even if your buddy doesn't have any symptoms, he could still be carrying the fungus that will make you miserable. Athlete's foot occurs even among those whose only physical exertion is Monday morning quarterbacking; it occurs in preadolescents as well as high school athletes.[3]

Fungal infections can mimic several other skin conditions such as eczema, impetigo, insect bites, plain old dandruff, and allergic reactions. Special tests may be needed to make the right diagnosis. Some fungi glow under black lights; your doctor may use a special light (known as a Wood's lamp) to see if the infected skin glows in the dark. Alternatively, she may scrape a tiny bit of skin onto a slide and examine it under a microscope to be sure it's a fungus and not an imitator. Sometimes a culture is necessary to be certain. Culture results can take several weeks. Most folks are eager to take action much sooner, so you may start therapy even without these diagnostic tests.

WHAT'S THE BEST WAY TO TREAT FUNGAL INFECTIONS?

All therapies take several weeks to eradicate fungus; there are no quick cures. Let's tour the Therapeutic Mountain to find out what works best. If you want to skip to my bottom-line recommendations, flip to the end of the chapter.

BIOCHEMICAL THERAPIES: MEDICATIONS, HERBS, NUTRITIONAL SUPPLEMENTS

Medications

Medical treatments are similar for most fungal infections *except* for those affecting the scalp. Scalp infections require medication that reaches deep beneath the skin surface because they usually involve the deep hair shafts. Most other fungal infections on the skin respond to medicated creams.

NONPRESCRIPTION MEDICATIONS FOR FUNGAL INFECTIONS

- Undecylenic acid: (Desenex, Pedi-Dri, Cruex)
- Miconazole: (Micatin, Monistat)
- Clotrimazole: (Lotrimin, Mycelex)
- Tolnaftate: (Tinactin, Desenex, and others)
- Selenium sulfide shampoo: (Selsun and others)

Undecylenic acid (Desenex and other brands) has been used to treat athlete's foot for over thirty years. The most commonly recommended antifungal agents in our clinic are undecylenic acid, clotrimazole, and miconazole because they have proven safety and effectiveness and are inexpensive. They are applied twice daily until after the rash has been gone for at least one week to ensure that all the fungi have been eliminated. I prefer creams and lotions to powders and sprays because they tend to stay on better, but you can experiment to find out what works best for your child.

Tolnaftate (Tinactin) is another effective antifungal medication. It is traditionally used to treat athlete's foot and jock itch, and it is effective against ringworm, too. Tolnaftate is also applied twice daily. Improvement is usually apparent within ten days, although complete cure may take a month or more.

Selenium sulfide shampoo (Selsun, Exsel) is an adjunctive therapy to treat fungal infections in the scalp. It does not eradicate the infection, but it helps prevent it from spreading to others.[4] Nonprescription strength (1%) selenium sulfide shampoo appears to be as effective as the more expensive 2.5% prescription formulations.[5]

PRESCRIPTION MEDICATIONS FOR FUNGAL INFECTIONS

- Griseofulvin (Fulvicin, Grisactin, Grifulvin V)
- Imidazoles: ketoconazole (Nizoral), oxiconazole (Oxistat), Econazole (Spectazole)
- Allylamines: terbinafine (Lamisil) and naftifine (Naftin)

For fungal infections in the scalp (*tinea capitis*), the oral medicine *griseofulvin* is the treatment of choice because of its low toxicity and low cost. It must be taken daily for at least six to eight weeks to eradicate fungal infections. Like penicillin, griseofulvin is derived from our old friend, the *Penicillium* mold. It is one of the rare medicines that actually works better if it is taken with food, especially fatty foods. Try giving it to your child with a glass of whole milk.

Ketoconazole is a unique prescription antifungal medication that kills yeast and fungus throughout the body. However, it can cause an upset stomach, suppress the body's own production of steroid and sex hormones, and interfere with the actions of several other medications.[6] It is *not* approved for use in children less than two years old. *Econazole* works quickly; it is effective within two weeks against ringworm and within one month against athlete's foot. *Oxiconazole* is another effective antifungal medication that is very safe. All of the prescription imidazole medications are effective, but they are significantly more expensive than their nonprescription relatives.

The *allylamines,* terbinafine and naftifine, are the newest and most effective antifungal medications. *Terbinafine* (Lamisil) is very effective in treating even difficult cases of athlete's foot and tinea capitis.[7, 8, 9, 10] However, terbinafine in large doses has been blamed for causing cancer in laboratory animals, and it has *not* been approved for use by children under twelve years of age. *Naftifine* is another very powerful antifungal medication for treating athlete's foot.[11] Like all fungal medicines, it can cause burning and stinging when applied to already irritated skin.

The most cost-effective medical approach to the typical fungal infection of the skin is to start with an inexpensive but effective nonprescription medication (such as miconazole); if there is no improvement after a month of twice daily use, see your physician about a more expensive and powerful prescription medication.[12]

Herbs

Tea tree oil has antibacterial and antifungal properties and has been recommended as a treatment for fungal infections. In an Australian study it was compared to tolnaftate for the treatment of athlete's foot. Although patients reported improved symptoms with both preparations, tea tree oil failed to kill the fungi.[13] Tea tree oil is safe when applied to nonirritated skin. You can try it if you are reluctant to use medication. As with any treatment, if the skin becomes more irritated, stop using it.

Garlic extracts have proven antifungal effects in test-tube studies.[14, 15, 16] However, they have not yet been tested against fungal skin infections in children. Garlic poultices can cause burns and severe skin irritation if left on too long.

Some herbalists recommend teas to help the immune system fight fungal infections. Teas reputed to have this effect are burdock, cleavers, dandelion root, echinacea (also available as a tincture), nettles, peppermint, and red clover. Teas used as washes for fungal infections are agrimony, burdock, and marigold. There are no studies evaluating the effectiveness of any of these teas or tinctures as treatments for fungal infections. I do *not* recommend them.

Preliminary studies in Mexico have identified an herb that appears to be as effective as miconazole in treating ringworm.[17] This herb, Solanum chrysotrichum, is not yet widely available in the United States. It would be premature to recommend it before further long-term studies of its safety and effectiveness have been completed.

Several essential oils have shown effectiveness against fungal infections in guinea pigs and test-tube studies: Artemisia nelagrica, Artemisia afra, Caesulia axillaris, Chenopodium ambrosioides, Cymbopogon citratus (lemon grass), and Mentha arvensis.[18, 19] These studies are promising, but until results are duplicated in human beings, I do *not* recommend these herbs as proven remedies for fungal infections.

On the Indian subcontinent there is very little tinea capitis (ringworm of the scalp) and a high use of hair dressings containing vegetable oil. A recent test-tube study showed that the most popular Indian hair oils (mustard oil, coconut oil, and Amla oil) had antifungal properties.[20] Although these results are too preliminary to claim that vegetable oils are effective treatments for human fungal infections, they are intriguing. These vegetable oils are safe and inexpensive and may be worth trying as preventive therapy, but do *not* forsake medications that have proven effectiveness for treating fungal infections that have already taken hold in the scalp.

Lemon juice and cider vinegar have both been recommended as ways to make the skin more acid (lower pH) and less hospitable for fungi. There are no scientific studies documenting their effectiveness in treating children with fungal infections, but they are inexpensive and safe. They may be worth trying as preventive therapies for athlete's foot.

Nutritional Supplements

Vitamin C in powder or crystal form has been recommended as topical treatment for fungal infections of the skin, but there are no studies evaluating its use.

LIFESTYLE THERAPIES: EXERCISE, ENVIRONMENT

Exercise

Exercise common sense. If your child is in gym class at school and takes showers in a common area, make sure he has shower sandals to keep his feet out of direct contact with the inevitable fungus on the floor. If your child has an infection, it's even more important to wear shower shoes to prevent the infection from spreading to others. Have him dry his feet well after a shower to make them less hospitable for fungi. After showering is the perfect time to apply antifungal medication. Even if your child doesn't have athlete's foot, he may want to dust his feet with anti-fungal medication several times a week in the locker room to prevent picking up a case.

Environment

Fungi love to live in warm, damp environments. High-top sneakers are perfect breeding grounds for athlete's foot fungus. If your child is prone to athlete's foot, have him forget the high-tops for a while and go with more breathable shoes such as sandals or thongs when he's not playing basketball. It takes a day or so for regular shoes to dry out from normal sweat. Frequent changes of shoes and socks (daily or twice daily) help reduce moisture; try not to wear the same shoes two days in a row. Children *can* catch fungal infections from pets and farm animals.

If your pets or livestock have skin problems, have them checked by your veterinarian and treated promptly to reduce your child's chances of catching a fungal infection.

BIOMECHANICAL THERAPIES

None of these therapies has scientifically proved benefit in treating children with ringworm or other fungal infections. I do *not* recommend them.

BIOENERGETIC THERAPIES: HOMEOPATHY

Commonly used homeopathic remedies for fungal infections include *Calcarea, Dulcamara, Graphites, Sepia, Sulfur,* and *Tellurium.* None has proved effectiveness.

WHAT I RECOMMEND FOR FUNGAL INFECTIONS

PREVENTING FUNGAL INFECTIONS

1. *Lifestyle—environment.* Use good hygiene. Prevent athlete's foot by using shower shoes, sandals, or flip-flops in the gym showers and locker room. Keep the feet clean and dry. Avoid high-top sneakers. Change socks and shoes frequently. If your pets or livestock develop skin problems, have them evaluated and treated promptly to prevent possible spread to your children.

2. *Biochemical—herbs.* Consider rinsing your child's feet in lemon juice or vinegar after showering in public places to make the skin more acidic and less hospitable to fungi.

See Your Health Care Provider If

- You suspect a fungal infection of the scalp. This requires prescription medication. It may also benefit from regular shampooing with selenium sulfide shampoo.
- The rash is not improving after ten days of therapy or is getting worse with home treatment.
- The rash is spreading.
- The rash involves the toenails or fingernails.

TREATING FUNGAL INFECTIONS

1. *Biochemical—medications.* Treat twice daily with nonprescription antifungal medications containing clotrimazole (Lotrimin, Mycelex), miconazole (Monistat), tolnaftate (Tinactin), or undecylenic acid (Desenex, Cruex, Caldesene). Continue treatment for at least one week after all symptoms have resolved to make sure the fungi have been eradicated.

2. *Biochemical—herbs.* Consider tea tree oil applied to the rash twice daily for four weeks.

3. *Biochemical—medications.* If the rash is not gone within a month with nonprescription treatments, see your health care provider to evaluate the need for prescription medication.

24

SLEEP PROBLEMS

- GETTING YOUR INFANT TO SLEEP THROUGH THE NIGHT
- GETTING YOUR TODDLER TO SLEEP
- NIGHTMARES AND NIGHT TERRORS
- INSOMNIA

"Our baby is four months old and still waking up to nurse at 2 a.m. and 5 a.m. When will he outgrow the need for middle of the night feeds so we can get some sleep? He still sleeps with us. Is that OK? Will giving him rice cereal at bedtime help him sleep better?"

"Our three-year-old is driving us nuts. Every night it's the same thing. We put her to bed, and then she wants a glass of water; next it's a story; by that time she has to go to the bathroom again. We get her in bed and five minutes later she's up again; if we don't read her another story, she starts crying. Bedtime started out as a fifteen-minute process, and now it takes an hour. How can we get back to a reasonable routine?"

"Our four-year-old has been waking up a few hours after we put him to bed, screaming like someone is killing him. We rush into the room to find him sitting up in bed, staring blankly. He doesn't seem to know we're there and won't talk about the bad dream. In the morning, he doesn't even seem to remember it. This has happened several times. Should we take him to a psychiatrist?"

One of the most common and frustrating problems parents face is getting their children to sleep through the night. Babies' sleep patterns simply are not like adults'. They learn sleep and wakefulness cycles just as they learn hunger cycles, bladder control, language, and walking. Children's sleeping patterns change throughout infancy and early childhood, from initially waking every few hours to nurse, to sleeping several hours at a time, to intermittently waking again in later infancy, to a full night's sleep plus naps at toddler age, to adolescent sleep patterns that are very similar to adult sleep. It takes the average two-month-old over twenty-five minutes to fall asleep, while the average nine-month-old needs just over fifteen minutes to drift off. Most infants awaken every few hours to nurse until they are three to four months old. By six months of age, over 80% of infants sleep at least five hours in a row.

TYPICAL SLEEP PATTERNS

AGE	TOTAL SLEEP	NAPS
Newborn	16–17 hours	a.m. and p.m.
6–12 months	14–15 hours	a.m. and p.m.
Toddlers	12 hours	p.m.
School-age	10 hours	None
Older school-age	8 hours	None
Teenagers	8–10 hours	None

Almost all children give up naps by first grade; some outgrow naps by the time they are three years old. Adolescents often nap again and sleep more during periods of intense growth and maturation. During illnesses and recovery from injury, children sleep more. Each child is different.

The two main phases of sleep are rapid-eye-movement (REM) (dream) sleep and non-REM sleep. Non-REM sleep is quiet sleep during which the child moves from wakefulness into deeper sleep with slower brain waves and less physical movement. During deepest sleep the brain waves are very slow. This is when growth hormone secretion reaches its peak. Infants can enter REM sleep practically immediately after falling asleep. Older children sleep quietly (non-REM) for about seventy to ninety minutes before REM sleep starts. During REM sleep the child dreams, moves about, and may appear restless. Following REM sleep the child may briefly waken before returning to quiet sleep and repeating the cycle. A teenager who sleeps seven and a half to eight hours goes through about four or five repetitions of this cycle every night.

If you think your child has sleep difficulties, you are not alone. Neither is your child. In a survey of nearly 1,000 school children, 43% were reported to have some kind of sleep difficulty: 14% had a hard time falling asleep or awoke in the middle of the night at least once a week; 15% had frequent nightmares or night terrors; 5% walked in their sleep. Other problems included bed-wetting, teeth grinding, and talking during sleep. In a survey of toddlers' parents, approximately 30% reported problems at least three nights a week in getting their child to sleep.[1] Children's sleep problems frequently disrupt parents' sleep, resulting in fatigue, frustration, anger, and guilt.

WHAT INTERFERES WITH NORMAL SLEEP

- Illness, pain, allergies
- Anxiety, depression, tension, or stress
- Change in routine, travel
- Being overtired
- Difficult temperament
- Caffeine-containing beverages or foods
- Medications and alcohol

Ear infections are perhaps the best example of a *painful illness* that awakens children in the middle of the night. Diabetes and bladder infections increase urination and thereby increase nighttime awakening. The pain or irritation of teething or itchy rashes can keep a child from a sound sleep. Breathing problems from a stuffy nose or asthma can interfere with sleep, too. *Allergy* to cow's milk often interferes with sleeping as well.[2] There is at least one study showing that sleep dramatically improves when allergic children stop drinking milk and deteriorates when milk is reintroduced.[3] (See Chapter 4, Allergies.)

Like adults, children can suffer from *stress, anxiety, depression, or tension* that keeps them awake.[4] Preschool-age children may be concerned about parental disputes or disruptions in normal household routines. School-age children and adolescents may worry about upcoming tests, peer pressure, dates, or scary movies. Major catastrophes and natural disasters often trigger nightmares. Following the 1989 San Francisco earthquake nightmares were eight times more frequent among San Francisco students than among students living in Tucson, Arizona.[5] Try to keep evening time quiet and relaxed. Discuss family disagreements during the day when coping and communication are at their peak rather than before bed.

Paradoxically, being *overtired* is a common cause of sleep problems. When a child becomes overtired, he compensates for his fatigue by increasing levels of stress hormones (such as epinephrine) that keep him awake. It takes a certain calm focus to allow the events of the day to slide away and allow sleep to take over.

Infants and toddlers who have trouble falling asleep or who waken frequently in the middle of the night are more likely to be viewed as having *difficult temperaments* than are children who sleep soundly.[6, 7] Children with persistent sleep problems are also more likely to have temper tantrums and other behavior problems.[8]

It is difficult to sort out whether less adaptable children are more likely to have sleep problems or whether children who awaken their parents in the middle of the night are labeled as troublesome. It is interesting that children with attention deficit disorder and hyperactivity waken frequently in the middle of the night and also suffer more commonly than other children from night sweats and bed-wetting.[9] Behavior problems don't necessarily stop the minute a child gets into bed.

What is hopeful is that sleep patterns can be substantially improved with a few straightforward measures. In a study of breast-fed infants and their parents, one group was taught how to train their infant to sleep through the night; the other group was put on a waiting list and not given any special instructions on infant sleep until the baby was eight weeks old. Those who were taught the techniques were able to train their infants to sleep better through the night (100% were sleeping at least five consecutive hours by the time they were eight weeks old compared to only 23% of control group infants). The trained group also rated their babies' temperaments as significantly easier than the untrained group whose babies were still waking frequently.[10] Parents who are taught to train their infants to sleep through the night also report an increased sense of competence as parents.[11] This study raises the possibility that the advantages of early sleep training may extend beyond peaceful parental slumber to benefit infant temperament and parental confidence.

Adults are not the only ones who are kept awake by *caffeine*. Its stimulant effects are found in tea, cola, and chocolate as well as coffee. Common cold medications and herbal remedies also contain potent stimulants: ephedrine, pseudoephedrine, phenylpropanolamine, and ephedra (*Ma Huang*). If you are nursing your baby, check with your health care professional before taking nonprescription cold medications because some of them end up in breast milk and may keep your baby awake. *Alcohol* is another common ingredient in many nonprescription cold remedies. While alcohol may initially seem to knock your child out, it actually induces a relatively light sleep, a full bladder, and a rebound awakening after a few hours—not good therapy for a child suffering from a cold.

Infants who are put into bed after they have fallen asleep or who fall asleep in the presence of a parent are more likely to awaken in the middle of the night (and wake their parents) than infants who fall asleep by themselves in their crib.[12] This is a strong argument for putting your child down to sleep while he is still awake. If your child is already used to falling asleep while you are holding him or rocking him, try making the change first at nap time. When he learns to fall asleep on his own at nap time, try putting him down at night while he is still awake. By learning to fall asleep on his own at nap time and bedtime, he can later put himself to sleep when he awakens in the middle of the night without waking you.

Nightmares are most common between the ages of three and six years old. Children who awaken with nightmares are generally fully awake, can be comforted by parents, and can tell their parents details about the bad dream. Children who suffer from frequent nightmares are not maladjusted, more anxious, or under more stress than children who don't have nightmares as frequently.[13, 14] Nightmares are not due to behavior problems, seizures, or brain wave abnormalities.[15] They are simply bad dreams. Adults who suffer from nightmares tend to be more sensitive and creative than those who aren't beset by troubling images at night.[16] Children, of course, have more vivid imaginations than adults and have active fantasies about imaginary friends, ghosts, monsters, and all kinds

of creatures. It's no surprise that many of them turn up in dreams. Nightmares can be inspired by anything from television violence to shadows cast by a night light to actual scary experiences.

FREQUENT NIGHTMARE TOPICS

- Scary animals
- Monsters
- Strangers attacking or chasing them
- Being abandoned or helpless in a strange place
- Being shot (more common with increasing violence in media and daily life)

Night terrors occur most commonly in children between the ages of one and four years old. Unlike dreams or nightmares, they do not occur during REM sleep. Rather, they occur in the deepest stages of sleep. Night terrors tend to occur within the first two hours of sleep, whereas nightmares occur during dream sleep in the later part of the night (between 3 a.m. and 6 a.m.). During a night terror, the child utters terrifying screams, sits bolt upright, and stares ahead with a glassy gaze. His eyes are open and he appears to be awake, but he does not notice or respond to his parents. This is very unnerving for the parent who is trying to comfort an obviously distraught and unresponsive child. Often the child doesn't even recall the incident the following morning. The episodes typically last fewer than fifteen minutes. Children who start having night terrors before the age of four tend to have more frequent episodes than children who start having them later. No one knows why some children have night terrors and why they usually outgrow them by school age. They tend to run in families and they are *not* signs of a psychiatric problem.[17] However, if your child has frequent night terrors (more than twice a week), see your health care professional for advice. Some prescription medications are helpful for this condition.

WHAT IS THE BEST WAY TO TREAT SLEEP PROBLEMS?

The best treatments for all children's sleep problems are to:

- prevent them in the first place
- treat the underlying problem if there is one
- reassure yourself and your child that good sleep is attainable
- use proper sleep hygiene, such as bedtime routines, calm, quiet, and appropriate parental responses to specific sleep problems

Lifestyle therapies are the best bet. Let's tour the Therapeutic Mountain to make sure we cover all the bases. If you want to skip to my bottom-line recommendations, flip to the end of the chapter.

BIOCHEMICAL THERAPIES: MEDICATIONS, HERBS, NUTRITIONAL SUPPLEMENTS

I do *not* recommend biochemical therapies for children who simply don't want to go to bed when their parents want them to sleep. Nor are they appropriate therapy for infants who still waken in the middle of the night to nurse or feed. The only time I recommend such therapies is when children have undergone a significant life change or disruption in their sleep-wake cycle, such as those who have been in a natural disaster, witnessed a death, traveled across three or more time zones, or are hospitalized. Even under these

circumstances, biochemical remedies should supplement, not replace, parental reassurance and lifestyle therapies. Do *not* use any medication, herbal remedy, or nutritional supplement daily for more than five days without consulting your health care professional. Tolerance to sleeping medications begins to develop within a week, and higher doses may be needed to achieve the same effect.

Medications

The medication most commonly recommended for children suffering from temporary sleep disruption is diphenhydramine (Benadryl). Benadryl is an antihistamine that reduces itching and allergy symptoms; its main side effect is drowsiness. Benadryl given thirty minutes before bedtime significantly reduces the time it takes to fall asleep and decreases episodes of awakening in the middle of the night, but some children feel drowsy and "out of it" the next day.[18] These hangover effects typically disappear within a few days of using the medication regularly.

MEDICATIONS USED FOR CHILDREN'S SLEEP

Antihistamines: diphenhydramine (nonprescription Benadryl), hydroxyzine (prescription Vistaril), trimeprazine (prescription Temaril)

Benzodiazepines: diazepam (Valium), lorazepam (Ativan), alprazolam (Xanax)—all prescription only

Sedatives/barbiturates: phenobarbital, secobarbital, chloral hydrate, and others—all prescription only

Benadryl may be helpful for children who have undergone a significant disruption in their lives or who have traveled across several time zones. Many parents take Benadryl along on cross-country trips just in case. Some children have contrary reactions to Benadryl; they become more aroused and excitable. It's impossible to predict in advance if your child will react this way. Benadryl is very safe when taken as recommended.

Vistaril (hydroxyzine) is a prescription antihistamine similar to Benadryl. It is frequently used to help hospitalized children (and adults) fall asleep. Another prescription antihistamine, *trimeprazine* (Temaril), was studied in three-year-old children with sleep problems. The usual doses were not very helpful, but higher doses (three times the normal antihistamine dose) knocked the toddlers out and kept them out through the night.[19] The medication is not a long-term cure, but it has few side effects. Most physicians prefer behavioral (lifestyle) changes rather than relying on antihistamines for typical toddler sleep problems.

Stronger sleeping medications are available with a prescription from your health care professional. I do *not* recommend sleeping pills for children unless you have tried safe home remedies without success and you have your child thoroughly evaluated by a professional. Many sleeping pills make children feel groggy or hungover the next day. Some can lead to addiction. If children take them for several days in a row, they begin to depend on them to be able to fall asleep.

The most commonly prescribed sleep medications for adults are benzodiazepines such as *Valium, Ativan, and Xanax* and sedatives such as *phenobarbital and secobarbital.* The benzodiazepines help reset the biological clock for those suffering from jet lag. Benzodiazepines also suppress deep sleep, the time when sleep terrors are most likely to occur. Valium and imipramine, a medication commonly used to treat bed-wetting (enuresis), are also useful in treating children suffering

from night terrors. I do *not* routinely recommend them because of the risk of serious side effects, because safe alternatives (such as hypnosis) are available, and because most children outgrow night terrors without any treatment.

Herbs

Traditional folk medicine has long relied on herbs as sleep aids. Most are given as tea (see Appendix A). In Europe, a small fancy pillow known as a *sleep pillow* is tucked under a sleepless child's regular pillow. A sleep pillow filled with a combination of dried sedative herbs makes a lovely, aromatic gift. Alternatively, sedative herbs can be added to the child's evening bath to help him relax and feel drowsy before bed.

HERBS TRADITIONALLY USED FOR INSOMNIA

- Balm mint (also known as lemon balm) and catnip
- Chamomile
- Hops
- Lavender
- Passion flower, skullcap, and valerian
- Saint-John's-wort

Balm, also known as *lemon balm* because of its refreshing fragrance, is included in herbal tea blends used to treat insomnia, anxiety, and "nerves." It is also commonly used to calm an upset stomach. Balm is often cultivated in household gardens because it attracts bees. Balm leaves are also tasty additions to summer salads. *Catnip* is from the same family of plants. Not only is it attractive to cats, it is also said to be soothing and sedating, allaying anxiety and preventing nightmares.

Chamomile flowers are among the safest and most widely used herbal remedies for children. Chamomile is calming and soothing (and was given to Peter Rabbit following a harrowing escapade in Mr. MacGregor's garden). It is said to help prevent nightmares. Chamomile is widely available in the commercial herbal teas found in your local grocery store. It has a pleasant aroma and taste. It is easily grown in the garden and can often be found growing wild along roadsides.

Hops are proven sedatives that have been traditional sleep remedies as least as far back as Roman times.[20] They are genetically related to the Cannabis (marijuana) family of plants. Hops are traditional ingredients in European sleep pillows, having been used by King George III to cure his insomnia. Tea made from hops can also be added to bath water for a relaxing soak. Hops are best used soon after they are picked. Within a year after drying, they lose 90% of their effectiveness.

Lavender flowers are often included in bedtime herbal tea blends. A few drops of essential oil of lavender can also be added to the child's evening bath or to a massage oil to help him relax. Lavender has a very pleasant, soothing scent. *Passion flower* is a common sleep remedy that is included in several herbal tea blends. Its name is not derived from its use as an aphrodisiac but from the flower's imagined resemblance to the crucifixion (the passion of Christ). There are *no* studies evaluating its safety or effectiveness in children.

Despite its creepy name, *skullcap* is a common ingredient in herbal bedtime teas. It is a traditional sedative that was initially used to treat rabies! A potential problem with skullcap is liver toxicity.

The name *valerian* comes from the Latin word *valere*, to be strong or well. Valerian root was used as a sedative in ancient Greece, Rome, China, and Persia and was also used by American Indians. Studies in adults have shown that valerian decreases the length of time it takes to fall asleep and improves the quality of sleep without leaving that drowsy morning-after feeling that is common with many sleep medications.[21] In adults suffering from insomnia, it improves the quality of sleep and reduces nighttime awakening as effectively as several prescription sleep medicines.[22] One drawback of valerian is its unpleasant scent, which can be described as musky, stale, or like a plant on which a dog has relieved himself. Phew! A more serious drawback is valerian's reportedly toxic effect on the liver.[23] There is substantial variation in the amount of the sedative compounds in different varieties and preparations of valerian.[24]

The leaves and flowers of *Saint-John's-wort* were used in ancient Greece and remain one of the most commonly recommended herbal remedies for a variety of sleep disturbances, including nightmares. Saint-John's-wort is also believed to balance the central nervous system in cases of depression and "nerves" and is an excellent choice for children whose sleep is disturbed due to a recent loss, such as the death of a grandparent or pet. Saint-John's-wort is a common wildflower, whose yellow blossoms burst into bloom about the time of the summer solstice near Saint John's Day. One potential side effect of Saint-John's-wort is photosensitivity; that is, when a child takes tea made from this plant, his skin may become extra sensitive and he may be easily sunburned.

Combinations of the above herbs are widely available in commercial teas, such as Nighty Night, SleepyTime, Surrender to Sleep, Tension Tamer, Calming Tea, and others. This is certainly a convenient way to go because the herbs have been selected, combined, and are available in easy-to-use teabags. No matter what blend you choose, *avoid herbal teas before bed if your child is prone to bed-wetting*. Also avoid stimulating herbs before bedtime: coffee, tea (with caffeine), cocoa, chocolate, cola, ephedra (*Ma Huang*), guarana, and ginseng.

Nutritional Supplements

The amino acid *L-tryptophan* is an effective sleep promoter in both adults and children.[25, 26, 27] It was one of the most popular supplements sold until it was banned in 1989 due to its reported association with the deadly disease eosinophilia myalgia syndrome (EMS). Before it was banned, L-tryptophan was linked to over 5,000 cases of EMS, including twenty-seven deaths. Because all of the EMS cases could be traced to the L-tryptophan from a single manufacturer, a search was made for possible contaminants. It turns out that the problem was probably *not* due to L-tryptophan but to a contaminant introduced in the manufacturing process. Nevertheless, since the EMS outbreak, L-tryptophan supplements are no longer available in the United States.

L-tryptophan is a precursor to the brain chemical serotonin, which plays an important role in regulating sleep and minimizing depression. Studies in the 1960s and 1970s showed that L-tryptophan effectively reduces the time it takes for adults to fall asleep. In a controlled study, supplemental L-tryptophan also helped infants fall asleep faster.[28] Breast milk and cow's milk contain L-tryptophan. Rather than giving your child supplements, I recommend that you breast-feed or give your child a glass of milk thirty to sixty minutes before bedtime. Be sure he brushes his teeth after the milk to reduce the risk of cavities!

Calcium and magnesium supplements are frequently recommended to adult sufferers of insomnia. However, there are *no* scientific studies evaluating the usefulness of such supplements in children. Children generally get all the calcium they need from milk. If your child does not nurse or drink milk, make sure he gets plenty of calcium from other foods such as yogurt, tofu, fish, and calcium-supplemented soy milk and orange juice.

Vitamin B12 supplements have been reported to be useful in a few adults and teenagers suffering from sleep problems,[29, 30] but vitamin supplements have not been compared with other therapies as sleep aids for children. I do *not* recommend them.

LIFESTYLE THERAPIES: NUTRITION, EXERCISE, ENVIRONMENT, MIND-BODY

The primary treatment for childhood sleep problems is a healthy lifestyle. Paying attention to your child's diet, exercise patterns, and sleep environment are key to improving sleeping patterns.

Nutrition

FOODS TO HELP WITH SLEEP

- Milk: yes
- Rice cereal: no
- Sweets: yes, followed by brushing teeth

Formula-fed babies generally fall asleep faster and sleep longer between feedings than breast-fed babies.[31] This is because the fat in formula takes longer to digest and longer to empty from the stomach than the fat in human milk. Mother's milk completely empties from the stomach within two hours, while formula may take three to four hours to make the same transition. This means that nursing babies' stomachs empty sooner and they are hungry sooner than formula-fed babies. Children who breast-feed through the second year of life may awaken in the middle of the night to nurse, especially if they sleep with their parents[32]; this is not a problem for the child unless it is a problem for you. It is the norm in many parts of the world. You need to decide if this is what you want for your family.

Hot beverages are traditionally used before bedtime to induce a state of relaxed drowsiness in older children and adults. You might try a cup of *warm milk*. There is probably not enough L-tryptophan in a glass of milk to work as a sedative, but there are many other compounds in milk that may contribute to sleepiness.

Despite common myths to the contrary, adding *rice cereal* to your babies' evening bottle does *not* help him sleep better through the night. A randomized, controlled trial done at the Cleveland Clinic clearly demonstrated that adding rice cereal to the evening feeding did not improve infants' sleep.[33] A similar study done at Johns Hopkins had identical results.[34] It turns out that many parents become frustrated with night wakenings and add cereal just about the time the baby is learning to sleep through the night on his own anyway. The cereal erroneously receives the credit for the baby's accomplishment in learning to fall asleep and stay asleep.

Sweets have long been known to induce a pleasant torpor. Honey is a traditional ingredient in home sleep remedies. Try adding a teaspoon of honey to a cup of hot tea. To avoid the risk of botulism, do *not* give honey to infants under a year of age. If you give your child something sweet to help him sleep, do so *before* he brushes his teeth!

Do *not* put your child to bed with a bottle in his mouth. Falling asleep with a bottle of milk or juice will rot your baby's teeth. Decay can start as soon as the teeth begin to emerge (usually between five and seven months of age). If your child is already in the habit of going to bed with a bottle and can't seem to fall asleep without one, here's a trick that will eliminate that habit within a week. The first night, dilute the milk or juice (whatever the child has been taking to bed) with one-eighth water. The next night, go to one-fourth water; the third night, half water; the fourth night, three-fourths water. The fifth night, nothing but water in the bottle. Most children don't like the taste of water as much as whatever they were drinking before. Some may protest at the watering down, but many will not even be aware of the gradual change. By the time you've reached pure water, most children willingly release the bottle altogether. If not, you can at least be assured that the water will not harm your child's teeth.

Exercise

Many physicians (and grandmothers) recommend that vigorous exercise be avoided in the hour just before bedtime. Regular daytime exercise can certainly contribute to sound sleep, but avoid running, dancing, spinning, and other frenetic exercises in the hour before bed.[35] Better bets are reading stories, listening to quiet music, and taking a hot bath.

Environment

Bed and bedtime should be as pleasant as possible. Do *not* send your child to bed during the day as a punishment. Associating bedtime with punishment will only make him want to avoid it.

SLEEPING ENVIRONMENT

- Light (dark), sound (quiet), temperature (cool)
- With parents vs. alone
- Hot bath before bed
- Music: Bach vs. Barney
- Favorite stuffed animal, blanket, pacifier
- Sleep position (face up vs. face down)

Emphasize the day-night differences in the environment. Pay attention to light, sounds, and temperature. Most children sleep better in a *cool* environment. *Quiet and dark* are conducive to sleep but are not essential. Many children feel more comfortable with a night-light or having their bedroom door open so they feel safe.

Should a baby sleep with his parents or not? This question must be answered by parents according to their own values and beliefs.

COSLEEPING: BENEFITS

- Lower risk of sudden infant death syndrome (SIDS)
- Cultural norm
- Easier breast-feeding

The risk of sudden infant death syndrome (SIDS) is actually lower in those cultures in which infants routinely sleep with their parents for the first year of life. Parents do *not* roll over on their babies and crush them or smother them unless the parent is very drunk or takes a strong sedative drug. In many cultures it is unthinkable for a baby *not* to sleep with his parents.[36, 37] Most nursing mothers find it more convenient to have the baby in bed with them so when the child awakens to feed there is no need to get up.

COSLEEPING: DRAWBACKS

- Baby learns to depend on parental presence to fall asleep
- Parents awaken every time baby awakens
- More sleep problems reported by parents

One of the drawbacks of letting the baby sleep with you is that the baby learns to fall asleep only with you present and doesn't learn to fall asleep by himself; it is harder to get the baby to fall asleep by himself in his own bed later on when you want the privacy of your own bed back. Some parents are light sleepers who awaken every time the baby moves or awakens. For these parents, it may be preferable to have the baby in a crib nearby for the first few months when the baby requires a nighttime feed, and then move the baby's crib to another room when a night feeding is no longer needed. *Parents must be attuned to and honor their own needs as well as the baby's needs.* Parents who are exhausted and irritable from insufficient sleep are prone to making poorer parenting decisions than parents who are well rested.

Flexibility is important when the toddler or infant is acutely ill. Children with acute illnesses such as colds, sore throats, and ear infections often feel more comfortable with a parent nearby. Many parents choose to allow the child back in bed with them for a few nights. Be aware that children often want to continue this pattern after the illness has resolved. In these cases, the parents will need to help the child reestablish a bedtime routine for falling asleep in his own bed and staying there. Some parents bring a large mattress into the child's room when the child is ill so the parents can sleep on the floor near the child without having the child come into the parents' room.

A *hot bath* before bed is a time-honored way of relaxing for sleep. Again, make sure the bath time is relatively quiet and calm. Too much excitement can rev a child up just when you want him drowsy.

Music is a key component of many families' bedtime routine. Some families start with soothing classical music or lullabies when their child is still an infant. Keeping to a routine of the same music every night helps the child use it as a stimulus to sleep. One of the advantages of using the same taped music is that it can be brought along in the car or on trips so that at least that aspect of the bedtime routine can be maintained no matter where the family is. *What music works best?* There are no studies, but common sense says that if the music is calming for parents, it will contribute to a calm, relaxing atmosphere for the child. One of my physician colleagues who has a new baby swears that a recording of Gregorian chants has miraculous sleep-inducing effects on her infant daughter. Others prefer Bach, and some like Barney. You'll have to experiment to find out what works best for your family.

Many children grow attached to *certain objects* such as a favorite blanket, stuffed animal, pacifier, or pillow. Most toddlers' parents believe that their child needs a transitional object (blanket, pacifier, toy, thumb-sucking) to help them fall asleep. Having this object along can help ease the way to sleep when the family is in the car, visiting grandparents, or otherwise outside of the usual sleep environment.

Sudden infant death syndrome (SIDS) is the sudden, unexpected death during sleep of a baby, usually between one and five months old. It is the second leading cause of death among infants under one year old. The number of SIDS deaths could be cut in half if all babies were put to sleep on their backs (supine) rather than on their tummies (prone).[38] *Lay your baby down to sleep on his back or side,* not *face down.* There has already been a dramatic decline in the incidence of SIDS since widespread publicity has changed sleep habits from tummy sleeping to back or side sleeping.[39] The American Academy of Pediatrics, the National Institute of Child Health and Human Development, the Indian Health Service, the Consumer Product Safety Commission, and the Bureau of Maternal and Child Health *all* recommend that you put your baby to sleep on his back reduce the risk of SIDS.[40]

TO REDUCE THE RISK OF SUDDEN DEATH DURING SLEEP, DO *NOT*

- Smoke or use heroin, crack, or cocaine
- Overheat or overbundle your baby
- Put your infant to sleep on a sheepskin, water bed, or a natural fiber mattress

Parental smoking[41] and drug use markedly increase the risk of SIDS.[42] SIDS is most common during the winter months when concerned parents bundle up their babies and turn the thermostats up in babies' rooms. Several studies have shown an increased risk of SIDS among babies who are overbundled or who sleep in overly warm rooms.[43] Although sheepskin and lambskin are soft and cuddly, they may increase your child's risk of suffocation. Studies also show an increased risk of SIDS among infants who sleep on natural fiber mattresses. Water beds may also be problematic. Unlike firmer foam bedding, natural fibers and water beds tend to conform to the baby, making it difficult for the baby to turn his head away from possible suffocation if he lies on his tummy with his nose facing into the mattress.[44]

Mind-Body

The most important thing you can do to help your child learn to fall asleep at night is to establish a bedtime routine or ritual. The routine should suit your needs as a parent and be consistent with your family beliefs.

COMMON ELEMENTS OF A
BEDTIME ROUTINE

- Same bedtime every night
- Going through the same routine of bathing, brushing teeth, toileting, putting on pajamas, stories, songs, lights out, shades drawn every night
- Wearing special clothes (pajamas) to bed; bed clothes should not be the same as day clothes; warm the sleep clothes (but not daytime clothes) on the radiator or the dryer so they are warm and snuggly
- Special bedtime stories or prayers
- Special bedtime lullabies or other music
- Bedtime massage, such as back rubs, stroking the forehead, foot rubs
- Favorite blanket, stuffed animal, pacifier, or pillow in bed
- Same words for goodnight
- A hug and "I love you" from parents

By establishing the *same bedtime* and *same routine* every day, you help your child establish a regular sleep-wake cycle. Our innate circadian rhythms are actually slightly longer than twenty-four hours, so it is natural for all of us to stay up a bit later each night and wake a bit later each morning. If you allow your child to stay up later on weekends and sleep in the next morning, you may have a real struggle on Mondays when you try to revert to the old schedule and your child's body wants to continue the later pattern. The same thing can happen during vacations.

Children who go to sleep early tend to awaken early, and those who stay up later tend to sleep later. You may need to adjust your child's bedtime to reflect your family's needs. If you are a night owl and like to sleep late in the morning, you may want to establish a late bedtime for your child. On the other hand, if you have to be up early for work, you may want your child asleep earlier. Children who have long afternoon naps are less sleepy for early bedtimes than those whose afternoon naps are cut shorter. You may need to juggle bedtimes and nap times to find the schedule that works best for you. Try to follow the same pattern at least three days in a row. If you switch sleep patterns every day, your child will just be confused, and his irritability may reflect his confusion rather than a real reaction to the new schedule.

It is very important to *put the child down to sleep while he or she is still awake*. Studies using all-night time-lapse photography have shown that children as young as three weeks old who are put to bed while they are still awake can learn to put themselves to sleep. In fact infants who learn to put themselves to sleep in their crib learn to fall asleep more easily on their own when they waken in the middle of the night.[45]

If you allow the child to fall asleep in your arms, he will learn that he can *only* fall asleep in your arms. He will then fuss and cry until you come pick him up, and he will not fall asleep until you are holding him. Babies are often drowsiest right after a meal. Try putting your infant down as soon as you've finished the last nursing of the evening. Falling asleep is a skill and a habit. Teach your children early on that they can fall asleep on their own and you will save yourself many later struggles.[46]

Try to put your child to sleep in the *same place* every night. Going to sleep in your arms one night, in the crib the next, on the floor the next, and in the car seat the next night can be very confusing. If you are out visiting friends or family for the evening when your child's bedtime comes, try to put your child to sleep using as many of the same routines as possible—pajamas, story, song, favorite blanket or stuffed animal, etc.

WHAT TO DO WHEN YOUR BABY WAKES UP IN THE MIDDLE OF THE NIGHT

- Check the baby: Does he need to be fed? Does the diaper need changing? Is he in pain (e.g., an open diaper pin, a hair wrapped around a finger or toe, ill)?
- Attend to his needs for nourishment, hygiene, or pain relief.
- Reassure him that you love him and are nearby with a few brief words and a pat on the tummy, stroking his head or patting his hand.
- When you finish, leave the room.
- If he keeps crying, recheck him in five minutes, repeat the steps, then leave the room.
- If he keeps crying, recheck him in ten minutes; repeat the above, then leave the room.
- If he keeps crying, recheck him in fifteen minutes; repeat the above, then leave the room; etc.
- Reward yourself for hanging in there and teaching your child a new skill!

Make your middle-of-the-night visits as *brief* and *boring* as possible so your baby isn't interested or stimulated by them. Make sure your baby's basic needs are met. Reassure him by speaking a few loving words and patting him on his tummy or stroking his head. If you have a music tape that helps him fall asleep, turn it on. Make sure he has his favorite blanket or toy nearby where he can see and touch it. Do not get your baby out of bed except to change diapers or feed him. Do *not* rock, cud-

dle, and walk your baby back to sleep or he will grow dependent on your ministrations. If you teach him to need this kind of attention in the middle of the night, he will continue to demand it long after you want to go to sleep.

If your baby is used to you getting up and playing with him or holding him and rocking him back to sleep and you *stop* doing those things, *he will probably cry* so you will do them again. This is the most difficult part for parents, and the part requiring the most self-control. If you want him to fall asleep on his own, leave the room even though he cries for you to return. It seems very cruel to leave the baby there, crying plaintively for your attention, but remind yourself of your long-term goal. If he's still crying after five minutes (he probably will be), go back and recheck him. It may help for you to set a small timer for yourself so you know when five minutes are up. Go through the same routine of checking and brief reassurance. Then leave. Next time wait ten minutes. Repeat this procedure, waiting an extra five minutes each time before going back to recheck, so that the intervals between rechecking lengthen to fifteen minutes, then twenty minutes, then twenty-five minutes, etc. You don't need to recheck him if he's not crying. This technique is called *Ferberizing* in honor of Dr. Richard Ferber, the pediatrician who developed it. Ferberizing has been successfully used by thousands of parents.

The first few nights this process may take longer than it would have taken simply to go in, pick your child up, and rock him or cuddle him until he falls back asleep. That's OK. Within a week, there will be much less protest and fewer night wakenings that you are called for at all because your child will have learned to put himself back to sleep. Even after your child has learned this skill, things may briefly fall apart the next time he becomes ill. Children who are ill often have legitimate needs for their parents in the middle of the night, so feel free to go comfort your child as needed during illnesses. After your child has recovered, he may want to continue the habit of extra attention. Then you may be called upon to repeat this routine until he has relearned to put himself back to sleep.

Acknowledge yourself for having the discipline to teach your child to put himself to sleep. This is one of the most difficult parenting tasks; many parents give in night after night rather than listen to their child cry. Give yourself some small reward for hanging in there for the first five minutes, then ten minutes, and so forth. Go ahead and brag to your friends, family, and colleagues. You've earned it!

Many parents just can't stand to hear their baby cry, even for five or ten minutes. An alternative to help your infant learn to sleep through the night is called *scheduled waking*.

SCHEDULED WAKING

- Keep a diary of your child's night wakenings.
- Note what time your child usually wakes up.
- Set the timer for ten minutes *before* your child usually wakes.
- Awaken your child *before* he wakes himself.
- Feed and soothe him.
- Repeat for each of the usual night wakening times.
- Every few days, reduce the number of times you waken your child.

Scheduled awakenings may seem bizarre, but they work. It takes a bit longer than the first process of gradually waiting longer and longer to respond to your child's cries, but it generally works within six weeks.[47] It may be worth trying for parents who don't want to ignore their child's cries but who do want to

eliminate the nighttime wakenings. This strategy has also proved successful in reducing night terrors in children who tend to have them at the same time each night.[48]

WHAT TO DO IF YOUR TODDLER KEEPS GETTING OUT OF BED

- Follow bedtime ritual (be firm about good-night).
- Explain consequences of getting out of bed.
- Follow through with consequences.

For many parents of toddlers, the most difficult part of getting them to bed is the seemingly endless requests for more water, another story, another back rub, etc. What starts out as a fifteen-minute routine turns into a nightly hour-and-a-half battle. The parents wearily give in to each request, not wanting to be cruel and hoping that this is the last thing the child wants. Parents may warn the child, "This is the last . . ." but give in to one more thing to avoid a tantrum or crying. This is a tough situation. Fortunately, it responds well to tough love. Tough love in this situation means setting limits, establishing clear consequences, and then sticking to them. It sounds easy, but it is very challenging. If it were easy, you wouldn't be facing the problem now. Be firm, be consistent, and be willing to put up with (and ignore) some serious crying for the first few days.

First, establish a bedtime routine that all adults in the house can live with. Make sure all adults know what's going on and agree with the plan so the child can't play one against another. Decide in advance how long the routine will take. Plan ahead. If you want the real bedtime to be 9 p.m. and the routine involves a bath, brushing teeth, a story, and a prayer, you'll need to start the routine by 8:15.

Warn the child at 8 p.m. that it's time to start wrapping up the evening's activities and getting ready for bed. Go through the bedtime routine you have agreed on in advance. Praise your child for cooperating with each phase of the routine (e.g., bath, tooth-brushing, picking the bedtime story, lying quietly while the story is read, prayer). Positive reinforcement for following each part of the bedtime routine is very effective in getting children to cooperate with bedtime, reducing tantrums and staying in bed once lights are out.[49]

Decide in advance what the *consequences* of getting out of bed will be. For most parents, the consequence is simply leading the child back to bed, having him get into bed, and repeating that it is now bedtime and the child is expected to remain in bed. The consequence must be immediate (not after five more minutes of TV or cuddling), loving, and firm. You may decide that the consequence for getting out of bed a second time is that the child's bedroom door is closed or the music tape is turned off. You can anticipate that the child will get out of bed to test these limits, and most likely he will cry. This is normal. Your child is not being bad, he is simply testing the rule to see if it's a real rule or not. It's up to you to make it clear that it is a real rule and you will enforce it by an immediate return to bed. The consequence must be immediate to be effective. Telling a three-year-old that the consequence is no TV the following day is nearly meaningless; many adults can't remember a consequence for that long!

There are numerous studies showing that this technique is effective.[50, 51] Most children get the idea within a week. Be prepared to be firm for five to seven days in a row and be prepared for a temporary escalation in whining, complaining, and crying. Don't try to start this rule/consequences routine when you are dealing with another major stressor or disruption in routines such as a new baby in the house or you will doom yourself to frustration and failure. By and large, the only time this technique does not work is when parents are unable to follow through with enforcing the limits they wanted to set.

There is an alternative for getting your toddler to bed. This is a sneakier way of introducing limits. Instead of forcing your child to go to bed at your preset time immediately, let your child stay up as late as he wants (e.g., 11 p.m.). Go through your bedtime routine in a calm, relaxed fashion. The next night, start the routine fifteen minutes earlier. Be sure to give your child fifteen to twenty minutes of warning so that he can wrap up his activities and be ready for bedtime routines. Every few days, push the routine back fifteen minutes earlier so that your child's biological clock is gradually reset to your desired bedtime. This technique takes a bit longer, but it may save you a few tantrums, and it does have proven effectiveness.[52]

Nightmares and Night Terrors

Do not talk about your child's fears or anxieties right before bed. Talking about the monsters in the closet or anxieties about an upcoming test may reassure your child but may also keep the anxieties spinning in his mind as he tries to fall asleep. Instead, reassure your child that everything is all right and that you can talk about such issues in the morning. If you postpone talking about your child's concerns, make sure that you really *do* set aside time the following morning to discuss them. Alternatively, you can talk about them early in the evening, well before bedtime, so that fears are resolved before the child gets in bed.

Being wakened by a terrified, screaming child is a frightening event for most parents. First reassure yourself that the house is not on fire and there is no immediate emergency. *Remain calm* as you enter your child's room.

Ask to hear about the scary dream. Listen and be sympathetic, letting your child know that you hear him and understand his fears. While you listen, calmly stroke his back, forehead, or hand; then reassure him that you are there and he is loved. Many children are comforted by hearing that parents, too, have frightening dreams sometimes but that the dreams aren't real and that everything is really OK. Reassure the child that you can talk more about the dream in the morning if he would like to discuss it further.

Hypnosis can help reduce the frequency of insomnia, nightmares, and night terrors.[53, 54] The noted child hypnotherapist Dr. G. Gail Gardner describes a simple technique that parents can use to help children reduce the frequency of nightmares and improve self-esteem.[55] During the daytime when your child feels relaxed and comfortable, begin to discuss the nightmare. Have the child tell you the story of the bad dream from beginning to end. When he has finished, ask him to pretend that the nightmare is a scary story that you read together and that he can make up a new, happy ending. Have him start at the beginning of the dream again, and this time, when the scary part comes (e.g., big animals chase him), instead of feeling frightened and running, he can be brave (e.g., turn around and ask the animals why they chase him) or ask for help from a superhero or fairy godmother or see the situation transformed (the monsters turn into soft butterflies) and see how things turn out differently (e.g., the monster becomes his friend, he is a hero, or the butterflies fly away). When he has completed the story to his satisfaction, tell him that he can do the same thing with his dreams at night *while he is dreaming them*. It is true. Becoming involved with dreams and changing them at the time one is dreaming is called *lucid dreaming*. Children who learn to become involved in their dreams in this way develop a powerful sense of self-esteem. This technique of rewriting the nightmare is also known as *rehearsal*, and it has proven effective in adult sufferers of severe nightmares.[56]

Professional hypnotherapy has also been used to help children with night terrors. After getting the night terrors under control with medication, school-age children trained in self-hypnosis gradually learn to control their night wakening with hypnosis alone, eliminating the need for medication.[57] (See Appendix A for resources on Hypnosis.)

Another therapy, *recording*, developed at the University of New Mexico, has proved very effective in adults suffering from severe, recurrent nightmares.[58] In recording therapy, the child recalls the nightmare while he is relaxed and comfortable in a safe place. He then writes down the nightmare or draws it in great detail. Although this technique is very simple, it has proved effectiveness.

Several of these techniques can be combined for children who suffer from severe nightmares. One ten-year-old boy who suffered from recurrent nightmares after a car ran into his house benefited from such a combined program: progressive relaxation, reminding himself that "it is only a dream," and reconstructing positive endings for his nightmares. Within weeks he was able to sleep through the night without waking his parents.[59]

Insomnia

For insomnia in older children and teenagers, the problem is likely to be anxiety about upcoming events or overstimulation from activities or caffeine. Make sure the child uses his bed only for sleeping. Have him listen to music, talk on the phone, do his homework, and conduct other activities somewhere else. Have him engage in relaxing activities such as reading or listening to quiet music for the hour before he goes to bed.

Meditation has proved helpful for adults suffering from insomnia.[60]

Progressive relaxation is an easy technique for most older children and teenagers to learn, and it is remarkably effective in allowing a child to relax so he can fall asleep. With this technique, the child focuses on one part of the body at a time, starting with the feet. As he focuses on that part of the body, he intentionally tightens the muscles there as tight as he can, holds it for a few seconds, and then releases. Attention moves from the feet to the lower legs, upper legs, hips, belly, chest, lower back, upper back, hands, arms, neck, and head. By the time the child tightens and relaxes the facial muscles, the whole body is generally quite relaxed and ready to fall asleep. I have found this technique very useful when my mind was racing on the night before an important decision, allowing me to fall asleep easily.

Progressive relaxation and pleasant imagery have also proved useful in children who are afraid of the dark or who are reluctant to go to bed.[61] Confronting oneself with potentially scary thoughts (such as fear of the dark, monsters, or tests) while one is very relaxed gradually drains the fear from the scary thought. This technique is called *desensitization* when used by professional therapists. It is very effective in reducing fears of the dark and nightmares.[62]

Biofeedback training can help insomniacs learn to affect their brain wave activity. By giving patients information about their brain waves and muscle tension, biofeedback devices help them progress from normal waking rhythms (beta activity) through light relaxation (alpha rhythm) into the deep theta and delta states normally achieved only with deep sleep or meditation. Even young children can learn to use biofeedback to improve their sleep.[63] Biofeedback is taught initially in an office or institution, but devices are available for home use so the child can continue to practice at home in his own bed.

This chapter would not be complete without including my grandmother's favorite advice about falling asleep: *counting your blessings*. I know that the standard advice is to count sheep and that counting sheep has worked for thousands of people. It is very boring and therefore very effective. However, counting your blessings, enumerating all the things for which you are grateful, has the added benefit of generating feelings of gratitude. This is one of the most potent antianxiety and antidepressant techniques I know. Since we know that anxiety is a major contributor to sleep problems, I think my grandmother was really on to something. It hasn't been evaluated in the laboratories of modern science, but I suggest you try it yourself or with your teenage insomniac.

BIOMECHANICAL THERAPIES: MASSAGE, SURGERY

Massage

Many parents and children enjoy a relaxing massage before falling asleep. In a study of adolescent psychiatric patients, a nightly back rub was more effective than watching relaxing videotapes in helping the children fall asleep. The positive effects of massage carried over into the day, helping the children manage their anxiety and depression and decreasing their levels of stress hormones.[64] Massage can be as simple as a back rub, stroking a child's forehead, or gently rubbing his hands or feet. Elaborate rituals are unnecessary. Scented oils containing one or more of the essential oils described in the Herbs section may also help the child relax and feel drowsy.

Surgery

If your child suffers from *severe snoring*, consider taking him to an ear-nose-throat (ENT) doctor to be evaluated for sleep apnea. Sleep apnea affects about 10% of children with severe snoring. In this condition the child's adenoids and tongue block airflow during sleep, resulting in loud snoring, long, frequent pauses in breathing, and increased work to breathe that results in poor growth, daytime sleepiness, and hyperactivity.[65] After the obstruction is removed, the child's sleep returns to normal, resulting in improved wakefulness during the day and an improved appetite, growth, and general disposition.[66]

BIOENERGETIC THERAPIES: THERAPEUTIC TOUCH, HOMEOPATHY

Therapeutic Touch

Therapeutic Touch has proved benefits in helping patients relax[67, 68] and in decreasing anxiety. Case reports (anecdotes) in adults suggest that it helps patients fall asleep and rest easily.[69, 70] A study in nursing home patients showed that Therapeutic Touch significantly improved sleep in elderly residents.[71] (See Appendix A for additional resources on Therapeutic Touch; see Appendix B for a brief "how to do" section on Therapeutic Touch.)

Homeopathy

Traditional homeopathic remedies for sleep problems include *Arsenicum* (for nightmares or other symptoms worse after midnight), *Belladonna* (for sudden frights), *Calcarea carbonica* and *phosphorica, Chamomile* (for teething or irritable infants), *Coffea cruda* (treating sleeplessness with extremely dilute concentrations of coffee is another perfect example of the homeopathic principle of like cures like), *Ignatia* (for insomnia due to grief), *Kali phosphoricum* (for night terrors), *Lycopodium, Natrum muriaticum* (for nightmares), *Nux vomica* (for insomnia due to overindulgence in caffeine or overstimulation), *Passiflora* (for insomnia due to an overactive mind in older children and teenagers), *Pulsatilla, Rhus toxicum* (for restless sleep), *Silica,* and *Sulfur.* There are *no* scientific studies evaluating the effectiveness of homeopathic remedies as sleep aids in children. I do *not* recommend them.

WHAT I RECOMMEND FOR SLEEP PROBLEMS

Take Your Child to a Health Care Professional If

- Your child's sleep does not improve with lifestyle changes or home remedies
- Your child's nightmares interfere with daytime activities or his ability to sleep by himself
- Your child has other symptoms and you are concerned that something more serious is going on (such as an ear infection, diabetes, a bladder infection)
- You think your child may need medication (long travel, severe stress)
- You think your child may need surgery (sleep apnea)
- You are becoming increasingly frustrated by your child's wakefulness

---

1. To help an infant learn to go to sleep:

   - Feed thirty minutes before bed, not put to bed while nursing.
   - Put him to sleep in the same place every night while still awake.
   - Create a consistent bedtime routine. Put him to sleep on his back to minimize the risk of SIDS.

2. To help decrease awakenings in the middle of the night:

   - Check on your child to make sure he's not hungry or in pain.
   - Leave the room. If he still cries, recheck him at longer and longer intervals.

3. For children who won't go to bed on time:

   - Establish a brief, consistent bedtime routine
   - Set firm limits, state consequences, and stick to them; *or* let the child stay up as late as he wants, and gradually move bedtime earlier by fifteen minutes every few nights.

4. For children with nightmares:

   - *Lifestyle.* Prevent nightmares by minimizing your child's exposure to scary or violent movies, television, and news before bedtime.

- *Lifestyle*. Reassure your child at the time he awakens.
- *Lifestyle*. Briefly listen to him if he wants to describe the nightmare; discuss the nightmare with him the next day; have him record the details of the nightmare in a dream journal or draw a picture of the scary dream; give him the opportunity to rewrite the nightmare with a different ending.

5. For a child who has night terrors:

- Reassure yourself that your child is normal; most children outgrow them.
- Do not try to waken your child or to soothe him unless he wakens; do stay in the room with him in case he wakes up and wants you.

6. For school-age children or teenagers with insomnia:

- *Lifestyle*. Encourage vigorous exercise during the day, not before bed.
- *Lifestyle*. Try a warm bath before bed; relaxing music or activity before bed; using the bed only for sleep (not for homework, TV, telephone); counting blessings; practicing meditation, progressive muscle relaxation, or other relaxation technique.
- *Lifestyle*. Avoid caffeinated beverages and food. Consider a glass of warm milk.
- *Biochemical*. Consider a hot cup of herbal tea with honey before bed.
- *Lifestyle*. Discuss stresses during the day when coping skills are highest.
- *Biomechanical*. Consider a back rub before bedtime to help him relax.
- *Bioenergetic*. Consider a Therapeutic Touch treatment to help him relax.

RESOURCES

Books

Ferber, Richard. *Solve Your Child's Sleep Problems*. New York: Simon & Schuster, 1986.

Huntley, Rebecca. *The Sleep Book for Tired Parents: A Practical Guide to Solving Children's Sleep Problems*. Parenting Press, 1991.

Wiseman, Anne Sayre. *Nightmare Help*. Ten Speed Press, 1989.

More Information

American Sleep Disorders Association
1610 14th Street, NW, Suite 300
Rochester, MN 55901
1(507)287–6006

25

SORE THROATS

Peter Phillips brought in his daughter, Angela, first thing one cold winter morning for a shot of penicillin. Six-year-old Angela had been ill for a day with a very sore throat, swollen, tender glands in her neck, and a fever. Her throat was so sore she couldn't even drink orange juice. Peter had been suffering from laryngitis himself; his voice was raspy and faint. He had heard there was an aggressive flesh-eating strain of Strep that could cause severe illness and even death, so he wanted Angela treated as rapidly as possible. He also didn't want to miss a day of work, so he wanted to take her directly from the office to school.

WHAT CAUSES SORE THROATS?

Sore throats are the third most common cause for doctor visits in the United States. There are different kinds of sore throats and different causes for each kind.

WHERE IT HURTS

TYPE OF SORE THROAT	BODY PART AFFECTED	SYMPTOMS
Pharyngitis	Pharynx, back of throat	Pain, fever, redness, sometimes ulcers or red spots on palate or back of throat
Tonsillitis	Tonsils	Pain, fever, red, swollen tonsils, sometimes with pus or white spots
Laryngitis	Larynx, voice-box, lower throat and upper windpipe	Hoarseness, whisper-voice, cough, sometimes pain; usually sound worse than they feel

It sounded as though Peter had laryngitis and Angela had tonsillitis or pharyngitis.

Pharyngitis can be caused by viruses, bacteria, allergies, irritants, overuse, or emotions. *Tonsillitis* is usually caused by a viral or bacterial infection. Viruses, irritants, and overuse can also cause *laryngitis*.

CAUSES OF SORE THROATS

- Viruses: Epstein-Barr virus (infectious mononucleosis), adenovirus, coxsackievirus (hand-foot-mouth disease), herpes virus (cold sores), canker sores, others
- Bacteria: various kinds of *Streptococcus, Staphylococcus, Mycoplasma, diphtheria* (rare in vaccinated people), and other bacteria
- Allergies: to dust, pollen, animals, pollutants
- Irritants: tobacco smoke, air pollution
- Miscellaneous: overuse; grief, anger, and other strong emotions

The most famous sore throat *virus* is the *Epstein-Barr virus* (EBV), the cause of infectious mononucleosis, or Mono. Teenagers with Mono usually suffer from sore throats, swollen lymph glands, a swollen spleen (a giant way station for lymph cells in the upper left side of the abdomen), and fatigue. Mono usually lasts for two weeks. Unfortunately, the fatigue can last weeks or even months, causing kids to miss major amounts of school. The sore throat can be so severe and the tonsils so swollen that it is hard to swallow anything. This makes it easy for Mono sufferers to become dehydrated. Dehydration makes them feel worse and even less like drinking, a downward spiral of symptoms that is best avoided by drinking plenty of fluids throughout the illness. Mono is uncommon before school age. Despite its reputation, the "kissing disease" is rarely caught from kissing. Affectionate family members rarely catch Mono from kissing one another.

It didn't sound as if anyone in the Phillips family was suffering from Mono.

Preschoolers' and summer sore throats are usually caused by *adenovirus*. Adenovirus sore throats are often very painful and may be accompanied by conjunctivitis (see Chapter 11).

Adenovirus was not a likely cause for either of the Phillips's symptoms.

Coxsackievirus (hand-foot-mouth disease), *Type I Herpes virus* (cold sores), and *canker sores* can all cause red spots or blisters in the mouth and throat. Coxsackievirus also causes tiny blisters or red spots on the palms of the hands and the soles of the feet. Children typically feel ill and complain of pain a day or two before the blisters appear and for several days afterward.

Group A beta-hemolytic Streptococcal bacteria (Strep) are responsible for about one-third of sore throats in school-age children, usually in the winter and spring. They are very rare in children under three years old.[1] Infections are spread from one person to another by secretions from the nose and mouth. Symptoms appear within a week after exposure. Many people carry *Strep* bacteria without having any symptoms. *Strep* carriers are *not* at risk of developing the most feared consequences of *Strep* infection—rheumatic fever and kidney disease—but they can infect others who are at risk for these serious sequelae. *Strep* typically lasts about three days but can go on for a week. *Strep* infections are easily treated with antibiotics. Because we can prevent serious consequences, *Strep* infections are important to diagnose and treat.

Other kinds of *Strep* (*Group C* and *Group G beta-hemolytic Streptococcus*) cause sore throats that look just like Group A *Strep*.[2, 3] Infections caused by these kinds of *Strep* also yield to antibiotics. Group C and Group G *Strep* do not lead to rheumatic fever or kidney disease.

Mycoplasma pneumonia bacteria cause sore throat and "walking pneumonia" in school-age children. The symptoms caused by *Mycoplasma* look just like those caused by *Strep* except that *Mycoplasma* also causes coughing, while Strep rarely does.

Allergies (see Chapter 4) cause sore throats as well as itchy eyes and watery noses. The most common and easily avoided throat irritant is tobacco smoke. Ironically, in the 1950s menthol cigarettes were advertised as medically approved sore throat soothers. Now we know that nothing could be farther from the truth. The menthol may be soothing, but the tobacco smoke makes things much worse. Children whose mothers smoke have more frequent and more severe sore throats.[4] Other irritants include air pollution, fumes, smoke from wood stoves, dry air, mouth-breathing, and the nasal drainage that drips down the back of the throat from colds or allergies.

A sore throat secondary to *overuse* is a common affliction of cheerleaders, singers, and sports enthusiasts. Although adults may recognize that a "lump in the throat" is due to *grief, anxiety, anger, or other strong emotions,* children may not be able to interpret this feeling except to say they have a sore throat.

Peter admitted that he smoked about a pack a day. His wife had quit smoking about a month earlier and was trying to get him to quit, but he said he just didn't have time, and there was no lung cancer in his family anyway. Peter also said that since the furnace had been on this winter, the air in the house was very dry. They had a humidifier, but it was up in the attic, gathering dust. I advised him to stop smoking now.

Based on their symptoms, it seemed likely that Angela had a Strep throat and that Peter had a viral infection.

Although the symptoms of *Strep* throat and other sore throats are usually different, even experienced clinicians are accurate only about 50% of the time when they guess whether or not *Strep* is the culprit based on symptoms and physical exam alone.[5]

How Can You Tell a Strep Throat from Other Types of Sore Throat?

Symptoms	Strep[6]	Viruses	Irritants	Allergies
Fever	√	√		
Red throat	√	√	√	√
Pus or white patches on tonsils	√	√		
Swollen glands in neck	√	√		
Trouble swallowing	√	√	√	√
Headache	√			√
Nausea, vomiting	√			
Bad breath	√			
Red, sandpapery skin rash	√			
Hoarse voice		√	√	√
Cough		√	√	√
Watery or red eyes		√		√
Runny nose		√		√
Fatigue	√	√		√
Under three years old[7,8]		√	√	√

Diagnosis

Several tests aid in the assessment of sore throats. Most children who have other symptoms such as a runny nose or a cough do *not* have *Strep* or Mono and do *not* need any diagnostic tests.[9]

LABORATORY TESTS FOR SORE THROATS

- Infectious Mononucleosis—blood tests
- *Strep* throat—throat swab for rapid test and/or culture

Blood tests are useful for diagnosing certain viral infections such as *infectious mononucleosis*. The test doesn't become positive until the disease has been present at least four or five days. A negative test in the first day or two of illness could be wrong. Children who have Mono can also have a *Strep* infection.

The only way to be sure an infection is caused by *Strep* is with a laboratory test. This means your child will need a swab of the back of the throat and tonsils. The swab is tested either with a rapid test that checks for signs of *Strep* (like a tracker following an animal's footprints) or a throat culture that checks for the presence of the bacteria themselves (seeing the animal directly).

A rapid *Strep* test can be ready within minutes. If the test is positive (meaning *Strep* is present), you can start antibiotics the same day. The bad thing about rapid tests is that a negative result doesn't necessarily mean that your child doesn't have *Strep*. If a tracker doesn't see footprints, it doesn't mean there is no animal—just that the signs aren't visible. If the rapid test is negative, a throat culture should be done to make sure an infection isn't missed.[10]

Throat cultures are the gold standard for diagnosing *Strep* throats. They are very reliable. It takes a day or two for the results to come back. Do *not* treat your child with leftover antibiotics before getting a throat culture. If a child has had any antibiotics within two days before a throat culture, the test may not be able to detect the *Strep,* and the test will be negative even if the child really is infected. You *can* treat your child's discomfort with analgesics or other remedies. Because of 1988 federal regulations regarding office laboratory testing, fewer and fewer physicians are providing their patients with in-office throat cultures or rapid *Strep* tests.[11]

In my office, we do a rapid test initially and process the test while the patient is still in the office. If the test is positive, we start antibiotic therapy that day. If the test is negative, we do a throat culture and wait for the results before starting antibiotics. With this approach, most patients who need antibiotics get them right away. Those who don't need them avoid unnecessary antibiotics (allergic reactions, upset stomachs, medication costs).[12] This approach is more cost-effective than either treating everyone or culturing everyone.[13] The only exceptions are children who have:

- symptoms of scarlet fever as well as sore throat,
- the classic symptoms of a *Strep* infection during a *Strep* outbreak,
- had rheumatic fever.

These children all get a throat culture to confirm the diagnosis *and* antibiotics even before the culture results are back because of their high risk of disease. Early treatment (within the first two days of symptoms) helps children feel better significantly faster than delaying treatment for a day or two while waiting for the cultures to come back.[14]

The rapid Strep test for Angela was positive, so no culture was needed. Peter's rapid test and his throat culture were negative for Strep.

WHY IS A *STREP* THROAT WORSE THAN ANY OTHER KIND OF SORE THROAT?

The reason *Strep* throat is more serious than other kinds of sore throat can be easily summed up: *rheumatic fever* and *glomerulonephritis* (kidney disease). Rheumatic fever follows *Strep* infections about two to three weeks after the sore throat is gone. Just after World War II, before antibiotics were widely available, *Strep* throat was followed by rheumatic fever in 2 to 3 percent of young soldiers.[15] Treatment with ten days of antibiotics reduces this risk tenfold. Treatment can be delayed as long as nine days after the first sore throat symptoms appear and still be effective in preventing rheumatic fever.[16]

Many people think rheumatic fever is a disease of the past, but outbreaks still occur. In the 1980s, outbreaks were reported in Ohio, Pennsylvania, Salt Lake City, San Diego, New York, and Nashville.[17, 18, 19, 20] Most of the recent outbreaks have been in suburban or rural middle-class neighborhoods, and the initial illnesses were so mild that many people had not even visited their doctors.

One to three weeks after some strains of *Strep* infection, the immune reaction between the *Strep* bacteria and the child's antibodies (immune molecules) can settle in the kidneys, resulting in a serious kidney disease known as *post Streptococcal glomerulonephritis.*

If not treated, the bacteria from a *Strep* throat sometimes spread, leading to ear infections, lymph node infections, and abscesses in the tonsils and throat. *Strep* bacteria can also cause serious, life-threatening infections such as shock, septicemia, and infections of the skin, connective tissues, and muscles.[21] These complications, though well publicized, are extremely rare. Some strains of *Strep* are more aggressive than others. Some are also more contagious (easier to spread) than others. It is impossible to sort out all of these strains of *Strep* without special laboratory tests.

WHAT'S THE BEST WAY TO TREAT A SORE THROAT?

The best treatment depends on what's causing the sore throat. Let's tour the Therapeutic Mountain to find out what works. If you want to skip to my bottom-line recommendations, flip to the end of the chapter.

BIOCHEMICAL THERAPIES: MEDICATIONS, HERBS, NUTRITIONAL SUPPLEMENTS

Medications

MEDICATIONS USED TO TREAT SORE THROATS

- Analgesics: acetaminophen, ibuprofen (nonprescription)
- Throat lozenges (nonprescription), antacid gargles (nonprescription)
- Antibiotics (prescription only): penicillin, erythromycin, others

Analgesics treat sore throat pain while the body heals the underlying problem. The most widely used analgesics are *acetaminophen* (Tylenol and other aspirin-free pain relievers) and *ibuprofen* (Advil or Motrin). Because of its association with the sometimes fatal Reye's syndrome, aspirin is not recommended. Acetaminophen and ibuprofen are both effective pain remedies. Ibuprofen works a bit longer than acetaminophen (six hours vs. four hours) and may be slightly more effective against pain.[22]

Throat lozenges containing benzocaine (such as Cepastat) help numb sore throat pain, but they don't do anything to treat an underlying infection. Some children have had serious side effects from benzocaine.[23] I do not recommend lozenges for children under four years old because of the risk that they will choke on them. In a study of adults with sore throats, Chloraseptic liquid (containing 1.4% phenol) significantly reduced sore throat symptoms compared with a placebo liquid.[24] I use throat sprays when I have a severe sore throat.

Antacids (such as Maalox) coat and soothe not only the stomach lining but also the throat. For children with frequent mouth and throat irritation from cancer chemotherapy, canker sores, or fever blisters. I often recommend Magic Mouthwash—a combination of Tylenol, Maalox, and Benadryl. This is a soothing combination of safe ingredients that can be repeated several times daily. Ask your physician for the right dose for your child.

Antibiotic treatment reduces *Strep* throat symptoms, consequences, and the chance that the sufferer will pass the illness on to someone else.[25] Antibiotics are *not* useful for treating sore throats caused by viruses, allergies, irritants, overuse, or emotions.

ANTIBIOTICS TO TREAT *STREP* THROAT (ALL REQUIRE A PRESCRIPTION)

- Penicillin; amoxicillin (Amoxil)
- Erythromycin, azithromycin (Zithromax), clarithromycin (Biaxin)
- Combinations: amoxicillin-clavulanic acid (Augmentin) and erythromycin-sulfisoxazole (Pediazole)
- Cephalosporins: cefadroxil (Duricef), cefaclor (Ceclor), cefuroxime (Ceftin), cephalexin (Keflex), cefpodoxime (Vantin), and others
- Clindamycin (Cleocin)

Penicillin is the official treatment of choice for children with true *Strep* throats.[26] Penicillin decreases the length of symptoms by about a day. More important, it dramatically reduces the subsequent risk of developing rheumatic fever. Penicillin can be given as an injection, pills, or syrups. If taken by mouth, it must be given at least twice[27] and preferably three times daily for at least ten days to eradicate *Strep* bacteria.[28, 29] Most parents quit giving medication by the sixth day

because the child is better and the need for medication seems less pressing, but it is markedly less effective when taken less than ten full days.[30] Penicillin also requires refrigeration, which is a drawback for homeless families and for families about to go on camping trips. For maximal absorption and effectiveness, penicillin should *not* be given within an hour before or two hours after mealtime. I give parents the choice of whether they want their child to receive an injection or oral medication. As much as most people hate needles, I'm surprised how often families choose to "take the shot and get it over with."

Amoxicillin is a derivative of penicillin that is also inexpensive and effective. It tastes better than penicillin. Like penicillin, it requires refrigeration. If amoxicillin is given to patients with Mono, they break out in a rash. This is one of the reasons physicians don't just give antibiotics to everyone who has a sore throat.

For children who are allergic to penicillin, the antibiotic of choice has been *erythromycin*. However, more and more strains of *Strep* are becoming resistant to erythromycin.[31] It requires dosing three or four times daily, and it often causes an upset stomach. About a third of patients stop taking it because of side effects. New antibiotic relatives of erythromycin, *azithromycin* (Zithromax) and *clarithromycin* (Biaxin), are more effective treatments for *Strep* throat. Azithromycin is one of the few antibiotics that has been demonstrated to be effective with only five days of treatment.[32] Both of these new antibiotics are more costly ($15 to $30) than penicillin (about $5 to $10) or erythromycin (about $10).

The *combination antibiotics* and the *cephalosporins* (such as Duricef and Vantin) are also more effective and expensive than penicillin, amoxicillin, or erythromycin.[33] Some are more convenient because they only require dosing once or twice a day and they do not require refrigeration. Cefpodixime (Vantin) taken twice daily for five days or cefuroxime (Ceftin) taken twice daily for four days is as effective as penicillin taken three times daily for ten days.[34, 35] Their success is costly. Most combination medications or cephalosporins cost three to four times as much as penicillin or erythromycin. They can also cause upset stomach and diarrhea and wipe out the "good" bacteria in the bowels, leading to yeast infections.

Clindamycin is a powerful antibiotic that effectively eradicates *Strep.* Based on Swedish studies, it is my choice for *Strep* throats that are resistant to penicillin and cephalo-sporins.[36] Clindamycin also does an excellent job of clearing *Strep* from carriers who keep reinfecting family members.[37] Unfortunately, it also kills many of the "good" bacteria in the bowels, leading to diarrhea.

Trimethoprim-sulfamethoxazole (Bactrim or Septra), *tetracycline,* and *sulfa* drugs are *not* effective in eradicating *Strep* from the throat. They are *not* recommended for *Strep* throat, though they are very helpful in other infectious illnesses such as bladder infections, ear infections, and acne.

It doesn't hurt to wait a day or two to start antibiotics, but the sooner treatment starts, the sooner the child will feel better. Delaying treatment for twenty-four to forty-eight hours may allow the body to build up its own antibodies (immune defenses against this and future attacks) and prevent subsequent infections.[38] One study found that children who were treated immediately had an eight times higher risk of developing another *Strep* infection within the next four months than children whose treatment was delayed for two days.[39] Other studies have found *no* difference in recurrence risks between those treated immediately and those whose treatment is delayed by forty-eight hours.[40] I do *not* withhold antibiotic therapy from a child who is sick with a *Strep* throat. I also don't

rush to treat a child who has a sore throat before appropriate laboratory tests have established a diagnosis.

After weighing all the options (and at Peter's urging), Angela agreed that the best choice for her was a shot of penicillin. This way they didn't need to remember all the doses of medicine for the next ten days.

When can your child return to school or day care? Children are no longer contagious to others when they have completed twenty-four hours of antibiotic therapy.[41] Even children who have received an injection should wait twenty-four hours before returning to school or day care to make sure the medicine has had a chance to begin eradicating the *Strep* bacteria.

No antibiotic is 100% effective.

REASONS FOR ANTIBIOTIC FAILURE

- Failure to take medication
- Reinfection from other family member or peers
- Not a bacterial infection
- Resistant bacteria, requiring different antibiotic
- Susceptible immune system

The main reason antibiotics fail is that people fail to take them often enough and long enough. Even if the child takes all of her doses, if someone else in the family is infected and not treated, that person can reinfect the child. Infection can go back and forth between family members like a ping-pong ball. For repeated, recalcitrant infections, it's worth testing and treating every infected person in the household. Children can also get reinfected by close peers in school and day care. In some cases, a second, more powerful antibiotic is needed.[42] Antibiotics are *not* effective against viruses; if your child's sore throat is not due to bacteria, antibiotics won't help.

Some children's throats are just more susceptible to the Strep bacteria.[43] Antibiotics can't do the job alone; they require a healthy immune system to wipe out bacteria and keep them out. If antibiotics haven't worked for your child, see your health care provider to discuss alternative antibiotics or other measures to support the immune system.

Herbs

There are no scientific studies specifically evaluating the effectiveness of any herbal remedy in treating sore throats. I do *not* recommend that any herbal remedy replace antibiotics for treating *Strep* throat. However, herbal remedies have a long history of soothing irritated sore throats. Below are some of the most commonly used herbal remedies.

HERBAL REMEDIES FOR SORE THROATS

- Demulcents (throat soothers): *comfrey, horehound, licorice, mullein, slippery elm bark*
- Immune boosters: *echinacea, licorice root*
- Bacteria fighters: *goldenseal*
- Astringent: *gum myrrh, mullein*
- Miscellaneous: *honey, sage, thyme, oil of eucalyptus, mustard*

Horehound is a demulcent and expectorant (loosens mucus) ingredient in many cough drops and candies. I recommend horehound cough drops or hard candies for children over four to help soothe their sore throats. To avoid the risk of choking, younger children should not use any throat lozenge or hard candy.

Licorice root is another demulcent. It also stimulates the immune system to better fight viral infections. Licorice tea may be especially useful for sore throats due to cold sores or canker sores.[44, 45] *Mullein* tea is used in India and by American Indians for sore throats and respiratory problems because it is so soothing. *Slippery elm bark* is another of my favorite remedies because it is so soothing to mucous membranes. It is the main ingredient in Throat Coat tea available in grocery stores. Slippery elm bark lozenges are also available as sore throat soothers.

Purple coneflower (echinacea). A Nebraska farmer stole the idea for this remedy from local Indians who had long used it as a blood purifier and as an anti-infective agent. It is now widely used in Germany as a stimulant for the immune system, especially in treating the common cold and sore throats. Scientific studies indicate that it stimulates several components of the immune system. It is very safe, but it does *not* kill *Strep* effectively or help prevent rheumatic fever.[46]

Goldenseal root contains the active ingredient berberine, which kills many bacteria (including *Strep*) in test tubes.[47] It was used by the Cherokee Indians to treat ulcers and arrow wounds. Goldenseal also stimulates the immune system. There are *no* studies evaluating its effectiveness in treating people with *Strep* throat. *Gum myrrh* is the gum resin of trees indigenous to East Africa and Arabia. It has been used since ancient times as a perfume and incense. It is also an ingredient in mouth washes and gargles for its fragrance and its mildly astringent properties.

Though not technically an herb, *honey* is traditionally added to tea or lemonade to help soothe sore throats. To avoid the risk of botulism, do *not* give honey to infants under one year of age.

Other traditional herbal remedies: compresses of *sage* and *thyme*, flannel mufflers of *Eucalyptus* oil, and *mustard* poultices. Some families add oil of *chamomile, lavender,* and *thyme* to steam baths to soothe the mucous mem branes of the nose and throat. There are no scientific studies evaluating the effectiveness of these remedies, but I encourage parents to follow their families' safe healing traditions.

Peter decided he would get some slippery elm bark lozenges for Angela and make some hot licorice and slippery elm bark tea for both of them.

Nutritional Supplements

Sugar-free *vitamin C* lozenges or *zinc* lozenges may be helpful in relieving sore throat pain, but there are no studies comparing their effectiveness to that of other throat lozenges, horehound drops, or other hard candy. There is evidence that both help reduce symptoms of the common cold, so if sore throat is just one of several cold symptoms, vitamin C and zinc lozenges may be worth a try.

Raw garlic and *onions* have antibacterial properties,[48] though they have never been specifically tested as treatments for sore throats. You might try giving your child raw garlic blended with mashed potatoes or vegetable juices.

One of the most time-honored sore throat remedies is the salt water gargle:

- ½ teaspoon of salt (or ¼ teaspoon of salt plus ¼ teaspoon of baking soda)
- 8–16 ounces of warm water

Other home remedies are:

- Hot tea with honey
- Honey mixed with roasted onion
- Honey and lemon juice (or cider vinegar) in 6 to 8 ounces of hot water
- Apple juice and clove tea (spiced apple cider)

There are *no* scientific studies evaluating the effectiveness of any of these home remedies. Remember, *no* honey for infants under one year of age to avoid the risk of botulism.

LIFESTYLE THERAPIES: NUTRITION, EXERCISE, ENVIRONMENT

Nutrition

As with other infectious diseases, drinking *plenty of fluids* is the order of the day. Your child's fluid intake is sufficient if it necessitates diaper changes or visits to the bathroom every two to three hours.

Exercise

Rest allows the body to concentrate its energy on healing. Teenagers suffering from Mono may be fatigued for months after the acute infection has resolved. They should not participate in contact sports such as football or soccer for at least a month to protect their spleens. There's no point in forcing a fatigued teenager out onto the football field or gymnastics floor. Continue mild, regular exercise such as yoga, tai chi, or walking to keep the muscles from becoming weak and wasted. This is not the time for wind sprints.

Rest is the therapeutic mainstay for children whose throats are sore from too much talking, shouting, or singing.

Peter realized that Angela needed her rest. He decided that he would take the day off to stay home with her, rent comedy movies, and take naps.

Environment

For sore throats due to allergens and irritants, the best treatment is environmental:

avoid the irritant. Do *not* smoke and do not allow others to smoke around your child. Avoid other sources of smoke, exhaust, and chemical fumes.

Humidity reduces throat irritation caused by dry winter air.

I suggested Peter get the humidifier out of the attic, clean it off, and get it going.

Cold foods and drinks are also soothing to sore throats. Even kids who won't eat their normal food when they are sick can often be coaxed to try ice cream, sorbet, popsicles, or even plain ice cubes.

BIOMECHANICAL THERAPIES: SURGERY

Surgery

At one time, tonsillectomy was the most common operation performed on children. Thankfully those days are long gone. However, there still are times when tonsillectomy is beneficial. Some children with recurrent infections do benefit from surgery. Those who have seven or more culture-proven infections with *Strep* and undergo a tonsillectomy have only half the number of infections in the next year compared with similar children who do not have surgery. The benefits only last a year or two. Three years later, the number of infections is identical in both groups.[49] Tonsillectomy is a very safe procedure for children between the ages of two and twelve years; it is often done as an outpatient procedure without the need for overnight hospitalization.[50]

This was Angela's first Strep throat, so there was no need to discuss surgery.

BIOENERGETIC THERAPIES: ACUPUNCTURE, HOMEOPATHY

Acupuncture

There is a point in the muscle between the base of the thumb and first finger that is effective in reducing all kinds of pain in the head, mouth, and neck. You can find it on yourself by massaging the area deeply. It is the point where deep massage feels a bit uncomfortable or odd. You can try massaging this point on both of your child's hands for several minutes as an experiment to see if it helps decrease her pain. Do *not* use acupuncture as a substitute for antibiotics for *Strep* throat.

Homeopathy

The most commonly recommended homeopathic remedies for sore throats are *Aconitum, Apis, Belladonna, Bryonia, Hepar sulf, Lachesis, Lycopodium, Mercurius solubis* or *vivus, Pulsatilla, Rhus toxicum, Silica,* and *Sulfur.* There are *no* scientific studies evaluating the effectiveness of homeopathic remedies in treating sore throats. I do *not* recommend homeopathic treatment of *Strep* throats.

WHAT I RECOMMEND FOR SORE THROATS

PREVENTING SORE THROATS

1. *Lifestyle—environment.* Minimize throat irritants. Do not smoke and do not allow others to smoke around your child. Avoid allergens. Minimize your child's exposure to other children with sore throats.

2. *Lifestyle—exercise.* Avoid overusing the throat.

3. *Biochemical—medications.* Have your child immunized against diphtheria.

See Your Health Care Professional If You Suspect Strep or If Your Child

- Is not better within forty-eight hours of starting treatment
- Has trouble swallowing her own saliva or starts drooling
- Develops signs of dehydration (such as fewer than four wet diapers within twenty-four hours or no tears when crying)
- Has severe pain
- Has trouble breathing

TREATING SORE THROATS

1. *Biochemical—medications.* For sore throat pain, try analgesics (such as Tylenol, Advil, or Motrin), gargles with antacids (such as Maalox), anesthetic throat sprays or lozenges for children over four years old. If your child has a *Strep* infection, I recommend a full course of antibiotics.

2. *Lifestyle—nutrition.* Encourage your child to drink plenty of fluids. Salt water gargles may be helpful for children who are old enough to gargle.

3. *Biochemical—herbs.* Try sucking on horehound drops for children over four years old or sipping hot tea with lemon and honey (slippery elm bark, licorice, or comfrey tea). *No honey* for infants less than one year of age.

4. *Lifestyle—environment.* Offer cold noncarbonated drinks, popsicles, sorbet, ice cream, ice cubes, or frozen yogurt. Humidifiers may help those with laryngitis.

5. *Lifestyle—exercise.* Rest.

6. *Biochemical—nutritional supplements.* Consider vitamin C and zinc lozenges if your child's sore throat is one of many cold symptoms.

7. *Biomechanical—surgery.* If your child has had many recurrent *Strep* throats, having her tonsils out may be helpful.

26

VOMITING AND NAUSEA

Jack Burnside called me about his eighteen-month-old daughter, Patrice, who had started vomiting the day before. She had thrown up about three times, most recently in the car on the way to the grocery to get some cola to settle her stomach. Jack had stopped giving her milk and started giving her clear liquids such as cola and chicken broth. His wife was concerned that their baby, Anna, was also spitting up after nursing. He had several questions:

- *What caused the girls' vomiting?*
- *Should he bring in Patrice, Anna, or both for evaluations and treatment?*
- *What were the safest and most effective remedies for vomiting?*

WHAT CAUSES VOMITING?

Vomiting is a distinctly uncomfortable experience, but it can spare us worse illnesses by rapidly eliminating toxins before they do serious damage. Vomiting is generally preceded by nausea, the feeling that one is about to vomit. Children who are nauseated generally avoid food, although most will still sip liquids if they are offered. Children vomit more easily than adults.

Gastroenteritis is the most common cause of nausea, vomiting, diarrhea, and abdominal pain in children. Most people call it an intestinal flu. Technically, this illness is not a "flu," because it is not caused by the influenza virus, but this doesn't stop health care practitioners and parents alike from calling it the flu bug. Gastroenteritis is normally caused by a viral infection and is over within forty-eight hours.

Patrice's symptoms sounded as if they were due to plain old gastroenteritis. We agreed that

Jack would try some simple home remedies and would bring her in the next day if she was still vomiting or developed any signs of dehydration.

CAUSES OF VOMITING

- Gastroenteritis (intestinal flu)
- Spitting up (gastroesophageal reflux)
- Food poisoning
- Swallowed phlegm dripping into the throat from the nose or sinuses
- Overeating, food intolerance, or food allergies
- Side effect of severe coughing
- Side effect of other treatments (medications, herbs, vitamins, surgery)
- Motion sickness
- Pregnancy
- Symptom of other illnesses (e.g., appendicitis, Strep throat, bladder infection, migraine headache)

All babies spit up milk from time to time. Spitting up is common in babies who are fed too much too quickly. It usually looks as if a lot more is coming up than there is. If you are concerned about how much milk is being regurgitated, try this simple test. Take a measuring tablespoon of milk and spill it on the floor, an old rag, or a towel. You'll probably be as surprised as I was the first time I tried this experiment at how much milk it looks like even when you know perfectly well that it's only a tablespoon.

Gastroesophageal reflux is when the stomach (gastric) contents move backwards up into the swallowing tube (esophagus). Refluxing stomach acid can cause heartburn pain. Severe, persistent reflux leads to inadequate nutrition and poor growth. If severe vomiting occurs in the first few days of life, it may be due to intestinal obstruction, which requires immediate professional evaluation and treatment.

Anna had been drinking avidly. She was gaining weight normally and had no other symptoms. She was so eager to eat that she seldom paused to burp. She was so tired by her vigorous feeding that she often fell asleep immediately after eating; when she was laid down, she spit up undigested milk. When Jack and his wife actually measured the amount she was spitting up, it was only about one and a half teaspoons.

Vomiting can be a useful reaction for eliminating tainted food (*food poisoning*) before it is absorbed into the system. If your child is vomiting because of food poisoning, it is better not to suppress the symptoms but to allow Nature to get rid of the poisons.

Children also vomit if they *swallow a lot of phlegm.* Children suffering from colds, ear infections, bronchitis, and particularly *Strep* throat and sinus infections are prone to vomiting because the phlegm from the infection irritates the stomach. The best way to reduce this kind of vomiting is to treat the underlying condition and remove extra phlegm from the nose with frequent nose blowing, a bulb syringe, or a nasal aspirator.

Overeating frequently causes indigestion, heartburn, and nausea, but it rarely causes vomiting in adults. Children seem to be more sensitive than adults to this manifestation of overindulgence. A trip to the ballpark or circus, complete with hot dogs, candy, soda pop, etc., sometimes ends unpleasantly in a rushed trip to the bathroom. *Certain foods,* such as green apples, have a well-deserved reputation for causing nausea and stomach aches. *Food allergies,* such as cow's milk and egg allergy, can also manifest as vomiting. Vomiting is seldom the only sign of a food sensitivity (see Chapter 4, Allergies).

Severe coughing can trigger vomiting. Vomiting triggers a reflex that actually relieves the coughing spasm. In the old days, ipecac (the medicine used to induce vomiting in cases of accidental poisoning) was used to treat children with asthmatic coughs. Nowadays effective asthma medicines don't necessarily cause vomiting.

Speaking of ipecac, many common *medications, herbs,* and *vitamins* and even the anesthetics used during *surgery* induce nausea and vomiting. Aspirin and ibuprofen commonly cause a queasy stomach. The antibiotic erythromycin frequently causes nausea and vomiting. Chemotherapy for cancer is notorious for causing such severe nausea and vomiting that some patients refuse continued treatment. Several Chinese herbs, notably *chuanwu* and *caowu* (the roots of aconitum), used as anti-inflammatory therapy, and *bajiaolian* (used to treat snake bite, tumors, and swollen lymph glands) have caused serious nausea and vomiting.[1, 2] African herbal remedies have also been reported to have serious side effects, including vomiting and dehydration.[3] Vitamin A overdoses (doses of at least 300,000 international units or 60 milligrams) and excessive vitamin D can cause vomiting, headaches, and other serious neurological problems. Anyone who has had major surgery can tell you that one of the worst parts of an operation is feeling sick to your stomach right after you wake up from the anesthesia. Depending on the type of operation, anywhere from 30 to 80 percent of children experience nausea and vomiting within twenty-four hours of surgery.

Children are also more susceptible than adults to *motion sickness*. Motion sickness can be brought on by the motion of a car, boat, airplane, or amusement park ride. Exhaust fumes and overexcitement make motion sickness worse.

Other conditions also include vomiting and nausea as key symptoms. Morning sickness is a classic early sign of *pregnancy*—an all too common condition in American teenagers. If *constipation* continues long enough, a child may become nauseated and may even vomit. Children suffering from *migraines* often

experience nausea and vomiting as cardinal symptoms of their "sick headaches" (see Chapter 20, Headache). Abdominal pain, nausea, and vomiting are also symptoms of severe *lead poisoning*.

TAKE YOUR BABY OR CHILD TO BE EVALUATED IF SHE

- Spits up more than a tablespoon of milk with each feeding
- Is losing weight or not gaining weight as well as predicted
- Is less than ten weeks old and has very forceful (projectile) vomiting
- Is vomiting even small amounts (less than a tablespoon) of water
- Has violent retching
- Has a yellowish tinge to her skin or eyes (jaundice)
- Vomits up bile (greenish fluid) or blood or coffee-ground looking material
- Has a temperature over 100.5°F if she is less than two months old
- Has a temperature over 103.9°F at any age
- Has severe abdominal pain, especially the lower right side (could be appendicitis)
- Vomits for more than three times or more than an hour following a head injury
- Vomits continuously for more than twenty-four hours
- Seems uninterested in drinking or appears to be dehydrated
- Or if you are concerned about her symptoms or appearance

Other serious causes of vomiting include appendicitis, bladder or kidney infections, and meningitis. Rare genetic diseases such as hereditary fructose intolerance or severe vitamin B12 deficiency can also cause vomiting. Vomiting is also one of the signs of hepatitis (liver disease). Children who have suffered a head injury often vomit once or twice within the first hour following the injury.

If your child has any of these symptoms, she may have something more complicated than simple gastroenteritis or spitting up and may need more therapy than you can provide at home.

Dehydration can occur within a day, especially if your child has diarrhea as well as vomiting. If your child has any of these signs, she needs to be evaluated by a health care professional to determine the cause of the vomiting and the potential need for fluids by vein (intravenous).

SIGNS OF DEHYDRATION

IF YOUR CHILD:

- voids (pees/urinates) less than four times per day or less than half of what is normal for her
- doesn't have tears when she cries
- loses weight
- has sunken eyes or a sunken fontanel (soft spot on baby's head)
- has dry lips and tongue or stringy saliva
- has hands and feet that are much cooler than her arms and legs

WHAT CAN BE DONE TO PREVENT VOMITING?

Prevent food poisoning and bacterial infections by keeping hot foods hot and cold foods cold. Cook all meat and poultry thoroughly to kill bacteria that cause vomiting and diarrhea. Wash all poultry products well before cooking to remove *Salmonella* bacteria. Wash the cutting board, knives, other utensils, and your hands after preparing poultry. Do not leave foods prepared with mayonnaise (such as chicken salad or tuna salad) out of the refrigerator for more than an hour before eating them.

Avoid motion sickness by having the child sit in the front seat, keeping a window open, and encouraging her to look out at the horizon rather than reading.

Avoid spreading infectious gastroenteritis by frequently washing your hands and your child's hands. Treat underlying illnesses promptly. Keep your child's nose cleaned out when she has a cold or sinus infection to keep her from swallowing lots of phlegm.

Prevent spitting up by slowing feedings, frequent burping, thickening feedings with rice cereal, or keeping your child upright for twenty to thirty minutes after feeding.

I suggested that Jack and his wife try slowing down Anna's feedings, having her burp at least twice each feeding and once afterward. I also suggested that they keep her upright for half an hour after she fed to give the milk a chance to pass on through the stomach, making it less likely that it would come back up when she lay down. Anna continued to grow well and stopped spitting up at about five months of age.

WHAT IS THE BEST WAY TO TREAT VOMITING?

The best way to treat vomiting depends on what is causing it. The treatments for motion sickness are not necessarily the same as for food poisoning or chemotherapy-induced vomiting. Let's tour the Therapeutic Mountain to find out what works for different kinds of vomiting. If you want to skip to my bottom-line recommendations, flip to the end of the chapter.

BIOCHEMICAL THERAPIES: MEDICATIONS, HERBS, NUTRITIONAL SUPPLEMENTS

Medications

Because vomiting is often the body's way of eliminating toxins from the system and because young children are more prone to suffering side effects, medications to suppress nausea and vomiting are *not* recommended for children under two years old. If your young child is undergoing chemotherapy or requires some other therapy that causes nausea, ask your health care provider about safe treatments to minimize symptoms.

NONPRESCRIPTION ANTINAUSEA MEDICATIONS

- Meclizine (Antivert)
- Diphenhydramine (Benadryl)
- Dimenhydrinate (Dramamine)
- Emetrol; Coca Cola syrup
- Pepto Bismol

Antivert (meclizine) is commonly used to prevent and treat motion sickness. It starts working within one hour and lasts for twelve to twenty-four hours. It is *not* recommended for children under twelve years old. It can cause drowsiness, restlessness, blurred vision, and a drop in blood pressure. It should *not* be taken if the teenager is planning to drive or operate dangerous equipment. Overdoses can cause seizures. Although it sounds scary, meclizine is actually safe enough to be used during pregnancy to treat morning sickness.[4]

Benadryl (diphenhydramine) is one of the most commonly used medications for motion sickness, nausea, and vomiting. It is often used in combination with other more powerful drugs to prevent nausea due to chemotherapy. Benadryl is fairly safe even for young children. It causes drowsiness, increased thirst, and dry mouth in most children, and irritability and excitement in a few.

Dramamine (dimenhydrinate) is the classic medication to prevent motion sickness. It is chemically very similar to Benadryl and has similar side effects: drowsiness or irritability, confusion, and dry mouth. It is *not* approved for children under two years old.

Emetrol, Nausetrol, and *Naus-A-Way* are all carbohydrate (sugar) solutions with phosphoric acid. Although they are marketed as antinausea medications, they are actually pretty similar to *Coca Cola syrup.* There is no scientific evidence that any of these medications are any more effective than flat soft drinks in reducing nausea and vomiting.

Pepto-Bismol is a great stomach soother. Because of the risk of Reye's syndrome, it should *not* be given to children with chicken pox or influenza.

PRESCRIPTION MEDICATIONS FOR VOMITING

- Prochlorperazine (Compazine), Promethazine (Phenergan), Chlorpromazine (Thorazine)
- Metoclopramide (Reglan)
- Trimethobenzamide (Tigan), Hydroxyzine (Vistaril)
- Scopolamine (Transderm Scop)
- Others

Compazine, phenergan, and *thorazine* are chemically related, powerful treatments for vomiting due to other medications and surgery. They can be very sedating. Phenergan helps prevent motion sickness.

Reglan is used to treat infants' gastroesophageal reflux and, in combination with other medications, to prevent chemotherapy-induced vomiting. It should *not* be used in babies who simply spit up a bit after feeding if they are growing well and do not have other problems.

Tigan and *Vistaril* are sedating medications related to nonprescription Benadryl and Dramamine. Tigan is commonly used in hospitalized adults and is approved for use in children as young as two years old. Vistaril is often given in combination with other antinausea medications and is safe for young children.

Transdermal scopolamine is available as an adhesive patch to prevent motion sickness. Because younger children are more susceptible to its side effects (dry mouth, drowsiness, blurred vision), it is *not* recommended for children under twelve years old.

Other effective medications that treat the serious nausea and vomiting accompanying cancer chemotherapy are steroids, sedatives,[5] droperidol,[6] and ondansetron.[7] These medicines are sometimes combined with Reglan and Benadryl to enhance their antiemetic (antivomiting) effect. These combinations have the risk of severe sedation and other side effects. They should be used *only* under the supervision of a physician with extensive experience in treating children with chemotherapy.

Medications are not *indicated for the vast majority of children suffering from gastronenteritis, spitting up, or food poisoning. Neither Patrice nor Anna needed medication for their symptoms.*

Herbs

Traditional tummy-settling teas contain chamomile and peppermint. You can find this combination ready made at your grocery store under several brand names (such as Celestial Seasonings' Grandma's Tummy Mint tea). Sometimes catnip and other members of the mint family are added or substituted for peppermint. Common additions include anise, dill, fennel, lemon balm, lime flowers, and meadowsweet. Some herbalists recommend

bitter herbs (such as gentian) to treat stomach upsets and stimulate appetites. These herbs don't taste very good and may not be helpful if the child is also having diarrhea. The combination of chamomile, vervain, licorice, and balm-mint has proven useful in treating infants suffering from colic (see Chapter 10), a common newborn condition often attributed to an upset stomach.[8]

My favorite herbal tea combination is chamomile, lemon balm, and peppermint because of its pleasant taste. This is the combination that Jack chose for Patrice.

Ginger has long been used to treat upset stomachs. Recent studies have shown it to be helpful in treating the morning sickness of pregnancy, sea sickness, and nausea caused by chemotherapy.[9, 10, 11] In a study of postoperative nausea, ginger was as effective as the powerful medicine Reglan.[12] Ginger functions both as a carminative (promoting elimination of intestinal gas) and to reduce intestinal spasms. Although it has not been tested in children suffering from nausea and vomiting, it is safe and worth a try. The total dose of powdered ginger root should be divided into four doses over the course of a day.

GINGER ROOT—DIVIDE INTO FOUR DOSES DAILY

- Over twelve years old: 1 gram (1,000 milligrams) daily or 250 milligrams per dose
- Six to twelve years old: 500 milligrams daily or 125 milligrams per dose
- Three to six years old: 250 milligrams daily or 50 to 75 milligrams per dose
- Under three years old: 100 milligrams daily or 25 milligrams per dose

You can also prepare homemade ginger tea.

- 1 cup of water
- 2 slices of ginger root

Simmer together for five minutes.

You can also try ginger soda, but check to make sure that the ginger ale you buy contains real ginger and not just ginger flavoring. You can also add freshly grated ginger (1/4 teaspoon at a time) to your child's juice, applesauce, or hot cereal.

Jack decided to change from root beer to real ginger ale for Patrice; this is the remedy his mother had used when he was ill as a child. We agreed that he would alternate ginger ale with chicken broth so that Patrice would get the even balance of salt (from chicken broth) and sugar (from ginger ale) that her body needed.

Clove tea (10 cloves in 12 ounces of boiling water, steeped ten minutes and strained) and cinnamon tea (1 to 2 sticks of cinnamon to 1 cup of boiling water, steeped ten minutes and drained) are also traditional, tasty remedies for nausea. You can experiment and combine different amounts of ginger, clove, and cinnamon. Basil tea (1/2 ounce of dry basil plus one cup of boiling water, steeped for five minutes and strained) is an old English remedy for nausea.

Goldenseal (Hydrastis canadensis) and barberry (Berberis vulgaris) tinctures are frequently recommended for diarrhea and may be helpful if the child is suffering from gastroenteritis—both vomiting and diarrhea. The dose of either tincture is 2 to 3 drops diluted in 4 ounces of water, sipped slowly over an hour.

Nutritional Supplements

Vitamin B6 (pyridoxine) has proven effective in reducing the nausea and vomiting of pregnancy.[13] The dose is 10 to 25 milligrams every eight hours until symptoms improve.[14] Although it is not clear exactly how pyridoxine works, it is an ingredient in a European medication used to treat morning sickness, Debendox.[15] Pyridoxine has also been used to treat the nausea caused by radiation therapy.[16] There are *no* studies evaluating the effectiveness of B6 in treating gastroenteritis, reflux, or other causes of nausea and vomiting in children. Because pyridoxine is generally safe, you can try giving your child 10 milligrams of vitamin B6 an hour before traveling to help minimize motion sickness.

LIFESTYLE THERAPIES: NUTRITION, EXERCISE, ENVIRONMENT, MIND-BODY

Nutrition

Giving *small amounts* of *clear fluids frequently* is the mainstay of treatment for vomiting. Small amounts means 1 to 2 tablespoons at a time. Frequently means every five to fifteen minutes. To give your child's stomach a chance to settle, wait for fifteen to thirty minutes after a vomiting spell before trying again. Avoid large volumes at one time. Often a child who vomits after 4 ounces of soda guzzled in two minutes can easily tolerate a tablespoon repeated every five minutes over an hour—which is equivalent to the same 4 ounces.

To replace fluid losses, especially if your child has diarrhea as well as vomiting, use a commercially prepared rehydration fluid (such as Pedialyte) or make your own.

HOME-MADE REHYDRATION SOLUTION

- 1 quart clean water
- ½ teaspoon salt
- 8 teaspoons of sugar *or* 1 cup of infant rice cereal

Use measuring spoons to measure precisely. Mix thoroughly. If you prefer to avoid straight sugar, you can substitute rice cereal.

A traditional Japanese home remedy for upset stomach is miso soup. Some children love it, but others really don't care for the flavor. You can find miso soup in most health food stores. A more American version is chicken bouillon or chicken broth.

If your baby is breast-feeding, continue to do so, even if the baby spits up every time she nurses. If she becomes uninterested in breast-feeding or has fewer wet diapers than usual, she needs to be evaluated professionally for dehydration and possible additional therapy.

Avoid solid food until the vomiting has stopped for at least two to four hours. Most children won't be hungry for solids until their stomachs have settled a bit anyway. Start cautiously with small amounts. Resume with bland foods such as rice, bananas, dry toast, Cheerios, teething biscuits, and crackers. Start with small amounts given frequently rather than one large meal. For at least a day or two, avoid greasy foods such as meats, fried eggs, or anything else that is fried. If your child is prone to motion sickness, give her a few crackers or some toast before leaving on a trip. An empty stomach can actually make her nausea *worse* than having a little something on board.

Avoid very cold foods and beverages as these can slow stomach emptying.[17]

Avoid very sweet beverages. Studies in cyclists showed that lower sugar solutions (6% glucose) were better absorbed and caused less nausea than higher sugar beverages (12% glucose).[18]

Thickening feedings may help minimize spitting up in babies with mild to moderate reflux.[19] You can thicken feedings by adding 1 tablespoon of infant rice cereal to each ounce of formula. Thickened feedings are most effective in combination with keeping the baby upright for twenty to thirty minutes following a feeding.

Exercise

Although exercise helps build strong muscles, lungs, and heart, it has some side effects on the intestines. Most long-distance runners are familiar with runner's diarrhea. Vomiting is also common after long runs or intense bicycle rides, possibly because the blood that normally supplies the stomach and intestines is diverted away to supply the muscles, interfering with normal gut function. Exercise also sometimes induces gastro-esophageal reflux, resulting in heartburn and nausea.[20] Your child is not likely to suffer these symptoms unless she is exercising very vigorously as part of a track or cross-country team. If your child does have heartburn with exercise, consider cutting back on the intensity of her workout.[21] Light exercise actually encourages the stomach to empty. Adequate training minimizes diarrhea, cramping, and nausea associated with intense exercise.[22]

As with most illnesses, rest is beneficial. If your child is tired, encourage her to rest. Try lying down with her to read a story or listening to quiet, soothing music.

Environment

Avoid stale, stuffy air. Do not let your child become chilled, but do keep fresh, cool air flowing around your child's face.

Keep an empty receptacle (a pot, bowl, or basin) near your child's bed or wherever she is resting so that if the urge strikes, she does not need to run all the way to the bathroom and worry about losing it on the way.

Some children are soothed by a cool, damp cloth placed on the forehead and over the eyes or the back of the neck. Gently clean your child's face after she vomits. If she is old enough, have her swish some water in her mouth and spit it out afterward to clean the taste of vomit out of her mouth.

Keep your baby upright after eating for at least thirty minutes. Sleeping on her tummy (prone) may result in less spitting up than sleeping on her back (spine). If she has serious problems with spitting up or reflux, you can consult a physical therapist about making a special foam wedge or sling to keep your baby's head and chest elevated while she sleeps, or you can buy one ready made [Infant Reflux Wedge, available from Pedicraft, 4134 St. Augustine Road, Jacksonville, FL 32207. 1(800)223–7649].

Mind-Body

Several studies have shown that hypnosis can be helpful in reducing intractable vomiting,[23] for children struggling with the severe nausea and vomiting due to cancer chemotherapy,[24, 25] for cutting back on the gagging children sometimes have when trying to swallow pills,[26] and for eliminating habitual vomiting.[27] Desensitization therapy, relaxation therapy, and biofeedback have also proved useful in treating air sickness in pilots and nausea in

patients undergoing chemotherapy.[28, 29] If your child has recurrent vomiting from chemotherapy or motion sickness, it is probably worthwhile to consult a hypnotherapist. If your child has a simple case of food poisoning or gastroenteritis, the vomiting will probably be over by the time you get an appointment to see a therapist.

For most people, there is something vaguely shameful about vomiting. It is important to reassure your child that you love her and will stay with her, that it's OK to vomit if she needs to, and that vomiting will help clear the toxins from her system.

BIOMECHANICAL THERAPIES: MASSAGE, SURGERY

Massage

Massaging the belly could trigger more nausea in sensitive children. Rather than massage the abdomen directly, you may try an old folk remedy: soak a cotton flannel cloth in castor oil and lay the cloth over your child's abdomen. Cover with a towel, and let the child rest for an hour or so before gently rinsing off with a baking soda and water solution. There are *no* scientific studies evaluating this remedy, but it is safe and inexpensive.

Surgery

Surgery is unnecessary to treat the flu, but it can be lifesaving if vomiting is due to appendicitis. If your child has severe abdominal pain, especially if it localizes on the right lower side where the appendix is located, please seek medical care immediately.

BIOENERGETIC THERAPIES: ACUPUNCTURE, HOMEOPATHY

Acupuncture

There are numerous studies evaluating the effectiveness of acupuncture and acupressure in treating nausea and vomiting. The point most often used is Pericardium 6 (P6), located about 1 inch above the wrist crease, between the two tendons leading to the palm. This is about where your watch clasp falls on your wrist.

In several comparison studies, acupuncture therapy given before surgery significantly reduced postoperative nausea and vomiting in adults for up to six hours after surgery.[30] Real acupuncture or acupressure is more effective than sham (placebo) acupuncture in preventing postsurgical nausea and reducing the need for antinausea medication in adults.[31, 32, 33] In fact, acupuncture stimulation is as effective as antiemetic medication.[34, 35] Applying pressure to the P6 point intermittently following the initial acupuncture treatment prolongs its antiemetic effect for up to twenty-four hours.[36]

Acupuncture treatment at the P6 point has also proved useful in treating morning sickness. Comparison studies have shown that daily pressure (using wrist bands) at the P6 point was more effective than sham or placebo acupressure in reducing nausea.[37, 38] Acupressure wrist bands may also reduce the anxiety, depression, and other emotional discomforts that accompany morning sickness.[39] While acupressure therapy is effective, it may need to be repeated as often as every two hours to achieve consistent control of symptoms.[40]

Stimulation of the P6 point has even proved effective in treating nausea due to cancer chemotherapy.[41] Like medications, acupuncture improves symptoms but does not cure the underlying cause. Treatment may need to be repeated every few hours.[42]

Unfortunately, there have been few studies of acupuncture in children. Several studies have shown that acupuncture therapy is *not* helpful in treating children suffering from postoperative nausea and vomiting.[43, 44] Acupuncture is extremely safe and low in side effects compared with antiemetic medications.[45] *All needling and injections should be done by a licensed health care provider*; acupressure massage can be done by nonlicensed persons such as parents.

Homeopathy

As expected from the homeopathic principle of "like cures like," all of these remedies actually *cause* vomiting if taken in higher, nonhomeopathic doses: *Aconitum* (aconite), *Antimonium tartaricum* (tartar emetic), *Arsenicum album* (arsenic), *Bryonia alba* (white bryony), *China officianalis* (Cinchona officianalis), *Ferrum metallicum* (iron), *Ipecac, Nux vomica* (poison nut), *Phosphorus,* and *Pulsatilla.* There are *no* scientific studies evaluating the effectiveness of homeopathy in treating children with nausea or vomiting. I do not recommend them.

WHAT I RECOMMEND TO TREAT VOMITING

> ### Take Your Baby or Child to be Evaluated If She
>
> - Spits up more than a tablespoon of milk with each feeding
> - Is losing weight or not gaining weight as well as predicted
> - Is less than ten weeks old and has very forceful (projectile) vomiting
> - Is vomiting when she drinks even small amounts (less than a tablespoon) of water
> - Has violent retching
> - Has a yellowish tinge to her skin or eyes (jaundice)
> - Vomits up bile (greenish fluid) or blood or coffee-ground looking material
> - Has a temperature over 100.5°F if she is less than two months old
> - Has a temperature over 103.9°F at any age
> - Has severe abdominal pain, especially in the lower right side (could be appendicitis)
> - Vomits more than three times or more than an hour following a head injury
> - Vomits continuously for more than twenty-four hours
> - Seems uninterested in drinking or appears to be dehydrated
> - Or if you are concerned about her symptoms or appearance

For Babies Who Spit Up (or Have Reflux)

1. *Lifestyle—nutrition.* Small, frequent feedings, frequent burping; consider thickening feedings by adding 1 tablespoon of dry rice cereal to each ounce of formula.

2. *Lifestyle—environment.* Keep the baby's head elevated during sleep; keep the baby's head elevated while feeding and for at least thirty minutes afterward.

For Gastroenteritis

1. *Lifestyle—nutrition.* Small amounts of rehydration fluid, Pedialyte, ginger soda, miso soup, broth, rice water, or herbal tea containing chamomile, lemon balm, and mint sipped frequently; avoid solid foods and milk until the child has had at least two to four consecutive hours without vomiting; start with bananas, crackers, toast, and rice. Avoid very cold or very sweet fluids.

2. *Biochemical—medications.* Avoid them unless you have consulted a health care professional.

For Motion Sickness

1. *Lifestyle—environment.* Fresh air (keep the window open or stay on deck); ride in the front seat; focus on the horizon (count telephone poles or other distant objects); don't let the child read or focus on objects close up inside the car or boat.

2. *Biochemical—herbs.* Consider ginger supplements (can chew on ginger root or sip ginger soda).

3. *Biochemical—nutritional supplements.* Consider pyridoxine (B6) supplements— 10 milligrams an hour or two before the ride.

4. *Lifestyle—nutrition.* Eat a light snack before traveling so the stomach isn't completely empty.

5. *Bioenergetic—acupuncture.* Consider acupressure or massage to the P6 point on the inside of the wrist.

6. *Biochemical—medications.* Consider medications such as Benadryl or Dramamine before the trip. If home remedies are unsuccessful, see your physician for stronger prescription medications.

7. *Lifestyle—mind-body.* If home remedies have not worked, consider professional hypnotherapy to prevent severe, recurrent motion sickness.

For Morning Sickness

1. *Biochemical—nutritional supplements.* Vitamin B6 (pyridoxine): 10–25 milligrams one to three times daily.

2. *Biochemical—herbs.* Ginger: tablets, soda, or freshly grated.

3. *Bioenergetic—acupuncture.* Acupuncture or acupressure at the P6 point (1 inch above the wrist crease between the tendons leading to the palm of the hand).

4. *Lifestyle—mind-body.* If home remedies have not worked, consider professional hypnotherapy, relaxation therapy, or biofeedback.

For vomiting due to other causes, treat the underlying problem.

27
WARTS

Nick Evans brought his six-year-old daughter, Amy, to be treated for warts. Amy had had a few warts on her knees for the last two months, but over the last week or so she had developed four new warts on her hands. The warts didn't hurt, but Amy kept picking at them and biting them, making them bleed. Nick had heard about having warts burned or frozen off, but he wondered if there wasn't some less drastic but still effective treatment.

WHAT CAUSES WARTS?

For one thing, frogs and toads don't! There are several kinds of warts, and all are caused by human papilloma viruses (HPV). This chapter covers the two kinds of warts that most often affect kids: *common warts* (usually found on the hands, face, knees, or elbows) and *plantar warts* (painful warts on the soles of the feet).

Common warts are bumpy and firm with a dry surface. Plantar warts grow into the skin on the soles of the feet and look flat. Warts can be skin color, pink, tan, yellow, gray, black, or brown. Warts often contain brown dots and do not contain the whorls and ridges of fingerprints. If the top is cut off, warts bleed because tiny blood vessels grow into their center. Warts seldom appear before the age of two or after the age of forty. Over the course of a lifetime, 75% of people develop warts. Warts are second to acne as the leading reason for visits to dermatologists.

Warts are not very contagious, but swimmers and other athletes who use communal showers are slightly more likely than those who don't use locker rooms to catch plantar warts.[1] If your child uses communal showers or locker rooms, have her wear flip-flop, sandals, or other shower shoes to prevent direct contact between her feet and the floor, which may be harboring wart viruses.

WHAT IS THE BEST WAY TO TREAT WARTS?

Most warts go away by themselves without any therapy other than patience. Interestingly, kids with overactive skin immunity (eczema) have fewer warts than normal kids.[2] A healthy immune system gets rid of 80% of warts within two to three years.

Warts that have been present for several months and big warts (more than 1/4 inch) are less likely to go away by themselves. They might need professional treatment. Even when warts do go away, they often recur throughout childhood. With apologies to Tom Sawyer fans, spunk water (from an old tree stump) and ritualized handling of dead cats have no proven efficacy in treating warts. Let's tour the Therapeutic Mountain to find out what does work; if you want to skip to my bottom-line recommendations, flip to the end of the chapter.

BIOCHEMICAL THERAPIES: MEDICATIONS, HERBS, NUTRITIONAL SUPPLEMENTS

Medications

The British call topical medicines (those applied directly to the skin) "wart paint." The most commonly used topical medication to treat warts is salicylic acid (the active ingredient in Compound W and Duofilm). It is available as a liquid, gel, or in "plasters" that can be placed directly on the wart. Plasters contain higher concentrations of medication and are the least messy to apply. For best results with topical wart medicine:

1. Soak the wart in warm water to soften it.
2. Peel away the loose skin on top of the wart or pare down plantar warts until you get to the tender part.[3]
3. Apply the wart medicine. Don't let it get on healthy skin.

4. Cover the medication with a dressing such as a Band-Aid or piece of tape.
5. Repeat daily until the wart is gone—up to three months.

These medications may cause some burning or blistering on healthy skin. Be careful.

Professionally applied medications may include stronger acids or silver nitrate.[4] Silver nitrate doesn't burn and is safe even on babies' tender skin. Some dermatologists have been using the ulcer medication cimetidine to treat recalcitrant warts because of cimetidine's effects on the immune system. Although there are several case reports of remarkable success with cimetidine, it has not been tested in comparison studies and has not been approved for use in young children.[5] I do *not* recommend it.

Nick decided to treat Amy's warts with Compound W every day.

Herbs

Common herbal remedies applied to warts include the juice of dandelion stalks, tincture of thuja (white cedar), milk of bitter root herbs, milk weed juice, tea tree oil, and fresh elderberry juice. None of these remedies has undergone scientific study.

Nutritional Supplements

Some folks advocate the application of vitamin A, vitamin E oil, or a paste of baking soda and castor oil to the wart several times daily until the wart is gone. Some crush a vitamin C tablet or an aspirin, mix it with water to make a paste, and apply it to the wart. Others advise rubbing the wart with a cut raw potato and burying the potato under a tree in the backyard under a full moon. Vitamins A, C, and E, castor oil, crushed aspirin, and raw potatoes have not been scientifically studied as wart treatments, but they are inexpensive and safe. Cover the wart with a Band-Aid after any treatment to minimize messiness.

LIFESTYLE THERAPIES: ENVIRONMENT, MIND-BODY

Environment

Keep warts in the *dark*. Cover the wart tightly with a piece of adhesive tape or a Band-Aid. Some people use duct tape; use whatever is handy. Keep the wart covered for a week. Take the tape off to check the wart, wash it well, and let it air out. Recover it for another week and take another peek. Many warts disappear in six weeks with this simple cover-up treatment. This technique seems to prompt the immune system to attack the wart, perhaps by increasing the temperature or humidity at the site. I could not find any scientific studies evaluating this technique, but several pediatricians I know say that this is their favorite wart remedy because it is so inexpensive and free of side effects.

A recent study showed that by *heating* warts to 50°C for thirty to sixty seconds, warts disappeared twice as well as in an untreated group.[6] Special equipment is needed to get this high temperature at the precise spot without burning healthy skin. You can try soaking warts in hot water (careful not to scald the child!) for five to ten minutes, three to four times daily. Heat seems to slow down reproduction of the wart virus.

Mind-Body

Hypnosis can be very effective in getting rid of warts.[7] In one study ten patients with warts on both the right and left sides of their body were given the hypnotic suggestion that the warts would disappear from just one side. Nine out of ten patients had warts disappear just on that one side (without any other treatment); the tenth lost warts on both sides.[8] Children have especially good imaginations, and hypnosis or suggestion can work very well in removing warts for them. Hypnosis can sometimes cure warts that have failed to respond to conventional medical therapies such as liquid nitrogen or salicylic acid.[9, 10] Involving the child in making the wart go away is more effective than simply telling him that a placebo will work.[11] Hypnosis is even effective in children whose immune systems are suppressed by illness or chemotherapy.[12]

I often use the technique my childhood doctor used with me: I tell the child that she can tell her warts to go away and that when she comes back in a month, I will give her a quarter for every wart she has made disappear. You can help your child imagine the wart disappearing, feeling the warmth or tingling as the blood carries it away. The more vivid the imagery, the more effective the treatment. Hypnotherapy or suggestion works best if the child is *convinced* that the wart will go away, *involved* in the cure, and something is *done* to the wart.[13]

No one knows whether hypnosis works by shrinking the blood vessels supplying the wart or by stimulating the immune system to fight the wart-causing virus.[14] This would be a fascinating area for additional research because, either way, there are important implications for other, more serious illnesses such as cancer.

Before applying the Compound W to Amy's warts, Nick planned to have her soak them in hot water for five minutes. After applying the Compound W, they covered each wart with a Band-Aid. Amy received a sticker each day she soaked, put the medicine on, and covered it with a Band-Aid. If she accumulated five stickers in a week, she could pick out her own video to rent on the weekend. I asked Amy to return to the clinic in a month so we could count the warts. For every wart she got rid of, I'd pay her a quarter. We repeated this routine once. Within three months all of Amy's warts had disappeared, without a single scar, and she was very proud of herself.

BIOMECHANICAL THERAPIES: SURGERY

Most doctors are trained in surgical methods for wart removal. The most common surgical treatment is freezing the wart with liquid nitrogen. The treatment consists of soaking the wart (to soften it), paring it down (especially for warts on the feet), and then applying cold liquid nitrogen until it freezes the wart. The liquid nitrogen is applied with a cotton swab or sprayed directly on the wart. Treatments are repeated every one to three weeks until the wart is gone. This works well for warts on the hand but is often painful and ineffective for warts on the sole of the foot.

Most of the time when parents come to me asking to have the wart frozen, they have tried a nonprescription treatment for a week or so, and the wart is still there. Usually it takes at least a month for any home remedy to work. I generally reserve liquid nitrogen or other surgical treatments for children who have already tried a mind-body technique (suggestion or hypnosis), home therapy with wart paint, and covering the wart with a Band-Aid or tape. If the warts survive one to three months of this treatment, I'll go ahead and use liquid nitrogen. It is inexpensive and has few side effects.

Warts can also be electrically cauterized (zapped), lasered, or cut off. I don't recommend these treatments unless all else has failed, because they are painful and can leave scars.

BIOENERGETIC THERAPIES: HOMEOPATHY

In a controlled trial in Canada, a combination homeopathic remedy was no more effective than a placebo in treating plantar warts. In both the treatment and the comparison placebo group, about 25% of patients were cured eighteen weeks after starting treatment.[15] I do *not* recommend homeopathic remedies as wart therapy.

WHAT I RECOMMEND FOR TREATING WARTS

Be patient. Most warts go away by themselves.

Seek Professional Help If

- The wart becomes infected (red, painful, swollen)
- The wart is on the face
- The wart doesn't disappear within three months with home therapy
- You are concerned about the wart

---

1. *Lifestyle—environment.* Keep the wart in the dark. Cover it with a Band-Aid or piece of adhesive tape for a week at a time. Many warts go away in six to eight weeks with this remedy alone.

2. *Lifestyle—mind-body.* Give your child the suggestion that she can make the warts go away. Help her develop vivid imagery about her immune system fighting the warts, the warts melting away, and how the skin might feel tingly or warm as it's working. Consider an incentive for her success (a quarter, a sticker, or a book for every wart she eliminates).

3. *Biochemical—medications.* If suggestion and darkness don't work, try a nonprescription salicylic acid preparation such as Compound W or Duofilm. Apply the medication daily, and keep it covered with a Band-Aid or adhesive tape.

4. *Biomechanical—surgery.* If warts have not disappeared with three months of home therapy, see your doctor about zapping the wart with liquid nitrogen.

ADDITIONAL RESOURCES

When requesting information by mail, please enclose a self-addressed, stamped envelope.

BIOCHEMICAL THERAPIES: HERBS

For answers to basic questions about herbs, or for a list of associations that can provide referrals to health providers familiar with herbs, contact:

Herb Research Foundation
1007 Pearl Street, Suite 200
Boulder, CO 80302
1(303)449–2265

For a free information packet or to order a newsletter, articles, or books, contact:

HerbalGram
American Botanical Council
PO Box 201660
Austin, TX 78720
1(800)373–7105

To order herbs, contact:

Merz Apothecary
4716 N Lincoln Avenue
Chicago, IL 60625
1(800)252–0275

Books on Herbal Medicine

McIntyre, Anne. *The Herbal for Mother and Child.* Element, 1992.

Murray, Michael T. *The Healing Power of Herbs: The Enlightened Person's Guide to the Wonders of Medicinal Plants.* Prima Publishing, 1992.

Tyler, V.E. *The Honest Herbal: The Sensible Guide to the Use of Herbs and Related Remedies.* 3rd ed. Pharmaceutical Products Press, 1993.

LIFESTYLE THERAPIES: NUTRITION, EXERCISE, MIND-BODY

Nutrition

For information on a vegetarian diet, contact:

Physician's Committee for
Responsible Medicine
PO Box 6322
Washington, DC 20015
1(800)US LIVES

For journals or newsletters, contact:

Nutrition Action Health Letter
Center for Science in the Public Interest
1875 Connecticut Avenue NW
Washington, DC 20009
1(202)332–9110, ext. 391

Vegetarian Times
1140 Lake Street, Suite 500
Oak Park, IL 60301
1(800)435–9610

Books on Nutrition

Barnard, Neal D. *The Power of Your Plate*.
   1990.

Carper, Jean. *Food, Your Miracle Medicine*.
   HarperCollins, 1993.

David, T.J. *Food and Food Additive Intolerance
   in Childhood*. Blackwell Scientific
   Publications, 1993.

Exercise

To find a yoga teacher in your area, contact:

Himalayan Institute of Yoga, Science
   and Philosophy
RR 1 Box 400
Honesdale, PA 18431
1(800)822–4547

Iyengar Yoga Institute
2404 27th Avenue
San Francisco, CA 94116
1(415)753–0909

Contact your local YMCA and YWCA for exercise programs in your community.

Books on Exercise

Prudden, Bonnie. *How to Keep Your Child Fit
   from Birth to Six*. Ballantine Books, 1986.

Reginer, Susan. *Exercises for Baby and Me*.
   Simon & Schuster, 1990.

Rosen-Sawyer, Fran, Malthy, Bonnie. *Yoga and
   Meditation for Children*. Fivefold Path, 1983.

Stewart, Mary, Phillips, Kathy. *Yoga for
   Children*. A Fireside Book. Simon &
   Schuster, 1992.

Mind-Body

Hypnosis

For more information about practitioners in
your area, contact:

Society for Clinical and Experimental
   Hypnosis
6728 Old McLean Village Drive
McLean, VA 22101–3906
1(800)214–1738

For more information about healing imagery,
contact:

Menninger Clinic
Biofeedback Department
PO Box 829
Topeka, KS 66601–0829
1(913)273–7500, ext. 5375

Books about Hypnosis and Imagery

Achterberg, Jeanne, Dossey, Barbara,
   Kolkmeier, Leslie. *Rituals of Healing: Using
   Imagery for Health and Wellness*. Bantam
   Books, 1994.

Hilgard, Josephine, LeBaron, Samuel.
   *Hypnotherapy of Pain in Children with
   Cancer*. Brunner-Mazel, 1991.

Simonton, Carl, Matthews-Simonton,
   Stephanie. *Getting Well Again*. Jeremy P.
   Tarcher, 1982.

Biofeedback

For local referrals and general information about biofeedback, contact:

Association for Applied Psychophysiology
 and Biofeedback
10200 West 44th Avenue, Suite 304
Wheat Ridge, CO 80033
1(303)422–8436

Books on Biofeedback

Norris, Patricia, Porter, Garrett. *Why Me? Harnessing the Healing Power of the Human Spirit*. Stillpoint Publishing, 1985.

Meditation

For information or referrals to similar clinics around the country, contact:

Stress Reduction Clinic
University of Massachusetts Medical Center
55 Lake Avenue North
Worcester, MA 01655–0267
1(508)856–1616

Mind-Body Medical Institute
Deaconess Hospital
185 Pilgrim Road
Boston, MA 02215
1(617)632–9530

For information about a Transcendental Meditation Center in your area, call:
 1(800)843–8332

For referrals to meditation centers and related products, contact:

Maharishi Ayur-Ved Products,
 International, Inc.
PO Box 49667
Colorado Springs, CO 80949–9667
1(800)255–8332

Books on Meditation

Benson, Herbert. *The Relaxation Response*. Outlet Books, 1993.

Borysenko, Jean. *Minding the Body, Mending the Mind*. Bantam Books, 1988.

Chopra, Deepak. *Perfect Health: The Complete Mind-Body Guide*. Crown, 1991.

Garth, Maureen. *Starbright: Meditations for Children*. Harper & Row, 1991.

Kabat-Zinn, Jon. *Full Catastrophe Living*. Doubleday, 1990.

Langford, Anne. *Meditation for Little People*. DeVorss, 1975.

Rozman, Deborah A. *Meditating with Children: The Art of Concentration and Centering*. Planetary Publications, 1994.

Counseling/Psychotherapy

For more information about pediatric psychologists in your state, contact:

American Psychological Association
750 First Street NE
Washington, DC 20002–4242
1(202)336–5500

Books on Mind-Body Medicine

Goleman, Daniel, Gurin, Joel. *Mind/Body Medicine: How to Use Your Mind for Better Health*. New York: Consumer Reports Books, 1993.

BIOMECHANICAL THERAPIES: MASSAGE, SPINAL MANIPULATION

Massage

For a referral to a local therapist, contact:

American Massage Therapy Association
820 Davis Street, Suite 100
Evanston, IL 60201–4444
1(312)761–2682 or 1(708)864–0123

Books about Massage

McClure, Vimala Schneider. *Infant Massage: A Handbook for Loving Parents*. Bantam Books, 1989.

Sinclair, Marribetts, Fingiand, Randy, Nelson, Stan. *Massage for Healthier Children*. Wingbow Press, 1992.

Thomas, Sara. *Massage for Common Ailments*. Fireside Books, 1989.

Spinal Manipulation

Chiropractic

For more information about chiropractors in your area, contact:

American Chiropractic Association
1701 Clarendon Boulevard
Arlington, VA 22209
1(800)986-INFO (4636)

Article on Chiropractic

Chiropractors. *Consumer Reports*, June 1994, pp. 383–90.

Osteopathic Manipulation

For information on locating a doctor of osteopathy, contact:

American Academy of Osteopathy
3500 DePauw Boulevard, Suite 1080
Indianapolis, IN 46268
1(317)879–1881

BIOENERGETIC THERAPIES: ACUPUNCTURE, THERAPEUTIC TOUCH, PRAYER, HOMEOPATHY

Acupuncture

Request a list of accredited practitioners from:

American Association of Acupuncture and
    Oriental Medicine
433 Front Street
Catasauqua, PA 18032
1(610)433–2448

National Committee for the Certification of
    Acupuncturists
1424 16th Street NW, Suite 501
Washington, DC 20036
1(202)232–1404

American Academy of Medical Acupuncture
    Physician Referral Line
1(800)521–2262

Article on Acupuncture

Acupuncture. *Consumer Reports*, Jan. 1994, pp. 54–9.

Therapeutic Touch, Healing Touch, Reiki, or *Qi Gong*

For information on how to find a trained Therapeutic Touch practitioner, contact:

Nurse Healers–Professional Associates, Inc.
PO Box 444
Allison Park, PA 15101–0444
1(412)355–8476

Books on Therapeutic Touch, Qi Gong, and Healing Touch

Brennan, Barbara Ann. *Hands of Light: A Guide to Healing Through The Human Energy Field*. Bantam Books, 1988.

Connor, Danny, Tse, Michael. *Qigong: Chinese Meditation and Movement for Health.* Weiser, 1992.

Krieger, Dolores. *The Therapeutic Touch: How to Use Your Hands To Help or Heal*, 1979.

Krieger, Dolores. *Accepting Your Power to Heal: The Personal Practice of Therapeutic Touch.* Bear & Co., 1993.

Tsu Kuo Shih. *Qi Gong: The Chinese Art of Healing with Energy.* Station Hill Press, 1992.

Weinman, Ric A. *Your Hands Can Heal: Learn to Channel Healing Energy.* New York: Viking/Penguin, 1992.

Prayer

An excellent recent review about the healing power of prayer is:

Dossey, Larry. *Healing Words: The Power of Prayer and the Practice of Medicine.* New York: HarperCollins, 1993.

Homeopathy

For a national directory of homeopaths and other information, contact:

Homeopathic Educational Services (also a source of homeopathic remedies)
2124 Kittredge Street
Berkeley, CA 94704
1(800)359–9051

For more information about practitioners in your area, contact:

National Center for Homeopathy
801 N. Fairfax Street, Suite 306
Alexandria, VA 22314
1(703)548–7790

International Foundation for Homeopathy
2366 Eastlake Avenue East, Suite 301
Seattle, WA 98102
1(206)324–8230

To obtain homeopathic products, contact:

Boericke and Tafel, Inc.
2381 Circadian Way
Santa Rosa, CA 95407
1(800)876–9505

Boiron
PO Box 449
#6 Campus Boulevard-Building A
Newtown Square, PA 19073
1(800)258–8823

Washington Homeopathic Products, Inc.
4914 Del Ray Avenue
Bethesda, MD 20814
1(800)336–1695

Standard Homeopathic Co.
154 W. 131st Street
Los Angeles, CA 90061
1(800)624–9659

Dolisos Homeopathic Co.
1(800)365–4767

Books and Articles on Homeopathy

Castro, Miranda. *Homeopathy for Pregnancy, Birth and Your Baby's First Year.* St. Martin's Press, 1993.

Homeopathy—Much Ado About Nothing? *Consumer Reports*, March 1994, pp. 201–6.

Kleijnen, J., Knipschild, P., Gerben, ter Riet. Clinical trials of homeopathy. *British Medical Journal* 302(1991):316–23.

Morgan, Lyle W, III. *Homeopathy and Your Child.* Healing Arts Press, 1992.

Ullman, Dana. *Homeopathic Medicine for Children and Infants.* Los Angeles: Jeremy P. Tarcher, 1992.

HOLISTIC MEDICINE

For a list of doctors in your area who are interested in holistic medicine, contact:

American Holistic Medical Association
4101 Lake Boone Trail, Suite 201
Raleigh, NC 27606
1(919)787–5181

Books and Articles on Holistic Medicine

Altenberg, Henry Edward. *Holistic Medicine: A Meeting of East and West*. Japan Publications, 1992.

Alternative Medicine. *Good Housekeeping*, March 1994, pp. 99–121.

Alternative Medicine: The Facts. *Consumer Reports*, Jan. 1994, pp. 51–3.

Guinness, Alma E, editor. *Family Guide to Natural Medicine: How to Stay Healthy the Natural Way*. Reader's Digest, 1993.

Holistic Health: Directory and Resource Guide, 1994–1995. *New Age Journal,* 1994.

Margen, Sheldon, editor. *The Wellness Encyclopedia: The Comprehensive Family Resource for Safeguarding Health and Preventing Illness*. Houghton Mifflin, 1991.

Strohecker, James, editor. *Alternative Medicine: The Definitive Guide*. Future Medicine Publishing, 1993.

University of California at Berkeley Wellness Letter. School of Public Health, PO Box 420148, Palm Court, FL 32142 ($24.00 per year).

To support research in holistic care for children, send donations to:

Foundation for Pediatric Holistic Health Research
4803 Phinney Ave. N.
Seattle, WA 98103

fax: (206) 789-7300

NATUROPATHY

For information and referrals, contact:

American Association of Naturopathic Physicians
2366 Eastlake Avenue E., Suite 322
Seattle, WA 98122
1(206)323–7610

Books on Naturopathy

Murray, Michael, Pizzorno, Joseph. *Encyclopedia of Natural Medicine*. Prima Publishing, 1991.

Riggs, Marcea. *Encyclopedia of Natural Health and Healing for Children*. Prima Publishing, 1992.

Weber, Maribeth. *Natural Child Care*. Harmony Books, 1989.

AYURVEDIC MEDICINE

Ayurvedic physician referrals may be obtained through:

Maharishi Ayur-Ved Products, International, Inc.
PO Box 49667
Colorado Springs, CO 80949–9667
1(800)255–8332

The Raj
RR 4, Box 503
Fairfield, IA 52556
1(800)248–9050

Books about Ayurvedic Medicine

Chopra, Deepak. *Quantum Healing: Exploring the Frontiers of Body-Mind Medicine.* Bantam Books, 1990.

Lad, Vasant. *Ayurveda: The Science of Self-Healing—A Practical Guide.* Lotus Light Publications, 1984.

Tiwari, Maya. *Ayurveda: A Life of Balance: The Complete Guide to Ayurvedic Nutrition and Body Types with Recipes and Remedies.* Inner Traditions, 1994.

TRADITIONAL CHINESE MEDICINE

Beinfeld, Harriet, Korngold, Efrem. *Between Heaven and Earth: A Guide to Traditional Chinese Medicine.* Ballantine Books, 1991.

Kaptchuk, Ted J. *The Web That Has No Weaver: Understanding Chinese Medicine.* Congdon & Weed, 1983.

OTHER RESOURCES
Breast-Feeding

For additional information about breast-feeding, contact:

La Leche League International
PO Box 4079
1400 N. Meacham Road
Schaumburg, IL 60168
1(800)LA LECHE [525–3243]

International Lactation Consultant
Association
201 Brown Avenue
Evanston, IL 60202–3601
1(708)260–8874

Books on Breast-Feeding

La Leche League International Staff. *The Womanly Art of Breastfeeding.* NAL Dutton, 1983.

Mason, Diane, Ingersoll, Diane. *Breastfeeding and the Working Mother: The Complete Guide for Today's Nursing Mother.* St. Martin's Press, 1986.

Chronic Illnesses and Disabilities

For information on a support network that connects people who are dealing with a similar illness, handicap, or injury, send a self-addressed, stamped legal-size envelope to:

Long Distance Love (LDL)
PO Box 114
New Brunswick, NJ 08903
1(908)249–9894

A $10 fee is requested but may be waived. Please indicate whether you want to correspond with someone who has the same illness or if you have a child with an illness.

Or contact:

Mothers United for Moral Support
150 Custer Court
Green Bay, WI 54301–1243
1(414)336–5333

National Parent Network on Disabilities
1600 Prince Street, # 115
Alexandria, VA 22314
1(703)684–6763

Association for the Care of Children's Health
7910 Woodmont Avenue, Suite 300
Bethesda, MD 20814
1(301)654–6549

National Information Center for Children and
    Youth with Disabilities
PO Box 1492
Washington, DC 20013
1(800)695–0285

Magazines

*The Exceptional Parent: Parenting Your Child
    or Young Adult with a Disability*
PO Box 3000, Dept. EP
Denville, NJ 07834
1(800)247–8080

Death and Dying

For more information on support, contact:

The Compassionate Friends
PO Box 3696
Oak Brook, IL 60522–3696
1(708)990–0010

The SIDS Alliance
10500 Little Patuxent Parkway, Suite 420
Columbia, MD 21044
1(800)221-SIDS

Supplies, General

The Natural Baby Company
816 Silvia Street, 800 B-S
Trenton, NJ 08628–3299
1(609)771–9233

Insurance Alternatives

Alternative Health Group
PO Box 6279
Thousand Oaks, CA 91359
1(805)494–7818

HOW TO . . .

MEDICATIONS

Always read package labels and instructions for the proper dose for your child. If you have any questions, call your health care professional. All medications carry risks of allergic reactions and other side effects. If your child takes an overdose of any medication, herb, or nutritional supplement, call your Poison Control Center immediately.

HERBS

Herbal teas can be taken straight, added to bath water, soaked in compresses, or used as washes for irritated skin. They can be consumed warm or cool. There are two ways to prepare herbal teas: infusions and decoctions. Infusions are best for soft herbs such as chamomile and peppermint. Decoctions are used to prepare hard or woody plants such as licorice, sarsaparilla or comfrey root, fennel seed, or willow bark.

HERBAL INFUSION

- 1 cup of boiling water
- 1 teaspoon of *dried* stems, leaves, or flowers *or* 3 teaspoons of *fresh** stems, leaves, or flowers

Pour the water over the herbs in a porcelain, glass, or stainless steel container.

Steep for ten to fifteen minutes in a covered pot and strain.

Herbal teas can be sweetened as desired. Discard any tea not used within seventy-two hours. Keep herbal teas refrigerated between doses.

* Because fresh herbs contain a lot of water compared to the active ingredient, more herb is needed to achieve the same effect as with a smaller amount of dried herb.

HERBAL DECOCTION

- 1½ cups of water
- 1 teaspoon of *dried* stems, leaves, or flowers *or* 3 teaspoons of *fresh* stems, leaves, or flowers

To extract as much goodness as possible, break the dried material into very small pieces. Combine the water and herbs in a glass, ceramic, or stainless steel pot, bring to a boil, and simmer for ten to fifteen minutes. Strain. Cool. Decoctions can be sweetened as desired and taken hot or cold. Discard any tea not used within seventy-two hours. Keep refrigerated between doses.

DOSAGE GUIDELINES FOR HERBAL TEAS

Age of child	Dose
Under a year	No more than 1 teaspoon three to four times daily
1 to 3 years old	Up to 1 ounce four times daily
4 to 6 years old	Up to 2 ounces four times daily
7 to 12 years old	Up to 3 ounces four times daily
Teenagers and adults	3 to 4 ounces every four to six hours

How to Make an Herbal Poultice or Compress

- Use 1 ounce of each dried herb or 3 ounces of fresh herbs (such as comfrey and eucalyptus or plantain).

- Bruise the herbs by pounding them on a chopping board or in a bowl (using the bottom of a coffee cup to grind them against the inside of the bowl).

- Cover with 4 cups of boiling water.

- Steep for ten minutes.

- Cool until the herbs are warm to touch.

- Place the herbs in a cotton cloth, folded over so the herbs don't fall out. Place the poultice on the child's chest. You may alternate placing the poultice on the chest and the back (between the shoulder blades).

Poultices are most soothing when they are hot, but should not be hot enough to burn the child's skin. Test the temperature on the inside of your wrist.

To make a *compress*, make an herbal tea, soak the cotton cloth in the tea, wring it out, and place on the child's skin.

How to Make a Castor Oil Poultice (for Upset Stomach, Constipation)

Castor oil poultices are used in many parts of the country and were recommended by the American psychic Edgar Cayce as a remedy for many illnesses. Castor oil is very soothing, so it can be applied directly to the skin. Alternatively, you can soak a piece of flannel in it and place the flannel over the chest, abdomen, or back. Cover it with a dry towel and some plastic wrap to keep castor oil from dripping on your clean sheets. Cover the whole poultice and wrap with a heating pad set on low for twenty minutes. Again, be careful not to burn your child. Wash off the oil with a paste of baking soda and water.

NUTRITIONAL SUPPLEMENTS

If you give your child nutritional supplements:

- Give them with meals to enhance absorption.
- Break up large doses into several smaller doses given throughout the day to balance blood levels and reduce side effects.

MIND-BODY TECHNIQUES

Remain calm yourself. Use whatever techniques work best for you to relax: for example, breathing, counting, imagining what a trusted friend or advisor would say.

The more *vivid* your child's imagery, incorporating colors, sounds, smells, and the way things feel or taste, the more effective the imagery technique will be. Here are some of my favorites:

Imagery Techniques You Can Use with Your Child

1. Have your child pretend he is in his favorite place at home or in his favorite vacation place.
2. Have your child pretend she is her favorite character in a movie, story, or song.
3. Have your child pretend he is having a conversation with his favorite character in a movie, story, or song or with his favorite cartoon character or animal.
4. Have your child pretend she is in a wonderful new imaginary place or having a conversation with an imaginary friend.
5. Have your child imagine he can see a switch, dial, or thermometer that indicates how much discomfort there is. Ask him what color it is and what it looks like. Now have him turn the dial down or watch the numbers go down, reducing the discomfort as the dial goes down.
6. Help your child count something over and over. The more boring this one is, the better. You can try counting:

   - breaths in, breaths out; very big breaths; very soft breaths; etc.
   - sheep
   - blessings
   - seconds on a clock or simply numbers up to five and repeating. I have done this using a syringe marked with numbers in an emergency room. I moved the plunger to each number as we counted out loud. This was an amazingly effective distraction for the five-year-old who was receiving stitches at the time.

7. Blowing bubbles is another wonderful distraction technique. Bring some bubbles with you the next time you come to the doctor's office. Blow them away, pretending to blow away any discomfort during uncomfortable procedures such as immunizations or blood tests.

Autogenic Training

This technique was devised by a German physician, Dr. Johannes Schultz, in 1932 as a home practice technique for his hypnotherapy patients. The child repeats six simple phrases over and over (you can record these phrases on a tape with quiet music in the background to help keep your child focused on the phrases):

1. I am quiet, relaxed, and comfortable.
2. My arms and hands are heavy, relaxed, and warm.
3. My legs and feet are heavy, relaxed, and warm.
4. My heartbeat is calm and regular.
5. My breathing is deep, easy, calm, and regular.
6. My forehead is cool, relaxed, and comfortable. I am comfortable and at ease.

These key phrases are repeated over and over. I recommend that children who use autogenic training practice twice daily. Optimally, each practice session lasts as long in minutes as the child is old in years. For example, a six-year-old would practice six minutes twice daily. A fifteen-year-old would practice fifteen minutes twice daily. After the child has repeated the phrases, he or she can imagine himself as healed and strong, playing happily in a favorite place with strong, happy friends.

Deep Breathing Relaxation Exercise

Concentration on taking deep breaths is very relaxing and is helpful in a variety of conditions. Here's one series of exercises that may help your child. It's often easiest to do these while lying down and resting in bed.

Stage 1–Relax all the tummy muscles. It may help to bend the knees or put a pillow under the knees so the tummy muscles can relax more easily. Notice the air coming in through your nose and filling up your lungs so much that the tummy starts to rise. Let all the air back out. This is called a belly balloon breath.

Stage 2–After a few belly balloon breaths, notice how the air fills up the lungs and pushes the lower and middle ribs out to the sides. Imagine an accordion expanding and contracting in your lungs and ribs with each breath. This is the mighty middle breath.

Stage 3–After a few mighty middle breaths, begin to notice how your breath just normally fills the upper part of the chest. Let it back out. This is the upper expander breath.

Now you can put all three breaths together. Start by feeling the belly balloon breath; then feel the breath expand into the mighty middle breath, finally filling the upper expander breath. Feel belly, lower chest, and upper chest as you breathe in. As you breathe out, notice how the air goes out in the same order, relaxing the belly, lower chest, and finally the upper chest.

THERAPEUTIC TOUCH

Paradoxically, Therapeutic Touch does not involve actually touching your child. Rather it relies on transmitting the healing intent and energy of the parent (or other health care provider) to the ill child. The following steps are merely an outline. You will feel more comfortable and more effective providing Therapeutic Touch if you read a book or two and take a workshop before trying it on your own. I am providing these points to demystify the process, *not* to be a comprehensive course. The key elements to successful Therapeutic Touch are as follows.

1. The intent to be helpful. Try to put other, distracting thoughts out of your mind.
2. The practitioner or provider must be centered and calm. Think of a pleasant place or some inspiring imagery such as a tree, a mountain, or a waterfall to help you feel your best. We all know how upsetting it can be to be around someone who is upset. You will do your child the most good by feeling your best, most tranquil, and serene.

These first two steps are the most important. Throughout the rest of the steps, remember to remain calm and focused.

1. Holding your hands an inch or two away from your child's body, move them slowly over the body from head to toe. I go over the head with one movement, then over the arms, the chest, and abdomen, the thighs, and then the lower legs and feet in subsequent movements. Your child can be sitting up or lying down or in your lap. It doesn't matter what position the child is in as long as she is comfortable. The child can keep all her clothes on. You don't have to go over both the front and the back, but you can if it is convenient. The point of this is to try to sense through your hands any areas of asymmetry, heat, cold, tingling, or other sensations that don't feel "just right" to you.

2. Now go over the child's body/energy field again (an inch or two away from the skin) as if you were petting a cat or a dog, with soothing, stroking, calming motions. This is called *unruffling*. Many recipients comment that it feels very nice, like having someone comb their hair.
3. Go over the child's body/energy field a third time. This time, focus on smoothing out whatever asymmetry you noticed during step 3. For example, if your son has a bruised knee, concentrate on soothing the knee, sending it healing energy and drawing away the pain and irritation.
4. When it feels as if you've finished, stop. It may take thirty seconds or it may take ten minutes, but you'll know when you've finished. You can go back and use your hands to reassess how things feel different from when you started.
5. *Release.* This step is very important. Once you have stopped, remember that your child is full of healing energy and the power to get well. His recovery is not up to you; it is up to him. You have done everything you can. It is time to release the healing process to your child, knowing that all will work out for the best. This step is very important in preventing burnout and lingering feelings of guilt and "if only I'd done. . . ."

HOMEOPATHIC REMEDIES

Homeopathic remedies are very safe. If you want to try them yourself at home, professional practitioners recommend that you stick to the 6X, 6C, 12C, and 30C dilutions. The 6X and 6C are available through health food stores and mail order (see Appendix A). The 12C and 30C are considered more potent than 6X and 6C. The more intense the symptoms, the more potent the remedy used (e.g., for more severe symptoms, use 30C; for mild symptoms, use 6X). Start with one dose every fifteen to thirty minutes; as your child improves, you can give the remedies less often (every thirty to sixty minutes, then every few hours) until the symptoms resolve. The more severe the symptoms are initially, the more frequently you give the remedy. As symptoms subside, doses are given less frequently. Only give one remedy at a time. Do *not* mix remedies except on the advice of a homeopathic practitioner. Avoid giving your child anything to eat or drink (except water) within fifteen minutes of a homeopathic remedy. Avoid treating your child with camphor, camphorated products, mint, or menthol while giving homeopathic remedies; strongly aromatic compounds are thought to reduce their effectiveness. Children may have a brief period in which symptoms seem to get worse just before they get better. If your child has more serious symptoms or is not better in a day or two, seek professional assistance.

GENERAL ADVICE FOR HELPING YOUR CHILD DURING A MEDICAL PROCEDURE

Sooner or later, many parents end up taking their child for stitches, a blood draw, or other painful medical procedure. Most parents want to stay with their child and comfort him, but they often aren't sure exactly what to do. Here are some tips for what you can do to be most helpful to your child during a painful procedure.

1. Stay with your child. Most children prefer to have a calm parent present during a procedure. If you feel that it would be very difficult for you to remain calm or you think you might pass out, go ahead and take a break and get someone else to stay with your child. Ask for a chair so you can sit down next to your child.
2. Stay near the child's head or hand during the procedure. Talk with your child and hold his hand or stroke him in some way to physically reassure him you are present. Do *not* assist in holding your child down. You are the good guy in this situation. Let the medical personnel be the bad guys. You are there as a comforter, not an enforcer.
3. You may want to tell stories or talk about vacations or other things to help distract your child. On the other hand, if your child really wants to be involved in the procedure, you can calmly tell him what's going on, pointing out things in the room that are neutral and familiar—the clock on the wall, the sink, the paper towels, the doctor's shoes.
4. You do *not* need to tell your child to be brave, and you do *not* need to tell him it won't hurt. Be honest. It does hurt, but only for a little while. It is OK to cry. Be honest with your child; expect him to behave like a child, not like an adult.
5. Give him a hug and comfort him when it's over.

TABLES

Table 1
Herbal Remedies for Specific Conditions

Table 2
Nutritional Supplements for Specific Conditions

Table 3
Homeopathic Remedies for Specific Conditions

Table 1: Herbal Remedies for Specific Conditions

HERBS

COMMON NAME (LATIN NAME)	Acne	Allergies	Asthma	Bed-Wetting	Burns	Chicken Pox	Colds
Agrimony							
Aloe (Aloe socotrina)	T				Y		
Angelica (Angelica archangelica)		T	T				T
Anise seed (Pimpinella anisum)							
Balm, lemon (Melissa officianalis)							
Barberry (Berberis vulgaris)							T
Basil (Ocimum basilicum)							
Bayberry (Myrica cerifera)							T
Bitter root (Apocynum androsaemifolium)							
Bitters (Angostura or gentian)							
Black haw bark (Viburnum prunifolium)			T				
Boneset (Eupatorium perfoliatum)							
Borage (Borago officinalis)							
Burdock root (Arctium lappa)	T					T	
Calendula (Calendula officinalis)	T	T			T	T	
Caraway (Carum carvi)							
Cardomom (Elettaria cardamomum)							T
Carob							
Cascara (Rhamnus purshiana) or Buckthorn							
Castor (Oleum ricini)							
Catnip or Catmint (Nepeta cataria)	T					T	
Chamomile (Anthemis nobilis)	T			T		T	T
Chickweed (Stellaria media)							
Cinnamon (Cinnamomum zeylanicum)							T
Cleavers							
Clove (Syzygium aromaticum)							T
Coleus root		T	T				

This is a summary table. See individual chapters for details. Allergies and side effects are a potential hazard of all remedies. Y=Yes, there are scientific studies to support this use; T=Traditional use; N=No, do not use, may aggravate condition.

ILLNESSES

Colic	Conjunctivitis	Constipation	Cough	Cradle Cap	Diaper Rash	Diarrhea	Ear Infections	Eczema	Fever	Headache	Hyperactivity	Jaundice	Ringworm	Sleep Problems	Sore Throat	Vomiting	Warts
					N							T					
		Y						T			T						
			T						T								
T			T													T	
Y								T	T				T			T	
						T		T								T	
																T	
																	T
								T									
								T									
		T															
			T					T					T				
	T				T		T	T									
T																	
					N												
		Y			N							T					
T			T			T			T		T			T		T	
T	T	T	T	T	T	T	T	T	T	T	T			T		T	
	T				T												
		T			T											T	
													T				
		T														T	
						T											

HERBS

COMMON NAME (LATIN NAME)	ACNE	ALLERGIES	ASTHMA	BED-WETTING	BURNS	CHICKEN POX	COLDS
Coltsfoot (Tussilago farfara)			T				
Comfrey (Symphytum officinale)	T		T	T	T		T
Cowslip (Primula officinalis)							
Dandelion (Leontodon taraxacum)							
Dill (Anethum graveolens)							
Dong quai		T	T				
Echinacea (Echinacea purpurea)	T						T
Elderberry (Sambucus canadensis)							
Elderflower (Sambucus nigra)							
Elecampane (Inula helnium)						T	
Ephedra sinica		Y	T				T
Eucalyptus (Eucalyptus globulus)							T
Eyebright (Euphrasia officinalis)		T					
Fennel (Foeniculum vulgare)							
Feverfew (Pyrethrum parthenium)							
Fo-ti							
Garlic (Allium sativum)					N		
Gentian							
Ginger (Zingiber officinale)			T				T
Ginseng (Panax quinquefolium)							
Goldenrod (Solidago canadensis)		T					
Goldenseal (Hydrastis canadensis)	T	T					T
Gotu kola (Centella asiatica)					T		
Ground ivy (Glechoma hederacea)							
Gum myrrh							
Gum plant (Grindelia sqaurrosa)						T	
Hawthorn							

This is a summary table. See individual chapters for details. Allergies and side effects are a potential hazard of all remedies. Y=Yes, there are scientific studies to support this use; T=Traditional use; N=No, do not use, may aggravate condition.

ILLNESSES

Colic	Conjunctivitis	Constipation	Cough	Cradle Cap	Diaper Rash	Diarrhea	Ear Infections	Eczema	Fever	Headache	Hyperactivity	Jaundice	Ringworm	Sleep Problems	Sore Throat	Vomiting	Warts
			N														
	T	T	T	T	T										T		
			T							T							
			T					T				T	T				T
T																	
Y																	
			T			T	T	T				T			T		
																	T
	T			T			T		T								
			T														
										N				N			
			T												T		
	T																
T		T	T													T	
										Y							
			T		N	T	T				T						
									T							T	
T		T	T		T											Y	
			T							T				N			
							T		T								
	T	T		T	T	T	T	T							T	T	
								T									
								T									
							T										
															T		
									T								

HERBS

COMMON NAME (LATIN NAME)	Acne	Allergies	Asthma	Bed-wetting	Burns	Chicken Pox	Colds
Hops (Humulus lupulus)				N		T	
Horehound (Marrubium vulgare)							T
Hyssop (Hyssopus officinalis)							T
Juniper (Juniperus communis)	T			T			
Lavender (Lavandula)	T						
Lemon balm (Melissa officinalis)							
Lemon grass							
Licorice (Glycyrrhiza glabra)		T	T				T
Lime or Linden flowers (Tilia europaea)							
Lobelia (Lobelia inflata)			T				T
Ma huang		T	T				T
Magnolia		T					
Marigold (Calendula officinalis)							
Marsh mallow root (Althaea officinalis)			T		T		
Meadowsweet (Filipendula ulmaria)							
Milk thistle							
Milkweed (Asclepias syriaca)							
Mugwort (Artemisia vulgaris)							
Mullein (Verbascum thapsus)			T		T		
Nettle (Urtica dioca or U. urens)		T	T				
Oregon grape	T						
Parsley (Petroselinum sativum)			T				
Passion flower (Passiflora incarnata)				N		T	
Peppermint (Mentha piperita)			T			T	
Picrorhiza kurroa							
Plantain (Plantago major)		T				T	T
Red clover (Trifolium pratense)			T				

This is a summary table. See individual chapters for details. Allergies and side effects are a potential hazard of all remedies. Y=Yes, there are scientific studies to support this use; T=Traditional use; N=No, do not use, may aggravate condition.

ILLNESSES

Colic	Conjunctivitis	Constipation	Cough	Cradle Cap	Diaper Rash	Diarrhea	Ear Infections	Eczema	Fever	Headache	Hyperactivity	Jaundice	Ringworm	Sleep Problems	Sore Throat	Vomiting	Warts
							T			N				T			
		T													T		
		T					T										
				T			T			T	T		T				
	T							T								T	
											T						
Y	T	T				T	T	T							T	T	
		T														T	
		T				T											
		T		T								T					
	T	T	T														
			T	T												T	
											T	T					
																	T
		T															
		T				T									T		
		T						T					T				
					T			T								T	
												T					
						T								T			
Y		T				T	T		T	T			T			T	
	T	T	T			T	T										
						T					T		T				

HERBS

Common Name (Latin Name)	Acne	Allergies	Asthma	Bed-wetting	Burns	Chicken Pox	Colds
Red raspberry leaf (Rubus idaeus)							
Rose (Rosa)							
Rosemary (Rosmarinus officinalis)							
Sage (Salvia officinalis)						T	
Saint-John's-wort (Hypericum perforatum)				T			
Sandalwood	T						
Sarsaparilla (Aralia nudicaulis)							
Senega snakeroot (Polygala senega)							T
Senna (Cassia marilandica)							
Skullcap (Scutellaria lateriflora)		T	T	N		T	
Slippery elm bark (Ulmus fulva)					T		T
Strawberry leaves (Fragaria vesca)							
Swedish bitters							
Tea tree	Y				N		T
Thuja (white cedar)							
Thyme (Thymus vulgaris)	T		T				T
Turmeric (Curcuma longa)	T						
Valerian					N	T	
Vervain (Verbena officinalis)							
Violet (Viola odorata)							
White willow bark							
Wild cherry bark			T				
Wild indigo							
Wild yam (Dioscorea villosa)		T					
Wintergreen (Gaultheria procumbens)							
Witch hazel (Hamamelis virginica)						T	
Yarrow (Achillea millefolium)	T	T		T		T	
Yellow dock root (Rumex crispus)							
Yerba santa (Eriodictyon californicium)			T				

Colic	Conjunctivitis	Constipation	Cough	Cradle Cap	Diaper Rash	Diarrhea	Ear Infections	Eczema	Fever	Headache	Hyperactivity	Jaundice	Ringworm	Sleep Problems	Sore Throat	Vomiting	Warts
	T					T											
	T									T							
T	T				T					T							
			T					T							T		
							T	T						T			
			T					T									
			T														
		Y				N											
							T			T				T			
		T	T	T		T									T	T	
								T		T							
								N					Y				T
																	T
			T												T		
										T	N			T			
Y																T	
	T							T		T							
									T	Y							
			T														
			T														
		T															
						T											
					T	T											
									T								
						T											

Table 2: Nutritional Supplements for Specific Conditions

NUTRITIONAL SUPPLEMENTS	Acne	Allergies	Asthma	Burns	Chicken Pox	Colds
VITAMINS						
Vitamin A	Y*	?		Y		
Vitamin B3 (niacin)						
Vitamin B6 (pyridoxine)	?	?	Y			
Vitamin B12 (cyanocobalamin)	N	?				
Vitamin C (ascorbic acid)		?	?	Y		Y
Vitamin D						
Vitamin E		?			?	
Biotin						
MINERALS						
Calcium						
Chromium	?					
Iodine	N					
Magnesium			Y			
Selenium	?	?				
Zinc	?	?		?		?
MISCELLANEOUS						
Apple cider vinegar					?	
Baking soda					?	
Bromelains (enzymes)		?				?
Castor oil						
EFA (evening primrose oil)		?				
Garlic						?
Ginger						
Honey					Y	
Papaya (digestive enzymes)		?				
Bee pollen or propolis		?				
Onion			?			?
Peppers, hot (capsaicin)		?	?			?

*topical

ILLNESSES

Colic	Constipation	Cough	Cradle Cap	Diaper Rash	Diarrhea	Ear Infections	Eczema	Fever	Headache	Hyperactivity	Jaundice	Ringworm	Sleep Problems	Sore Throats	Vomiting	Warts
		?		?	?	?	?	N	N							?
											N					
															Y	
	Y	?											?			
	Y				N	?	Y	?		?		?		?		?
									N							
				?		?										?
			?			?										
													?			
	Y								?				?			
					Y	Y	?		?	N	?			?		
														?		
			T									?				
																?
		?														?
			?			?	Y									
?		?	N					?				?		?		
								?	?						?	
		?												?		
									?							
?		?												?		
		?						?								

?=Unknown or insufficient data for children; Y=Yes, proven effective; N=No, may worsen condition

Table 3: Homeopathic Remedies for Specific Conditions

ILLNESSES

REMEDIES

FORMAL NAME (COMMON NAME)	Acne	Allergies	Asthma	Bed-wetting	Burns	Chicken Pox
ABC						
Aconitum (aconite or monkshood)						
Allium cepa (red onion)		T				
Alumina (aluminum)						
Ambrosia (ragweed)		T				
Antimonium	T		T			
Apis (crushed bee)		T				
Arnica (arnica)					T	
Arsenicum album (white arsenic)			T			
Belladonna (deadly nightshade)				T		
Bryonia (wild hops)		T				
Calcarea Carbonica (calcium carbonate)						
Calendula (pot marigold)					T	
Cantharis (Spanish fly)						
Carbo animalis	T					
Causticum (potassium hydrate)				T	T	
Chamomilla (chamomile)			T			
Cinchona (Peruvian bark)						
Colocynthis (bitter cucumber or apple)						
Dioscorea (wild yam)						
Equisetum (horsetail)				T		
Euphrasia (eyebright)		T				
Ferrum metallicum (iron)						
Ferrum phosphorica (phosphate of iron)						
Gelsemium (yellow jasmine)						
Graphites (black lead)						
Hepar sulfur	T					
Housedust						

T=Traditional use. This is a summary table; see text for additional information.

Colds	Colic	Conjunctivitis	Constipation	Cough	Diaper Rash	Diarrhea	Ear Infections	Eczema	Fever	Headache	Jaundice	Ringworm	Sleep Problems	Sore Throat	Vomiting	Warts
							T									
T			T			T	T		T					T	T	
T			T													
			T													
															T	
		T												T		
				T												
T					T	T			T				T		T	
T		T		T	T		T		T	T			T	T		
T			T	T					T	T					T	
			T			T					T	T				
		T		T												
	T			T	T	T							T			
											T				T	
	T				T											
	T															
T		T		T												
															T	
									T							
T									T	T						
				T								T				
				T											T	
							T									

341

REMEDIES

FORMAL NAME (COMMON NAME)	Acne	Allergies	Asthma	Bed-wetting	Burns	Chicken Pox
Hypericum (Saint-John's-wort)					T	
Ipecac (ipecac root)			T			
Kali bichromicum (potassium bichromate)		T				
Kali bromatum	T					
Kreosotum (beechwood kreosote)				T		
Lachesis (venom of the bushmaster)						
Lobelia (Indian tobacco)		T				
Lycopodium (club moss)						
Magnesia Phosphorica (phosphate of magnesium)						
Medorrhinum						
Mercurius (mercury)						
Natrum muriaticum (sodium chloride)						
Natrum sulfuricum (sodium sulfate)						
Nux vomica (poison nut)		T	T			
Oleander						
Phosphorus (phosphorus)				T		
Podophyllum (podophyllum)						
Pulsatilla (wildflower)		T	T	T		
Rhus tox (poison ivy)		T				T
Rumex (yellow dock)						
Sabadilla (cevadilla seed)		T				
Sepia (cuttle fish)				T		
Silica						
Spongia (roasted sponge)						
Sulfur (sulfur)	T			T		
Tub bov						
Urtica urens (stinging nettle)		T			T	
Wyethia (poison wood)						

T=Traditional use. This is a summary table; see text for additional information.

ILLNESSES

Colds	Colic	Conjunctivitis	Constipation	Cough	Diaper Rash	Diarrhea	Ear Infections	Eczema	Fever	Headache	Jaundice	Ringworm	Sleep Problems	Sore Throat	Vomiting	Warts
		T		T												
			T		T										T	
T																
													T			
			T									T	T			
	T															
								T								
		T												T		
												T				
			T							T						
T	T		T						T	T		T			T	
								T								
T			T												T	
					T											
T	T	T	T		T	T	T	T				T		T	T	
													T	T		
			T													
											T					
													T	T		
			T													
					T		T	T				T	T	T		
							T									

REFERENCES

CHAPTER 1 — The Therapeutic Mountain

1. Paulsen, E., Andersen, K.E., Hausen, B.M. Compositate dermatitis in a Danish dermatology department in one year. *Contact Dermatitis* 29(1993):6–10.
2. Knight, T.E., Hausen, B.M. Melaleuca oil (tea tree oil) dermatitis. *Journal of the American Academy of Dermatology* 30(1994):423–7.
3. deGroot, A.C., Berretty, P.J., vanGinkel, C.J., et al. Allergic contact dermatitis from tocopheryl acetate in cosmetic creams. *Contact Dermatitis* 25(1991):302–4.
4. Dunn, C., Sleep, J., Collett, D. Sensing an improvement: an experimental study to evaluate the use of aromatherapy, massage and periods of rest in an intensive care unit. *Journal of Advanced Nursing* 21(1995):34–40.
5. Borkan, J., Neher, J.O., Anson, O., et al. Referrals for alternative therapies. *Journal of Family Practice* 39(1994):545–50.
6. Blumberg, D.L., Grant, W.D., Hendricks, W.R., et al. The physician and unconventional medicine. *Alternative Therapies* 1(1995):31–5.
7. Reilly, D.T. Young doctors' views on alternative medicine. *British Medical Journal* 287(1983):337–9.

CHAPTER 3 — Acne

1. Kraus, S.J. Stress, acne and skin surface free fatty acids. *Psychosomatic Medicine* 32(1970):503-7.
2. Morillas, I.M., Martinez, A.A., Lozano, L.S., et al. Is benzoyl peroxide an irritant or sensitizer? *Contact Dermatitis* 16(1987):232-3
3. Slaga, T.J., Klein-Szanto, A.J.P., Triplett, L.L., et al. Skin tumor-promoting activity of benzoyl peroxide, a widely used free radical-generating compound. *Science* 213(1981):1023-5.
4. Cartwright, R.A., Hughes, B.R., Cunliffe, W.J. Malignant melanoma, benzoyl peroxide and acne: a pilot epidemiological case-control investigation. *British Journal of Dermatology* 118(1988):239-42.
5. Zander, E., Weisman, S. Treatment of acne vulgaris with salicylic acid pads. *Clinical Therapeutics* 14(1992):247-53.
6. Fugere, P., Percival-Smith, R.K., Lussier-Cacan, S., et al. Cyproterone acetate/ethinyl estradiol in the treatment of acne: a comparative dose-response study of the estrogen component. *Contraception* 42(1990):225-34.
7. Stoughton, R.B., Leyden, J.J. Efficacy of 4 percent chlorhexidine gluconate skin cleanser in the treatment of acne vulgaris. *Cutis* 39(1987):551-3.
8. Shalita, A.R., Smith, E.B., Bauer, E. Topical erythromycin vs. clindamycin therapy for acne. *Archives of Dermatology* 120(1984):351-5.
9. Tucker, S.B., Tausend, R., Cochran, R., et al. Comparison of topical clindamycin phosphate, benzoyl peroxide, and a combination of the two for the treatment of acne vulgaris. *British Journal of Dermatology* 110(1984): 487-92.

10. Katsambas, A., Towarky, A.A., Stratigos, J. Topical clindamycin phosphate compared with oral tetracycline in the treatment of acne vulgaris. *British Journal of Dermatology* 116(1987):387-91.

11. Bassett, I.B., Pannowitz, D.L., Barnetson, R. A comparative study of tea-tree oil versus benzoyl peroxide in the treatment of acne. *Medical Journal of Australia* 153(1990):455-8.

12. Snider, B.L., Dieteman, D.F. Pyridoxine therapy for premenstrual acne flare [letter]. *Archives of Dermatology* 110(1974):130-1.

13. Michaelsson, G., Juhlin, L., Vahlquist, A. Effect of oral zinc and vitamin A in acne. *Archives of Dermatology* 113(1977):31-6.

14. Weimar, V.M., Puhl, S.C., Smith, W.H., et al. Zinc sulfate in acne vulgaris. *Archives of Dermatology* 114(1978):1776-8.

15. Kligman, A.M., Mills, O.H., Leyden, J.J., et al. Oral vitamin A in acne vulgaris: preliminary report. *International Journal of Dermatology* 20(1981):278-85.

16. Labadarios, D., Cilliers, J., Visser, L., et al. Vitamin A and acne vulgaris. *Clinical and Experimental Dermatology* 12(1987):432-6.

17. Michaelsson, G., Edqvist, L-E. Erythrocyte glutathione peroxidase activity in acne vulgaris and the effect of selenium and vitamin E treatment. *Acta Dermato-Venereologica (Stockholm)* 64(1984):9-14.

18. Dupre, A., Albarel, N., Bonafe, J.L., et al. Vitamin B-12 induced acnes. *Cutis* 24(1979):210-1.

19. Fulton, J.E., Plewig, G., Kligman, A.M. Effect of chocolate on acne vulgaris. *Journal of the American Medical Association* 210(1969): 2071-4.

20. Hoehn, G.H. Acne and diet. *Cutis* 2(1966): 389-94.

21. Wortis, J. Common acne and insulin hypoglycemia. *Journal of the American Medical Association* 108(1937):971.

22. Semon, H.C., Herrmann, F. Some observations on the sugar metabolism in acne vulgaris, and its treatment by insulin. *British Journal of Dermatology* 52(1940):123-8.

23. Bettley, F.R. The treatment of acne vulgaris with tolbutamide. *British Journal of Dermatology* 73(1961):149-51.

24. McCarty, M. High-chromium yeast for acne? *Medical Hypotheses* 14(1984):307-10.

25. Minkin, W., Cohen, H.J. Effect of chocolate on acne vulgaris [letter]. *Journal of the American Medical Association* 211(1970):1856.

26. Feldman, W., Hodgson, C., Corber, S., et al. Health concerns and health-related behaviors of adolescents. *Canadian Medical Association Journal* 134(1986):489-93.

27. Motley, R.J., Finlay, A.Y. How much disability is caused by acne? *Clinical and Experimental Dermatology* 14(1989):194-8.

28. Yihou, X. Treatment of acne with ear acupuncture: a clinical observation of 80 cases. *Journal of Traditional Chinese Medicine* 9(1989):238-9.

29. Yihou, X. Treatment of facial skin diseases with acupuncture: a report of 129 cases. *Journal of Traditional Chinese Medicine* 10(1990):22-5.

CHAPTER 4—Allergies

1. Odze, R.D., Wershil, B.K., Leichtner, A.M., Antonioli, D.A. Allergic colitis in children. *Journal of Pediatrics* 126(1995):163–9.

2. Newacheck, P.W., Taylor, W.R. Childhood chronic illness: prevalence, severity and impact. *American Journal of Public Health* 82(1992):364–71.

3. Wright, A.L., Holberg, C.J., Martinez, F.D., et al. Epidemiology of physician-diagnosed allergic rhinitis in childhood. *Pediatrics* 94(1994):895–901.

4. Wolthers, O.D. Use of alternative forms of treatment by patients attending a pediatric outpatient clinic: a questionnaire study. *Ugeskrift for Laeger (Copenhagen)* 151(1989):87–90.

5. Monro, J., Carini, C., Brostoff, J. Migraine is a food-allergic disease. *Lancet* 2(1984):719–21.

6. Egger, J., Graham, P.J., Carter, C.M., et al. Controlled trial of oligoantigenic treatment in the hyperkinetic syndrome. *Lancet* 1(1985):540–5.

7. Kahn, A., Mozin, M.J., Rebuffat, E., et al. Milk intolerance in children with persistent sleeplessness: a prospective double-blind crossover evaluation. *Pediatrics* 84(1989):595–603.

8. Berezin, S., Schwarz, S.M., Glassman, M., et al. Gastrointestinal milk intolerance of infancy. *American Journal of Diseases of Children* 143(1989):361–2.

9. Sampson, H.A., Mendelson, L., Rosen, J.P. Fatal and near-fatal anaphylactic reactions to food in children and adolescents. *New England Journal of Medicine* 326(1992):380–4.

10. Paulsen, E., Andersen, K.E., Hausen, B.M. Compositae dermatitis in a Danish dermatology department in one year. *Contact Dermatitis*, 29(1993):6–10.

11. Jalonen, T. Identical intestinal permeability changes in children with different clinical manifestations of cow's milk allergy. *Journal of Allergy and Clinical Immunology* 88(1991):737–42.

12. Sampson, H.A., Scanlon, S.M. Natural history of food hypersensitivity in children with atopic dermatitis. *Journal of Pediatrics* 115(1989):23–7.

13. Bock, S.A. Prospective appraisal of complaints of adverse reactions to foods in children during the first three years of life. *Pediatrics* 79(1987):683–8.

14. Hill, D.J., Firer, M.A., Ball, G., et al. Recovery from milk allergy in early childhood: antibody studies. *Journal of Pediatrics* 114(1989):761–6.

15. Shapiro, G.G., Anderson, J.A. Controversial techniques in allergy. *Pediatrics*, 82(1988):935–7.

16. Jewett, D.L., Fein, G., Greenberg, M.H. A double-blind study of symptom provocation to determine food sensitivity. *New England Journal of Medicine* 323(1990):429–33.

17. Kemp, J.P. Antihistamines: is there anything safe to prescribe? *Annals of Allergy* 69(1992):276–80.

18. Freier, S., Berger, H. Disodium cromoglycate in gastrointestinal protein intolerance. *Lancet* 1(1973):913–5.

19. Grossman, J., Banov, C., Bronsky, E.A., et al. Fluticasone propionate aqueous nasal spray is safe and effective for children with seasonal allergic rhinitis. *Pediatrics* 92(1993):594–9.

20. Busse, W.W. Action and effects of corticosteroids in allergic rhinitis. *Journal of Respiratory Disease* 12(1991):S36-8.

21. Valentine, M.D., Schuberth, K.C., Kagey-Sobotka, A., et al. The value of immunotherapy with venom in children with allergy to insect stings. *New England Journal of Medicine* 323(1990):1601–3.

22. Wood, R.A., Eggleston, P.A. Management of allergy to animal danders. *Pediatric Asthma, Allergy and Immunology* 7(1993):13–21.

23. Rooklin, A.R., Gawchik, S.M. Allergic rhinitis: it's that time again! *Contemporary Pediatrics* 11(1994):19–41.

24. Canadian Society of Allergy and Clinical Immunology. Guidelines for the use of allergen immunotherapy. *Canadian Medical Association Journal* 152(1995):1413–7.

25. Meltzer, E.O. Intranasal anticholinergic therapy of rhinorrhea. *Journal of Allergy and Clinical Immunology* 90(1992):1055–64.

26. Cavagni, G., Piscopo, E., Rigoli, E., et al. Food allergy in children: an attempt to improve the effects of the elimination diet with an immunomodulating agent (thymomodulin): a double-blind clinical trial. *Immunopharmacology and Immunotoxicology* 11(1989):131–42.

27. Marzari, R., Mazzanti, P., Cazzola, P., et al. Perennial allergic rhinitis: prophylaxis of acute episodes using thymomodulin. *Minerva Medica* 78(1987):1675–81.

28. Kasahara, Y., Hikino, H., Tsurufuji, S., et al. Antinflammatory actions of ephedrines in acute inflammations. *Planta Medica* 4(1985):325–31.

29. Sung, C.-P., Baker, A.P., Holden, D.A., et al. Effect of extracts of *Angelica polymorpha* on reaginic antibody production. *Journal of Natural Products* 45(1982):398–406.

30. Hikino, H. Recent research on Oriental medicinal plants. *Economic Medicinal Plant Research* 1(1985):53–85.

31. Kerouac, R., St-Pierre, S., Rioux, F. Forskolin inhibits histamine release by neurotensin in the rat perfused hind limb. *Research Communications in Chemical Pathology and Pharmacology* 45(1984):309–12.

32. Cyong, J., Otsuka, Y. A pharmacological study of the anti-inflammatory activity of Chinese herbs: a review. *Acupuncture and Electro-Therapeutics* 7(1982):173–202.

33. Kumagai, A., Nanaboshi, M., Asanuma, Y., et al.

Effects of glycyrrhizin on thymolytic and immunosuppressive action of cortisone. *Endocrinologia Japonica* 14(1967):39–42.

34. Armanini, D., Karbowiak, I., Funder, J.W. Affinity of liquorice derivatives for mineralocorticoid and glucocorticoid receptors. *Clinical Endocrinology (Oxford)* 19(1983):609–12.

35. Tsuruga, T., Ebizuka, Y., Nakajima, J., et al. Biologically active constituents of Magnolia salicifolia: inhibitors of induced histamine release from rat mast cells. *Chemical and Pharmaceutical Bulletin (Tokyo)* 39(1991):3265–71.

36. Bucca, C., Rolla, G., Oliva, A., et al. Effect of vitamin C on histamine bronchial responsiveness of patients with allergic rhinitis. *Annals of Allergy* 65(1990):311–4.

37. Lundberg, J.M., Saria, A. Capsaicin-induced desensitization of airway mucosa to cigarette smoke, mechanical and chemical irritants. *Nature* 302(1983):251–3.

38. Andre, C., Andre, F., Colin, L., et al. Measurement of intestinal permeability to mannitol and lactulose as a means of diagnosing food allergy and evaluating therapeutic effectiveness of disodium cromoglycate. *Annals of Allergy* 59(1987):127–30.

39. Fergusson, D.M., Horwood, L.J., Shannon, F.T. Early solid feeding and recurrent childhood eczema: a 10-year longitudinal study. *Pediatrics* 86(1990):541–6.

40. Paganus, A., Juntunen-Backman, K., Savilahti, E. Follow-up of nutritional status and dietary survey in children with cow's milk allergy. *Acta Paediatrica* 81(1992):518–21.

41. Heiner, D.C., Sears, J.N., Kniker, W.T. Multiple precipitins to cow's milk in chronic respiratory disease. *American Journal of Diseases of Children* 103(1962):40–60.

42. Dohi, M., Suko, M., Sugiyama, H., et al. Food-dependent, exercise-induced anaphylaxis: a study on 11 Japanese cases. *Journal of Allergy and Clinical Immunology* 87(1991):34–40.

43. Zuberbier, T., Bohm, M., Czarnetzki, B.M. Food intake in combination with a rise in body temperature: a newly identified cause of angioedema. *Journal of Allergy and Clinical Immunology* 91(1993):1226–7.

44. Martin-Munoz, F., Lopez-Cazana, J.M., Villas, F., et al. Exercise-induced anaphylactic reaction to hazelnut. *Allergy* 49(1994):314–6.

45. McDonald, L.G., Tovey, E. The role of water temperature and laundry procedures in reducing house dust mite populations and allergen content of bedding. *Journal of Allergy and Clinical Immunology* 90(1992):599–608.

46. Garrison, R.A., Robertson, L.D., Koehn, R.D., Wynn, S.R. Effect of heating-ventilation-air conditioning system sanitation on airborne fungal populations in residential environments. *Annals of Allergy* 71(1993):548–56.

47. Huang, S.-W. The effects of an air cleaner in the homes of children with perennial allergic rhinitis. *Pediatric Asthma, Allergy and Immunology* 7(1993):111–7.

48. Verhoeff, A.P., vanStrien, R.T., vanWijnen, J.H., Brunekreef, B. Damp housing and childhood respiratory symptoms: the role of sensitization to dust mites and molds. *American Journal of Epidemiology* 141(1995):103–10.

49. Brown, H.M., Merrett, T.G. Effectiveness of an acaricide in management of house dust mite allergy. *Annals of Allergy* 67(1991):25–31.

50. Sellinger, C.R. Immunotherapy for insect stings. *Pediatrics in Review* 14(1993):246.

51. Georgitis, J.W. Local hyperthermia and nasal irrigation for perennial allergic rhinitis: effect on symptoms and nasal airflow, *Annals of Allergy* 71(1993):385–9.

52. Zachariae, R., Bjerring, P. Increase and decrease of delayed cutaneous reactions obtained by hypnotic suggestions during sensitization: studies on dinitrochlorobenzene and diphenylcyclopropenone, *Allergy* 48(1993):6–11.

53. Laidlaw, T.M., Booth, R.J., Large, R.G. The variability of Type I hypersensitivity reactions: the importance of mood. *Journal of Psychosomatic Research* 38(1994):51–61.

54. Perloff, M.M., Spiegelman, J. Hypnosis in the treatment of a child's allergy to dogs. *American Journal of Clinical Hypnosis* 15(1973):269–72.

55. Belgrade, M.J., Solomon, L.M., Lichter, E.A. Effect of acupuncture on experimentally induced itch. *Acta Dermato-Venereologica (Stockholm)* 64(1984):129–33.

56. Chari, P., Biwas, S., Mann, S.B.S., et al. Acupuncture therapy in allergic rhinitis. *American Journal of Acupuncture* 16(1988):143–7.

57. Xinsheng, L., Ling, S., Re, J., et al. Acupuncture treatment of Type 1 allergic diseases: a clinical observation. *International Journal of Clinical Acupuncture* 3(1992):109–15.

58. Knipschild, P., Kleijnen, J., Rietter, G. Belief in the efficacy of alternative medicine among general practitioners in the Netherlands. *Social Science and Medicine* 31(1990):625–6.

59. Reilly, D.T., Taylor, M.A., McSharry, C., et al. Is homeopathy a placebo response? Controlled trial of homeopathic potency, with pollen in hayfever as a model. *Lancet* 2(1986):881–6.

60. Wiesenauer, M., Gaus, W. Double-blind trial comparing the effectiveness of the homeopathic preparation Galphimia potentisation D6, Galphimia dilution 10^{-6} and placebo on pollinosis. *Arzneimittelforschung(Drug Research)* 35(1985):1745–7.

61. Kleijnen, J., Knipschild, P., ter Riet, G. Clinical trials of homeopathy. *British Medical Journal* 302(1991):316–23.

CHAPTER 5 — Asthma

1. Halfon, N., Newacheck, P.W. Childhood asthma and poverty: differential impacts and utilization of health services. *Pediatrics* 91(1993):56–61.

2. Centers for Disease Control. Asthma-United States, 1982–1992. *MMWR. Morbidity and Mortality Weekly Report* 51(1995):952–5.

3. Crain, E.F., Weiss, K.B., Bijur, P.E., et al. An estimate of the prevalence of asthma and wheezing among inner city children. *Pediatrics* 94(1994):356–62.

4. Taylor, W.R., Newacheck, P.W. Impact of childhood asthma on health. *Pediatrics* 90(1992):657–62.

5. Yunginger, J.W., Reed, C.E., O'Connell, E.J., et al. A community-based study of the epidemiology of asthma: incidence rates, 1964–1983. *American Review of Respiratory Disease* 146(1992):888–94.

6. Weitzman, M., Gortmaker, S., Sobol, A. Racial, social, and environmental risks for childhood asthma. *American Journal of Diseases of Children* 144(1990):1189–94.

7. Orenstein, D.M. Exercise tolerance and exercise conditioning in children with chronic lung disease. *Journal of Pediatrics* 112(1988):1043–7.

8. Peat, J.K., van den Berg, R.H., Green, W.F., et al. Changing prevalence of asthma in Australian children. *British Medical Journal* 308(1994):1591–6.

9. May, C.D. Objective clinical and laboratory studies of immediate hypersensitivity reactions to foods in asthmatic children. *Journal of Allergy and Clinical Immunology* 58(1976):500–15.

10. Hill, D.J., Hosking, C.S. Cow's milk allergy. In David, T.J., editor. *Recent advances in pediatrics (Vol. 9)*. London: Churchill Livingstone, 1991, pp. 187–206.

11. Steinman, H.A., Weinberg, E.G. The effects of soft-drink preservatives on asthmatic children. *South African Medical Journal* 70(1986):404–6.

12. Freedman, B.J. Asthma induced by sulphur dioxide, benzoate and tartrazine contained in orange drinks. *Clinical Allergy* 7(1977):407–15.

13. McFadden, E.R., Gilbert, I.A. Exercise-induced asthma. *New England Journal of Medicine* 330(1994):1362–7.

14. Strauss, R.H., McFadden, E.R., Ingram, R.H., et al. Enhancement of exercise-induced asthma by cold air. *New England Journal of Medicine* 297(1977):743–7.

15. Paul, D.W., Bogaard, J.M., Hop, W.C. The bronchoconstrictor effect of strenuous exercise at low temperatures in normal athletes. *International Journal of Sports Medicine* 14(1993):433–6.

16. Johnston, S., Pattemore, P.K., Sanderson, G., et al. Community study of role of viral infections in exacerbations of asthma in 9–11 year old children. *British Medical Journal* 310(1995):1225–8.

17. Lemanske, R.F., Jr., Dick, E.C., Swenson, C.A., et al. Rhinovirus upper respiratory infection increases airway hyperactivity and late asthmatic reactions. *Journal of Clinical Investigation* 83(1989):1–10.

18. Vedanthan, P.K., Menon, M.M., Bell, T.D., et al.

Aspirin and tartrazine oral challenge: incidence of adverse response in chronic childhood asthma. *Journal of Allergy and Clinical Immunology* 60(1977):8–13.

19. Gustafsson, P.A., Bjorksten, B., Kjellman, N.I. Family dysfunction in asthma: a prospective study of illness development. *Journal of Pediatrics* 125(1994):493–8.

20. Barbee, R.A. National asthma education program guidelines for the management of asthma. *Resident and Staff Physician* 39(1993):35–46.

21. National Asthma Education Program; Expert Panel Report. *Executive Summary: Guidelines for the Diagnosis and Management of Asthma.* U.S. Dept. of Health and Human Services, Publication No. 91–3042A, June, 1991.

22. Hickey, R.W., Gochman, R.F., Chande, V. Albuterol delivered via metered-dose inhaler with spacer for outpatient treatment of young children with wheezing. *Archives of Pediatic and Adolescent Medicine* 148(1994):189–94.

23. Lin, Y.-Z., Hsieh, K.-H. Metered dose inhaler and nebuliser in acute asthma. *British Medical Journal* 72(1995):214–8.

24. Chou, K.J., Cunningham, S.J., Crain, E.F. Metered-dose inhalers with spacers vs nebulizers for pediatric asthma. *Archives of Pediatic and Adolescent Medicine* 149(1995):201–5.

25. Parkin, P.C., Saunders, N.R., Diamond, S.A., et al. Randomised trial spacer v nebuliser for acute asthma. *Archives of Disease in Childhood* 72(1995):239–40.

26. Croft, R.D. Two year old asthmatics can learn to operate a tube spacer by copying their mother. *Archives of Disease in Childhood* 64(1989):742–3.

27. Calpin, C., MacArthur, C., Parkin, P., et al. Effectiveness of prophylactic inhaled steroids in children with asthma: a review of the literature. *Archives of Pediatic and Adolescent Medicine* 148(1994):27.

28. Scarfone, R.J., Fuchs, S.M., Nager, A.L., et al. Controlled trial of oral prednisone in the emergency department treatment of children with acute asthma. *Pediatrics* 92(1993):513–8.

29. Brunette, M.G., Lands, L., Thibodeau, L.-P. Childhood asthma: prevention of attacks with short-term corticosteroid treatment of upper respiratory tract infection. *Pediatrics* 81(1988):624–9.

30. Perera, B.J.C. Efficacy and cost-effectiveness of inhaled steroids in asthma in a developing country. *Archives of Disease in Childhood* 72(1995):312–6.

31. Allen, D.B., Mullen, M.L., Mullen, B. A meta-analysis of the effect of oral and inhaled corticosteroids on growth. *Journal of Allergy and Clinical Immunology* 93(1994):967–76.

32. Connett, G.J., Warde, C., Wooler, E., et al. Prednisolone and salbutamol in the hospital treatment of acute asthma. *Archives of Disease in Childhood* 70(1994):170–3.

33. Klig, J.E., Hodge, D., Rutherford, M.W., et al. Symptomatic improvement following emergency department management of asthma: oral prednisone vs. intramuscular dexamethasone. *Archives of Pediatic and Adolescent Medicine* 148(1994):71.

34. D'Alonzo, G.E., Nathan, R.A., Henochowicz, S., et al. Salmeterol xinafoate as maintenance therapy compared with albuterol in patients with asthma. *Journal of the American Medical Association* 271(1994):1412–6.

35. Sullivan, P., Bekir, S., Jaffar, Z., et al. Anti-inflammatory effects of low-dose oral theophylline in atopic asthma. *Lancet,* 343(1994):1006–8.

36. Chow, O.K.W., Fung, K.P. Slow-release terbutaline and theophylline for the long-term therapy of children with asthma: a latin-square and factorial study of drug effects and interactions. *Pediatrics* 84(1989):119–25.

37. Schlieper, A., Alcock, D., Beaudry, P., et al. Effect of therapeutic plasma concentrations of theophylline on behavior, cognitive processing, and affect in children with asthma. *Journal of Pediatrics* 118(1991):449–55.

38. Rappaport, L., Coffman, H., Guare, R., et al. Effects of theophylline on behavior and learning in children with asthma. *American Journal of Diseases of Children* 143(1989):368–72.

39. Weldon, D.P., McGeady, S.J. Theophylline effects on cognition, behavior and learning. *Archives of Pediatric Adolescent Medicine* 149(1995):90–3.

40. Needleman, J.P., Kaifer, M.C., Nold, J.T., et al. Theophylline does not shorten hospital stay

for children admitted for asthma. *Archives of Pediatic and Adolescent Medicine* 149(1995):206–9.

41. Strauss, R.E., Wertheim, D.L., Bonagura, V.R., et al. Aminophylline therapy does not improve outcome and increases adverse effects in children hospitalized with acute asthmatic exacerbations. *Pediatrics* 93(1994):205–10.

42. Schuh, S., Johnson, D.W., Callahan, S., et al. Efficacy of frequent nebulized ipratropium bromide added to frequent high-dose albuterol therapy in severe childhood asthma. *Journal of Pediatrics* 126(1995):639–45.

43. Kreutner, W., Chapman, R.W., Gulbenkian, A., et al. Bronchodilator and antiallergy activity of forskolin. *European Journal of Pharmacology* 111(1985):1–8.

44. Collipp, P.J., Goldzier, S., Weiss, N., et al. Pyridoxine treatment of childhood bronchial asthma. *Annals of Allergy* 35(1975):93–7.

45. Sur, S., Camara, M., Buchmeier, A., et al. Double-blind trial of pyridoxine (vitamin B6) in the treatment of steroid-dependent asthma. *Annals of Allergy* 70(1993):147–52.

46. Anibarro, B., Caballero, T., Garcia-Ava, C., et al. Asthma with sulfite intolerance in children: a blocking study with cyanocobalamin. *Journal of Allergy and Clinical Immunology* 90(1992):103–9.

47. Moshenin, V., Dubois, A.B., Douglas, J.S. Effect of ascorbic acid on response to methacholine challenge in asthmatic subjects. *American Review of Respiratory Disease* 127(1983):143–7.

48. Schwartz, J., Weiss, S.T. Dietary factors and their relation to respiratory symptoms. *American Journal of Epidemiology* 132(1990):67–76.

49. Anderson, R., Hay, I., VanWyk, H.A., et al. Ascorbic acid in bronchial asthma. *South African Medical Journal* 63(1983):649–52.

50. Anah, C.O., Jarike, L.N., Baig, H.A. High dose ascorbic acid in Nigerian asthmatics. *Tropical and Geographical Medicine* 32(1980):132–7.

51. Britton, J., Pavord, I., Richards, K., et al. Dietary magnesium, lung function, wheezing and airway hyper-reactivity in a random adult population sample. *Lancet* 344(1994):357–62.

52. Skorodin, M.S., Tenholder, M.F., Yetter, B., et al. Magnesium sulfate in exacerbations of chronic obstructive pulmonary disease. *Archives of Internal Medicine* 155(1995):496–500.

53. Skobeloff, E.M., Spivey, W.H., McNamara, R.M., et al. Intravenous magnesium sulfate for the treatment of acute asthma in the emergency department. *Journal of the American Medical Association* 262(1989):1210–3.

54. Pabon, H., Monem, G., Kissoon, N. Safety and efficacy of magnesium sulfate infusions in children with status asthmaticus. *Pediatric Emergency Care* 10(1994):200–3.

55. Ciarallo, L., Sauer, A., Shannon, M. Clinical efficacy of intravenous magnesium in moderate to severe asthma: results of a randomized, placebo-controlled trial. *Archives of Pediatic and Adolescent Medicine* 148(1994):69.

56. Lee, T.H., Arm, J.P., Horton, C.E., et al. Effects of dietary fish oil lipids on allergic and inflammatory diseases. *Allergy Proceedings* 12(1991):299–303.

57. Dry, J. Effect of a fish oil diet on asthma: results of a 1-year double-blind study. *International Archives of Allergy and Applied Immunology* 95(1991):156–7.

58. Schwartz, J., Weiss, S.T. The relationship of dietary fish intake to level of pulmonary function in the first National Health and Nutrition Survey (NHANES I). *European Respiratory Journal* 7(1994):1821–4.

59. Stenius-Aarniala, B., Aro, A., Hakulinen, A., et al. Evening primrose oil and fish oil are ineffective as supplementary treatment of bronchial asthma. *Annals of Allergy* 62(1989):534–7.

60. Porro, E., Indinnimeo, L., Antognoni, G., et al. Early wheezing and breastfeeding. *Journal of Asthma* 30(1993):23–8.

61. Wright, A.L., Holberg, C.J., Taussig, L.M., et al. Relationship of infant feeding to recurrent wheezing at age 6 years. *Archives of Pediatric and Adolescent Medicine* 149(1995):758–63.

62. Dorsch, W., Wagner, H. New anti-asthmatic drugs from traditional medicine? *International Archives of Allergy and Applied Immunology* 94(1991):262–5.

63. Dorsch, W., Scharff, J., Bayer, T., et al. Antiasthmatic effects of onions. *International*

Archives of Allergy and Applied Immunology 88(1989):228–30.

64. Dorsch, W., Weber, J. Prevention of allergen-induced bronchial obstruction in sensitized guinea pigs by crude alcoholic onion extract. *Agents and Actions* 14(1984):626–9.

65. Schwartz, J., Weiss, S.T. Caffeine intake and asthma symptoms. *AEP* 2(1992):627–35.

66. Wilson N., Vickers H., Taylor G., et al. Objective test for food sensitivity in asthmatic children: increased bronchial reactivity after cola drinks. *British Medical Journal* 284(1982):1226–8.

67. Towns, S.J., Mellis, C.M. Role of acetyl salicylic acid and sodium metabisulfite in chronic childhood asthma. *Pediatrics* 73(1984):631–7.

68. Friedman, M.E., Easton, J.G. Prevalence of positive metabisulphite challenges in children with asthma. *Pediatric Asthma, Allergy and Immunology* 1(1987):53–9.

69. Wilson, N.M. Bronchial hyperactivity in food and drink intolerance. *Annals of Allergy* 61(1988):75–9.

70. Unge, G., Grubbstrom, J., Olsson, P., et al. Effects of dietary tryptophan restrictions on clinical symptoms in patients with endogenous asthma. *Allergy* 38(1983):211–2.

71. Lindahl, O., Lindwall, L., Spangberg, A., et al. Vegan regimen with reduced medication in the treatment of bronchial asthma. *Journal of Asthma* 22(1985):45–55.

72. Hoj, L., Osterballe, O., Bundgaard, A., et al. A double-blind controlled trial of elemental diet in severe, perennial asthma. *Allergy* 36(1981):257–62.

73. Haas, F., Bishop, M.C., Salazar-Schicchi, J., et al. Effect of milk ingestion on pulmonary function in healthy and asthmatic subjects. *Journal of Asthma* 28(1991):349–55.

74. Jain, S.C., Talukdar, B. Evaluation of yoga therapy programme for patients of bronchial asthma. *Singapore Medical Journal* 34(1993):306–8.

75. Singh, V. Effect of respiratory exercises on asthma: the pink city lung exerciser. *Journal of Asthma* 24(1987):355–9.

76. Nagarathna, R., Nagendra, H.R. Yoga for bronchial asthma: a controlled study. *British Medical Journal* 291(1985):1077–9.

77. Tiep, B.L., Burns, M., Kao, D., et al. Pursed lips breathing training using ear oximetry. *Chest* 90(1986):218–21.

78. Bar-On, O., Inbar, O. Swimming and asthma: benefits and deleterious effects. *Sports Medicine* 14(1992):397–405.

79. Olivia, C.K.W. Physical conditioning programme for children with bronchial asthma. *Acta Paediatrica Japonica* 32(1990):173–5.

80. Nelson, H.S., Hirsch, S.R., Ohman, J.L., et al. Recommendations for the use of residential air-cleaning devices in the treatment of allergic respiratory diseases. *Journal of Allergy and Clinical Immunology* 82(1988):661–9.

81. Hidden life of spider plants. *University of California at Berkeley Wellness Letter* 10(5)(1994):1–2.

82. Platts-Mills, T.A.E., deWeck, A.L. Dust mite allergens and asthma: a worldwide problem. *Journal of Allergy and Clinical Immunology* 83(1989):416–27.

83. Charpin, D., Kleisbauer, J.P., Lanteaume, A., et al. Asthma and allergy to house-dust mites in populations living at high altitudes. *Chest* 93(1988):758–61.

84. Harving, H., Korsgaard, J., Dahl, R. Clinical efficacy of reduction in house-dust mite exposure in specially designed, mechanically ventilated "healthy" homes. *Allergy* 49(1994):866–70.

85. Owen, S., Morganstern, M., Hepworth, J., et al. Control of house dust mite antigen in bedding. *Lancet* 1(1990):396–7.

86. Korsgaard, J. Preventive measures in mite asthma: a controlled trial. *Allergy* 38(1983):93–102.

87. Green, W.F., Nicholas, N.R., Salome, C.M., et al. Reduction of house dust mites and mite allergens: effects of spraying carpets and blankets with Allersearch DMS, and acaricide combined with an allergen reducing agent. *Clinical and Experimental Allergy* 19(1989):203–7.

88. Reiser, J., Ingram, D., Mitchell, E.B., et al. House dust mite allergen levels and an anti-mite mattress spray (natamycin) in the treatment of childhood asthma. *Clinical and Experimental Allergy* 20(1990):561–7.

89. Warner, J.A., Marchant, J.L., Warner, J.O. Double-blind trial of ionisers in children with

asthma sensitive to the house dust mite. *Thorax* 48(1993):330–3.

90. Godfrey, S., Silverman, M. Demonstration of placebo response in asthma by means of exercise testing. *Journal of Psychosomatic Research* 17(1973):293–7.

91. Khan, A.U., Staerk, M., Bonk, C. Hypnotic suggestibility compared with other methods of isolating emotionally-prone asthmatic children. *American Journal of Clinical Hypnosis* 17(1974):50–3.

92. Diamond, H.H. Hypnosis in children: the complete cure of 40 cases of asthma. *American Journal of Clinical Hypnosis* 1(1959):124–9.

93. Smith, J.M., Burns, C.L.C. The treatment of asthmatic children by hypnotic suggestion. *British Journal of Diseases of the Chest* 54(1960):78–81.

94. Collison, D.R. Which asthmatic patients should be treated by hypnotherapy? *Medical Journal of Australia* 1(1975):776–81.

95. Barbour, J. Self hypnosis seems to diminish asthma attacks. *American Family Physician* 21(1980):173.

96. Henry, M., DeRivera, J.L.G., Gonzalez-Martin, I.J., et al. Improvement of respiratory function in chronic asthmatic patients with autogenic therapy. *Journal of Psychosomatic Research* 37(1993):265–70.

97. Peper, E., Tibbetts, V. Fifteen-month follow-up with asthmatics utilizing EMG/incentive inspirometer feedback. *Biofeedback and Self Regulation* 17(1992):143–51.

98. Feldman, G.M. The effect of biofeedback training on respiratory resistance of asthmatic children. *Psychosomatic Medicine* 38(1976):27–34.

99. Scherr, M.S., Crawford, P.L. Three-year evaluation of biofeedback techniques in the treatment of children with chronic asthma in a summer camp environment. *Annals of Allergy* 41(1978):288–92.

100. Asher, M.I., Douglas, C., Airy, M., et al. Effects of chest physical therapy on lung function in children recovering from acute severe asthma. *Pediatric Pulmonology* 9(1990):146–51.

101. Morton, A.R., Fazio, S.M., Miller, D. Efficacy of laser-acupuncture in the prevention of exercise-induced asthma. *Annals of Allergy* 70(1993):295–8.

102. Fung, K.P., Chow, O.K.W., So, S.Y. Attenuation of exercise-induced asthma by acupuncture. *Lancet* 2(1986):1419–22.

103. Tashkin, D.P., Kroening, R.J., Bresler, D.E., et al. A controlled trial of real and simulated acupuncture in the management of chronic asthma. *Journal of Allergy and Clinical Immunology* 76(1985):855–64.

104. Kleijnen, J., ter Riet, G., Knipschild, P. Acupuncture and asthma: a review of controlled trials. *Thorax* 46(1991):799–802.

105. Attevelt, J.R.M. Research into paranormal healing. Ph.D. dissertation, University of Utrecht, 1988.

106. Reilly, D., Taylor, M.A., Beattie, N.G.M., et al. Is evidence for homeopathy reproducible? *Lancet* 344(1994):1601–6.

CHAPTER 6 — Bed-wetting

1. Jarvelin, M.R., Vikevainen-Tervonen, L., Moilanen, I., et al. Enuresis in seven-year-old children. *Acta Paediatrica Scandinavica* 77(1988):148–53.

2. Yazbeck, S., Schick, E., O'Regan, S. Relevance of constipation to enuresis, urinary tract infection and reflux: a review. *European Urology* 13(1987):318–21.

3. O'Regan, S., Yazbeck, S., Hamberger, B., et al. Constipation a commonly unrecognized cause of enuresis. *American Journal of Diseases of Children* 140(1986):260–1.

4. Zaleski, A., Shokeir, M.K., Gerrard, J.W. Enuresis: familial incidence and relationship to allergic disorders. *Canadian Medical Association Journal* 106(1972):30–1.

5. Haque, M., Ellerstein, N.S., Gundy, J.H., et al. Parental perceptions of enuresis: a collaborative study. *American Journal of Diseases of Children* 135(1981):809–11.

6. Foxman, B., Valdez, R.B., Brook, R.H. Childhood enuresis: prevalence, perceived impact, and prescribed treatments. *Pediatrics* 77(1986):482–7.

7. Moffatt, M.E., Kato, C., Pless, I.B. Improvements in self-concept after treatment of nocturnal enuresis: randomized controlled trial. *Journal of Pediatrics* 110(1987):647–52.

8. Fergusson, D.M., Horwood, L.J., Shannon, F.T.

Factors related to the age of attainment of nocturnal bladder control: an 8-year longitudinal study. *Pediatrics* 78(1986):884–90.

9. Tissier, G. Bedwetting at five years of age. *Health Visitor* 56(1983):333–5.

10. Starfield, B. Functional bladder capacity in enuretic and non-enuretic children. *Journal of Pediatrics* 70(1967):777–81.

11. Berger, R.M., Maizels, M., Moran, G.C., et al. Bladder capacity (ounces) equals age (years) plus 2 predicts normal bladder capacity and aids in diagnosis of abnormal voiding patterns. *Journal of Urology* 129(1983):347–9.

12. Rittig, S., Knudsen, U.B., Norgaard, J.P., et al. Abnormal diurnal rhythm of plasma vasopressin and urinary output in patients with enuresis. *American Journal of Physiology* 256(1989):F644–71.

13. Norgaard, J.P., Pedersen, E.B., Djurhuus, J.C. Diurnal anti-diuretic-hormone levels in enuretics. *Journal of Urology* 134(1985):1029–31.

14. Norgaard, J.P., Djurhuus, J.C. The pathophysiology of enuresis in children and young adults. *Clinical Pediatrics* Spec Ed(1993): 5–7.

15. Rauber, A., Maroncelli, R. Prescribing practices and knowledge of tricyclic antidepressants among physicians caring for children. *Pediatrics* 73(1984):107–9.

16. Fjellestad-Paulsen, A., Wille, S., Harris, A.S. Comparison of intranasal and oral desmopressin for nocturnal enuresis. *Archives of Disease in Childhood* 62(1987):674–7.

17. Post, E.M., Richman, R.A., Blackett, P.R., et al. Desmopressin response of enuretic children: effects of age and frequency of enuresis. *American Journal of Diseases of Children* 137(1983):962–3.

18. Stenberg, A., Lackgren, G. Desmopressin tablets in the treatment of severe nocturnal enuresis in adolescents. *Pediatrics* 94(1994):841–6.

19. Pedersen, P.S., Hejl, M., Kjoller, S.S. Desamino-D-arginine vasporessin in childhood nocturnal enuresis. *Journal of Urology* 133(1985):65–6.

20. Robson, W.L., Leung, A.K. Side effects and complications of treatment with desmopressin for enuresis. *Journal of the National Medical Association* 86(1994):775–8.

21. Beach, P.S., Beach, R.E., Smith, L.R. Hyponatremic seizures in a child treated with desmopressin to control enuresis: a rational approach to fluid intake. *Clinical Pediatrics* 31(1992):566–9.

22. Hjalmas, K., Bengtsson, B. Efficacy, safety and dosing of desmopressin for nocturnal enuresis in Europe. *Clinical Pediatrics* Spec No.(July) (1993):19–24.

23. Moffatt, M.E.K., Harlos, S., Kirshen, A.J., et al. Desmopressin acetate and nocturnal enuresis: how much do we know? *Pediatrics* 92(1993):420–5.

24. Lovering, J.S., Tallett, S.E., McKendry, J.B. Oxybutynin efficacy in the treatment of primary enuresis. *Pediatrics* 82(1988):104–6.

25. Egger, J., Carter, C.H., Soothill, J.F., et al. Effect of diet treatment on enuresis in children with migraine or hyperkinetic behavior. *Clinical Pediatrics* 31(1992):302–7.

26. Breneman, J.C. Allergic cystitis: the cause of nocturnal enuresis. *General Practitioner* 20(1959):85–98.

27. Esperanca, M., Gerrard, J.W. Nocturnal enuresis: comparison of the effect of imipramine and dietary restriction on bladder capacity. *Canadian Medical Association Journal* 101(1969):65–8.

28. Starfield, B., Mellits, E.D. Increase in functional bladder capacity and improvement in enuresis. *Journal of Pediatrics* 74(1968):483–7.

29. Netley, C., Khanna, F., McKendry, J.B., et al. Effects of different methods of treatment of primary enuresis on psychologic functioning in children. *Canadian Medical Association Journal* 131(1984):577–9.

30. Wagner, W., Johnson, S.B., Walker, D., et al. A controlled comparison of two treatments for nocturnal enuresis. *Journal of Pediatrics* 101(1982):302–7.

31. Wille, S. Comparison of desmopressin and enuresis alarm for nocturnal enuresis. *Archives of Disease in Childhood* 61(1986):30–3.

32. Devlin, J.B., O'Cathain, C. Predicting treatment outcome in nocturnal enuresis. *Archives of Disease in Childhood* 65(1990):1158–61.

33. Geffken, G., Johnson, S.B., Walker, D. Behavioral interventions for childhood nocturnal enuresis: the differential effect of blad-

der capacity on treatment progress and outcome. *Health Psychology* 5(1986):261–72.

34. Azrin, N.H., Thienes, P.M. Rapid elimination of enuresis by intensive learning without a conditioning apparatus. *Behavior Therapy* 9(1978):342–54.

35. Whelan, J.P., Houts, A.C. Effects of a waking schedule on primary enuretic children treated with full-spectrum home training. *Health Psychology* 9(1990):164–76.

36. Iester, A., Marchesi, A., Cohen, A., et al. Functional enuresis: pharmacological versus behavioral treatment. *Child's Nervous System* 7(1991):106–8.

37. Olness, K. The use of self-hypnosis in the treatment of childhood nocturnal enuresis: a report of forty patients. *Clinical Pediatrics* 14(1975):273–9.

38. Banerjee, S., Srivastav, A., Palan, B.M. Hypnosis and self-hypnosis in the management of nocturnal enuresis: a comparative study with imipramine therapy. *American Journal of Clinical Hypnosis* 36(1993):113–9.

39. Libo, L.M., Arnold, G.E., Woodside, J.R., et al. EMG biofeedback for functional bladder-sphincter dyssynergia: a case study. *Biofeedback and Self Regulation* 8(1983):243–53.

40. Reed, W.R., Beavers, S., Reddy, S.K., et al. Chiropractic management of primary nocturnal enuresis. *Journal of Manipulative and Physiological Therapeutics* 17(1994):596–600.

41. LeBoeuf, C., Brown, P., Herman, A., et al. Chiropractic care of children with nocturnal enuresis: a prospective outcome study. *Journal of Manipulative and Physiological Therapeutics* 14(1991):110–5.

42. Baoqin, X. 302 cases of enuresis treated with acupuncture. *Journal of Traditional Chinese Medicine* 11(1991):121–2.

43. Ionescu-Tirgoviste, C., Rodica, V., Ionescu, C., et al. The treatment of enuresis by acupuncture. *American Journal of Acupuncture* 11(1983):119–24.

44. Tuzuner, F., Kecik, Y., Ozdemir, S., et al. Electro-acupuncture in the treatment of enuresis nocturna. *Acupuncture and Electro-Therapeutics Research* 14(1989):211–5.

45. Zaiwen, C., Ling, C. The treatment of enuresis with scalp acupuncture. *Journal of Traditional Chinese Medicine* 11(1991):29–30.

46. Baozhu, S., Xiyou, W. Short-term effect in 135 cases of enuresis treated by wrist-ankle needling. *Journal of Traditional Chinese Medicine* 5(1985):27–8.

47. Chunpu, Y. Acupuncture of Guanyuan (Ren 4) and Baiui (Du 20) in the treatment of 500 cases of enuresis. *Journal of Traditional Chinese Medicine* 8(1988):197.

48. Minni, B., Capozza, N., Creti, G., et al. Bladder instability and enuresis treated by acupuncture and electro-therapeutics: early urodynamic observations. *Acupuncture and Electro-Therapeutics Research* 15(1990):19–25.

49. Capozza, N. Treatment of nocturnal enuresis: a comparative study between desmopressin and acupuncture used separately or in association. *Journal of the American Medical Association* 267(1992):1741.

CHAPTER 7 — Burns

1. McLoughlin, E., McGuire, A. The causes, cost and prevention of childhood burn injuries. *American Journal of Diseases of Children* 144(1990):677–83.

2. Seidel, J.S. The danger of scald burns during hair braiding. *Annals of Emergency Medicine* 23(1994):1388–9.

3. Feldman, K.W., Schaller, R.T., Feldman, J.A., et al. Tap water scald burns in children. *Pediatrics* 62(1978):1–7.

4. Erdmann, T.C., Feldman, K.W., Rivara, R.P., et al. Tap water burn prevention: the effect of legislation. *Pediatrics* 88(1991):572–7.

5. Walker, A.R. Fatal tapwater scald burns in the USA, 1979–1986. *Burns* 16(1990):49–52.

6. Katcher, M.L., Landry, G.L., Shapiro, M.M. Liquid-crystal thermometer use in pediatric office counseling about tap water burn prevention. *Pediatrics* 83(1989):766–71.

7. Nemethy, M., Clore, E.R. Microwave heating of infant formula and breast milk. *Journal of Pediatric Health Care* 4(1990):131–5.

8. Ebrahim, M.K., Bang, R.L., Lari, A.R., et al. Scald accidents during water aerosol inhalation in infants. *Burns* 16(1990):291–3.

9. Strock, L.L., Lee, M.M., Rutan, R.L., et al.

Topical Bactroban (mupirocin): efficacy in treating burn wounds infected with methicillin-resistant staphylococci. *Journal of Burn Care and Rehabilitation* 11(1990):454–9.

10. Kaplan, J.Z. Acceleration of wound healing by a live yeast cell derivative. *Archives of Surgery* 119(1984):1105–8.

11. Grindlay, D., Reynolds, T. The aloe vera phenomenon: a review of the properties and modern uses of the leaf parenchyma gel. *Journal of Ethnopharmacology* 16(1986):117–51.

12. Rodriguez-Bigas, M., Cruz, N.I., Suarez, A. Comparative evaluation of aloe vera in the management of burn wounds in guinea pigs. *Plastic and Reconstructive Surgery* 81(1988):386–9.

13. Gravel, J.A. Oxygen dressings and asiaticoside in the treatment of burns. *Laval Medicine* 36(1965):413–5.

14. O'Keefe, P. A trial of asiaticoside on skin graft donor areas. *British Journal of Plastic Surgery* 27(1974):194–5.

15. Bosse, J.P., Papillon, J., Frenette, G., et al. Clinical study of a new antikeloid agent. *Annals of Plastic Surgery* 3(1979):13–21.

16. Maquart, F.X., Bellon, G., Gillery, P., et al. Stimulation of collagen synthesis in fibroblast cultures by a triterpene extracted from Centella asiatica. *Connective Tissue Research* 24(1990):107–20.

17. Izu, R., Aguirre, A., Gil, N., et al. Allergic contact dermatitis from a cream containing Centella asiatica extract. *Contact Dermatitis* 26(1992):192–3.

18. Ivancheva, S., Manolova, N., Serkedjieva, J., et al. Polyphenols from Bulgarian medicinal plants with anti-infectious activity. *Basic Life Sciences* 59(1992):717–28.

19. Gegova, G., Manolova, N., Serkedzhieva, I., et al. Combined effect of selected antiviral substances of natural and synthetic origin: II. Anti-influenza activity of a combination of a polyphenolic complex isolated from Geranium sanguineum L. and rimantadine in vivo. *Acta Microbiologica Bulgarica* 30(1993):37–40.

20. Abeywickrama, K., Bean, G.A. Toxigenic Aspergillus flavus and aflatoxins in Sri Lankan medicinal plant material. *Mycopathologica* 113(1991):187–90.

21. Knight, T.E., Hausen, B.M. Melaleuca oil (tea tree oil) dermatitis. *Journal of the American Academy of Dermatology* 30(1994):423–7.

22. Villar, D., Knight, M.J., Hansen, S.R., et al. Toxicity of melaleuca oil and related essential oils applied topically on dogs and cats. *Veterinary and Human Toxicology* 36(1994):139–42.

23. Garty, B.Z. Garlic burns. *Pediatrics* 91(1993):658–9.

24. O'Neil, C.E., Hutsler, D., Hildreth, M.A. Basic nutritional guidelines for pediatric burn patients. *Journal of Burn Care and Rehabilitation* 10(1989):278–84.

25. Berger, M.M., Cavadini, C., Chiolero, R., et al. Influence of large intakes of trace elements on recovery after major burns. *Nutrition* 10(1994):327–34.

26. Gottschlich, M.M., Warden, G.D., Michel, M., et al. Diarrhea in tube-fed burn patients: incidence, etiology, nutritional impact, and prevention. *Journal of Parenteral and Enteral Nutrition* 12(1988):338–45.

27. Matsuda, T., Tanaka, H., Hanumadass, M., et al. Effects of high-dose vitamin C administration on post-burn microvascular fluid and protein flux. *Journal of Burn Care and Rehabilitation* 13(1992):560–6.

28. Haberal, M., Hamaloglu, E., Bora, S., et al. The effects of vitamin E on immune regulation after thermal injury. *Burns Include Thermal Injury* 14(1988):388–93.

29. Jenkins, M., Alexander, J.W., MacMillan, B.G., et al. Failure of topical steroids and vitamin E to reduce postoperative scar formation following reconstructive surgery. *Journal of Burn Care and Rehabilitation* 7(1986):309–12.

30. Shewmake, K.B., Talbert, G.E., Bowser-Wallace, B.H., et al. Alterations in plasma copper, zinc and ceruloplasmin levels in patients with thermal trauma. *Journal of Burn Care and Rehabilitation* 9(1988):13–7.

31. Subrahmanyam, M. Topical application of honey in treatment of burns. *British Journal of Surgery* 78(1991):497–8.

32. Subrahmanyam, M. Honey impregnated gauze versus polyurethane film (OpSite) in the treatment of burns: a prospective randomised study. *British Journal of Plastic Surgery*

46(1993):322–3.

33. Willix, D.J., Molan, P.C., Harfoot, C.G. A comparison of the sensitivity of wound-infecting species of bacteria to the antibacterial activity of manuka honey and other honey. *Journal of Applied Bacteriology* 73(1992):388–94.

34. Allen, K.L., Molan, P.C., Reid, G.M. A survey of the antibacterial activity of some New Zealand honeys. *Journal of Pharmacy and Pharmacology* 43(1991):817–22.

35. Efem, S.E., Udoh, K.T., Iwara, C.I. The antimicrobial spectrum of honey and its clinical significance. *Infection* 20(1992):227–9.

36. Postmes, T., van den Bogaard, A.E., Hazen, M. Honey for wounds, ulcers and skin graft preservation. *Lancet* 341(1993):756–7.

37. Mirkin, G. Side effects of raw honey. *Journal of the American Medical Association* 266(1991):2766.

38. Lampe, K.F. Rhododendrons, mountain laurel and mad honey. *Journal of the American Medical Association* 259(1988):2009.

39. Baxter, C.R. Metabolism and nutrition in burned patients. *Comprehensive Therapy* 13(1987):36–42.

40. Alexander, J.W., MacMillan, B.G., Stinnett, J.D., et al. Beneficial effects of aggressive protein feeding in severely burned children. *Annals of Surgery* 192(1980):505–17.

41. Parrott, M., Ryan, R., Parks, D.H., et al. Structured exercise circuit program for burn patients. *Journal of Burn Care and Rehabilitation* 9(1988):666–8.

42. Purdue, G.F., Layton, T.R., Copeland, C.E. Cold injury complicating burn therapy. *Journal of Trauma* 25(1985):167–8.

43. Carr-Collins, J.A. Pressure techniques for the prevention of hypertrophic scar. *Clinics in Plastic Surgery* 19(1992):733–43.

44. Wakeman, R.J., Kaplan, J.Z. An experimental study of hypnosis in painful burns. *American Journal of Clinical Hypnosis* 21(1978):3–12.

45. Patterson, D.R., Everett, J.J., Burns, G.L., et al. Hypnosis for the treatment of burn pain. *Journal of Consulting and Clinical Psychology* 60(1992):713–7.

46. Patterson, D.R., Questad, K.A., Boltwood, M.D. Hypnotherapy as a treatment for pain in patients with burns: research and clinical considerations. *Journal of Burn Care and Rehabilitation* 8(1987):263–8.

47. Kelley, M.L., Jarvie, G.J., Middleborrk, J.L., et al. Decreasing burned children's pain behavior: impacting the trauma of hydrotherapy. *Journal of Applied Behavior Analysis* 17(1984):147–58.

48. Kavanaugh, C., Freeman, R. Should children participate in burn care? *American Journal of Nursing* (May) (1984):601.

49. Lewis, S.M., Clelland, J.A., Knowles, C.J., et al. Effects of auricular acupuncture-like transcutaneous electric nerve stimulation on pain levels following wound care in patients with burns: a pilot study. *Journal of Burn Care and Rehabilitation* 11(1990):322–9.

50. Wirth, D.P. The effect of non-contact Therapeutic Touch on the healing rate of full thickness dermal wounds. *Subtle Energies* 1(1990):1–20.

51. Leaman, A.M., Gorman, D. Cantharis in the early treatment of minor burns. *Archives of Emergency Medicine* 6(1989):259–61.

CHAPTER 8 — Chicken Pox

1. Kohl, S. Risks of chickenpox in asthmatic children receiving inhalation steroids and therapeutic recommendations. *Pediatric Infectious Disease Journal* 12(1993):174–5.

2. Cowan, M.R., Primm, P.A., Scott, S.M., et al. Serious group A beta-hemolytic streptococcal infections complicating varicella. *Annals of Emergency Medicine* 23(1994):818–22.

3. Tucker, J.R., Linakis, J.G. Complications of varicella: varicella-associated cerebritis in a child. Case report and review. *Journal of Emergency Medicine* 11(1993):535–8.

4. Lantner, R., Rockoff, J.B., DeMasi, J., et al. Fatal varicella in a corticosteroid-dependent asthmatic receiving troleandomycin. *Allergy Proceedings* 11(1990):83–7.

5. Lieu, T.A., Finkler, L.J., Sorel, M.E., et al. Cost-effectiveness of varicella serotesting versus presumptive vaccination of school-age children and adolescents. *Pediatrics* 95(1995):632–8.

6. Huse, D.M., Meissner, H.C., Lacey, M.J., et al. Childhood vaccination against chickenpox: an

analysis of benefits and costs. *Journal of Pediatrics* 124(1994):869–74.

7. Lieu, T.A., Cochi, S.L., Black, S.B., et al. Cost-effectiveness of a routine varicella vaccination program for US children. *Journal of the American Medical Association* 271(1994):375–81.

8. Suga, S., Yoshikawa, T., Ozaki, T., Asano, Y. Effect of oral acyclovir against primary and secondary viremia in incubation period of varicella. *Archives of Disease in Childhood* 69(1993):639–42.

9. Committee on Infectious Diseases. *1994 Red Book.* Elk Grove Village, Ill: American Academy of Pediatrics, 1994, pp. 510–6.

10. Dunkle, L.M., Arvin, A.M., Whitley, R.J., et al. A controlled trial of acyclovir for chicken pox in normal children. *New England Journal of Medicine* 325(1991):1539–44.

11. Doran, T.F., De Angelis, C., Baumgardner, R.A., et al. Acetaminophen: more harm than good for chicken pox? *Journal of Pediatrics* 114(1989):1045–8.

12. Duckett, S. Plantain leaf for poison ivy. *Lancet* 303(1980):583.

CHAPTER 9—Colds

1. Naclerio, R.M., Proud, D., Kagey-Sobotka, A., et al. Is histamine responsible for the following symptoms of rhinovirus colds? a look at the inflammatory mediators following infection. *Pediatric Infectious Disease Journal* 7(1988):215–42.

2. Wald, E.R., Guerra, N., Byers, C. Upper respiratory tract infections in young children: duration of and frequency of complications. *Pediatrics* 87(1991):129–33.

3. Fleming, D.W., Cochi, S.L., Hightower, A.W., et al. Childhood upper respiratory tract infections: to what degree is incidence affected by day-care attendance? *Pediatrics* 79(1987):55–60.

4. Kogan, M.D., Pappas, G., Yu, S.M., et al. Over-the-counter medication use among U.S. preschool-age children. *Journal of the American Medical Association* 272(1994):1025–30.

5. Gaffey, M.J., Gwaltney, J.M., Jr., Sastre, A., et al. Intranasally and orally administered antihistamine treatment of experimental rhinovirus colds. *American Review of Respiratory Disease* 136(1987):556–60.

6. Howard, J.C., Jr., Kantner, T.R., Lilienfield, L.S., et al. Effectiveness of antihistamines in the symptomatic management of the common cold. *Journal of the American Medical Association* 242(1979):2414–7.

7. Gaffey, M.J., Kaiser, D.L., Hayden, F.G. Ineffectiveness of oral terfenadine in natural colds: evidence against histamine as a mediator of common cold symptoms. *Pediatric Infectious Disease Journal* 7(1988):223–7.

8. Bye, C.E., Cooper, J., Empey, D.W., et al. Effects of pseudoephedrine and triprolidine, alone and in combination, on symptoms of the common cold. *British Medical Journal* 281(1980):189–90.

9. Roth, R.P., Cantekin, E.I., Bluestone, C.D., et al. Nasal decongestant activity of pseudoephedrine. *Annals of Otology, Rhinology and Laryngology* 86(1977):235–42.

10. Akerlund, A., Klint, T., Olen, L., et al. Nasal decongestant effect of oxymetazoline in the common cold: an objective dose-response study in 106 patients. *Journal of Laryngology and Otology* 103(1989):743–6.

11. Taylor, J.A., Novack, A.H., Almquist, J.R., et al. Efficacy of cough suppressants in children. *Journal of Pediatrics* 122(1993):799–802.

12. Kuhn, J.J., Hendley, J.O., Adams, K.F., et al. Antitussive effect of guaifenesin in young adults with natural colds. *Chest* 82(1982):713–8.

13. Hirsch, S.R., Viernes, P.F., Kory, R.C., et al. The expectorant effect of glyceryl guaiacolate in patients with chronic bronchitis. *Chest* 63(1973):9–14.

14. Sperber, S.J., Hendley, J.O., Hayden, F.G., et al. Effects of naproxen on experimental rhinovirus colds: a randomized double-blind, controlled trial. *Annals of Internal Medicine* 117(1992):37–41.

15. Graham, N.M., Burrell, C.J., Douglas, R.M., et al. Adverse effects of aspirin, acetaminophen and ibuprofen on immune function, viral shedding and clinical status in rhinovirus-infected volunteers. *Journal of Infectious Diseases*

(1990)162:1277–82.

16. Hutton, N., Wilson, M.H., Mellits, D., et al. Effectiveness of an antihistamine-decongestant combination for young children with the common cold: a randomized, controlled clinical trial. *Journal of Pediatrics* 118(1991):125–30.

17. Weippl, G. Therapeutic approaches to the common cold in children. *Clinical Therapeutics* 6(1984):475–82.

18. Smith, M.B.H., Feldman, W. Over-the-counter cold medications: a critical review of clinical trials between 1950 and 1991. *Journal of the American Medical Association* 269(1993):2258–63.

19. Kumar, A., Rawlings, R.D., Beaman, D.C. The mystery ingredients: sweeteners, flavorings, dyes, and preservatives in analgesic/antipyretic, antihistamine/decongestant, cough and cold, antidiarrheal and liquid theophylline preparations. *Pediatrics* 91(1993):927–33.

20. Eccles, R., Jawad, M.S., Morris, S. The effects of oral administration of (-)-menthol on nasal resistance to airflow and nasal sensation of airflow in subjects suffering from nasal congestion associated with the common cold. *Journal of Pharmacy and Pharmacology* 42(1990):652–4.

21. Gadomski, A.M. Potential interventions for preventing pneumonia among young children: lack of effect of antibiotic treatment for upper respiratory infections. *Pediatric Infectious Disease Journal* 12(1993):115–20.

22. Barrow, G.I., Higgins, P.G., al-Nakib, W., et al. The effect of intranasal nedocromil sodium on viral upper respiratory tract infections in human volunteers. *Clinical and Experimental Allergy* 20(1990):45–51.

23. Dockhorn, R., Grossman, J., Posner, M., et al. A double-blind, placebo-controlled study of the safety and efficacy of ipratropium bromide nasal spray versus placebo in patients with the common cold. *Journal of Allergy and Clinical Immunology* 90(1992):1076–82.

24. Hendeles, L. Efficacy and safety of antihistamines and expectorants in nonprescription cough and cold preparations. *Pharmacotherapy* 13(1993):154–8.

25. Murray, S., Brewerton, T. Abuse of over-the-counter dextromethorphan by teenagers. *Southern Medical Journal* 86(1993):1151–3.

26. Graham, N.M., Burrell, C.J., Douglas, R.M., et al. Adverse effects of aspirin, acetaminophen and ibuprofen on immune function, viral shedding and clinical status in rhinovirus infected volunteers. *Journal of Infectious Diseases* 162(1990):1277–82.

27. Cowan, P.F. Patient satisfaction with an office visit for the common cold. *Journal of Family Practice* 24(1987):412–3.

28. Ryan, R.E. A double-blind clinical evaluation of bromelains in the treatment of acute sinusitis. *Headache* 7(1967):13–7.

29. Zhang, J.S., Tian, Z., Lou, Z.C. Quality evaluation of twelve species of Chinese ephedra (ma huang). *Yao Hsueh Hsueh Pao* 24(1989):865–71.

30. Ozaki, Y. Antiinflammatory effect of tetramethylpyrazine and ferulic acid. *Chemical and Pharmaceutical Bulletin (Tokyo)* 40(1992):954–6.

31. Abe, N., Ebina, T., Ishida, N. Interferon induction by glycyrrhizin and glycyrrhetinic acid in mice. *Microbiology and Immunology* 26(1982):535–9.

32. Roesler, J., Emmendorffer, A., Steinmuller, C., et al. Application of purified polysaccharides from cell cultures of the plant *Echinacea purpurea* to test subjects mediates activation of the phagocyte system. *International Journal of Immunopharmacology* 13(1991):931–41.

33. Mengs, U., Clare, C.B., Poiley, J.A. Toxicity of Echinacea purpurea: acute, subacute and genotoxicity studies. *Arzneimittel-Forschung* 41(1991):1076–81.

34. Denyer, C.V., Jackson, P., Loakes, D.M., et al. Isolation of antirhinoviral sesquiterpenes from ginger (Zingiber officianale). *Journal of Natural Products* 57(1994):658–62.

35. Pinnock, C.B., Douglas, R.M., Badcock, N.R. Vitamin A status in children who are prone to respiratory tract infections. *Australian Paediatric Journal* 22(1986):95–9.

36. Stansfield, S.K., Pierre-Louis, M., Lerebours, G., et al. Vitamin A supplementation and increased prevalence of childhood diarrhea and acute respiratory infections. *Lancet* 341(1993):578–82.

37. Kartasasmita, C.B., Rosmayudi, O., Soemantri, E.S., et al. Vitamin A and acute respiratory infections. *Paediatrica Indonesiana* 31(1991):41–9.

38. Chalmers, T.C. Effects of ascorbic acid on the common cold: an evaluation of the evidence. *American Journal of Medicine* 58(1975):532–36.

39. Baird, I.M., Hughes, R.E., Wilson, H.K., et al. The effects of ascorbic acid and flavonoids on the occurrence of symptoms normally associated with the common cold. *American Journal of Clinical Nutrition* 32(1979):1686–90.

40. Hemila, H. Vitamin C and the common cold. *British Journal of Nutrition* 67(1992):3–16.

41. Coulehan, J.L., Reisinger, K.S., Rogers, K.D., et al. Vitamin C prophylaxis in a boarding school. *New England Journal of Medicine* 290(1974):6–10.

42. Hemila, H. Does vitamin C alleviate the symptoms of the common cold?: a review of current evidence. *Scandinavian Journal of Infectious Diseases* 26(1994):1–6.

43. Eby, G.A., Davis, D.R., Halcomb, W.W. Reduction in duration of common colds by zinc gluconate lozenges in a double-blind study. *Antimicrobial Agents and Chemotherapy* 25(1984):20–4.

44. Farr, B.M., Conner, E.M., Betts, R.F., et al. Two randomized controlled trials of zinc gluconate lozenge therapy of experimentally induced rhinovirus colds. *Antimicrobial Agents and Chemotherapy* 31(1987):1183–7.

45. Godfrey, J.C., Sloane, B.C., Smith, D.S., et al. Zinc gluconate and the common cold: a controlled clinical study. *Journal of International Medical Research* 20(1992):234–46.

46. Chandra, R.K. Excessive intake of zinc impairs immune responses. *Journal of the American Medical Association* 252(1984):1443–6.

47. Potter, Y.J., Hart, L.L. Zinc lozenges for treatment of common colds. *Annals of Pharmacotherapy* 27(1993):589–92.

48. Focht, J., Hansen, S.H., Nielsen, J.V., et al. Bactericidal effect of propolis in vitro against agents causing upper respiratory tract infections. *Arzneimittel-Forschung* 43(1993):921–3.

49. Saketkhoo, K., Januszkiewicz, A., Sackner, M.A. Effects of drinking hot water, cold water, and chicken soup on nasal mucus velocity and nasal airflow resistance. *Chest* 74(1978):408–10.

50. Nieman, D.C. Exercise, upper respiratory tract infection, and the immune system. *Medicine and Science in Sports and Exercise* 26(1994):128–39.

51. Forstall, G.J., Macknin, M.L., Yen-Lieberman, B.R., et al. Effect of inhaling heated vapor on symptoms of the common cold. *Journal of the American Medical Association* 271(1994):1109–11.

52. Ophir, D., Elad, Y. Effects of steam inhalation on nasal patency and nasal symptoms in patients with the common cold. *American Journal of Otolaryngology* 3(1987):149–53.

53. Tyrrell, D., Barrow, I., Arthur, J. Local hyperthermia benefits natural and experimental common colds. *British Medical Journal* 298(1989):1280–3.

54. Macknin, M.L., Mathew, S., Medendorp, S.V. Effect of inhaling heated vapor on symptoms of the common cold. *Journal of the American Medical Association* 264(1990):989–91.

55. Cohen, S., Tyrrell, D.A.J., Smith, A.P. Psychological stress and susceptibility to the common cold. *New England Journal of Medicine* 325(1991):606–12.

56. Stone, A.A., Bovbjerg, D.H., Neale, J.M., et al. Development of common cold symptoms following experimental rhinovirus infection is related to prior stressful life events. *Behavioral Medicine* 18(1992):115–20.

57. Tan, D. Treatment of fever due to exopathic wind-cold by rapid acupuncture. *Journal of Traditional Chinese Medicine* 12(1992):267–71.

58. deLange-deKlerk, E.S.M., Blommers, J., Kuik, D.J., et al. Effect of homeopathic medicines on daily burden of symptoms in children with recurrent upper respiratory tract infections. *British Medical Journal* 309(1994):1329–32.

CHAPTER 10 — Colic

1. Brazelton, T.B. Crying in infancy. *Pediatrics* 29(1962):579–88.

2. Poole, S.R. The infant with acute, unexplained, excessive crying. *Pediatrics* 88(1991):450–5.

3. Rautava, P., Helenius, H., Lehtonen, L. Psychosocial predisposing factors for infantile

colic. *British Medical Journal* 307(1993):600–4.

4. Carey, W.B. Maternal anxiety and infantile colic: is there a relationship? *Clinical Pediatrics* 7(1968):590–5.

5. Miller, A.R., Barr, R.G., Eaton, W.O. Crying and motor behavior of six-week-old infants and postpartum maternal mood. *Pediatrics* 92(1993):551–8.

6. Barr, R.G., Kramer, M.S., Pless, I.B., et al. Feeding and temperament as determinants of early infant crying/fussing behavior. *Pediatrics* 84(1989):514–21.

7. Lothe, L., Ivarsson, S.A., Ekman, R., et al. Motilin and infantile colic. *Acta Paediatrica Scandinavica* 79(1990):410–6.

8. Moore, D.J., Robb, T.A., Davidson, G.P. Breath hydrogen response to milk containing lactose in colicky and noncolicky infants. *Journal of Pediatrics* 113(1988):979–84.

9. Berezin, S., Glassman, M.S., Bostwick, H., Halata, M. Esophagitis as a cause of infant colic. *Clinical Pediatrics*, 34(1995):158–9.

10. Thomas, D.W., McGilligan, K., Eisenberg, L.D., et al. Infantile colic and type of milk feeding. *American Journal of Diseases of Children* 141(1987):451–3.

11. Nelson, S.E., Ziegler, E.E., Copeland, A.M., et al. Lack of adverse reactions to iron-fortified formula. *Pediatrics* 81(1988):360–4.

12. Oski, F.A. Iron-fortified formulas and gastrointestinal symptoms in infants: a controlled study. *Pediatrics* 66(1980):168–170.

13. Barr, R.G., Elias, M.F. Nursing interval and maternal responsivity: effect on early infant crying. *Pediatrics* 81(1988):529–36.

14. Jakobsson, I., Lindberg, T. Cow's milk as a cause of infantile colic in breast-fed infants. *Lancet* 2(1978):437–9.

15. Iacono, G., Carroccio, A., Montalto, G., et al. Severe infantile colic and food intolerance: a long-term prospective study. *Journal of Pediatric Gastroenterology* 12(1991):332–5.

16. Jakobsson, I., Lindberg, T. Cow's milk proteins cause infantile colic in breast-fed infants: a double-blind crossover study. *Pediatrics* 71(1983):268–71.

17. Clyne, P.S., Kulczycki, A., Jr. Human breast milk contains bovine IgG: relationship to infant colic? *Pediatrics* 87(1991):439–44.

18. Lothe, L., Lindberg, T. Cow's milk whey protein elicits symptoms of infantile colic in colicky formula-fed infants: a double-blind crossover study. *Pediatrics* 83(1989):262–6.

19. Evans, R.W., Fergusson, D.M., Allardyce, R.A., et al. Maternal diet and infantile colic in breast-fed infants. *Lancet* 1(1981):1340–2.

20. Hide, D.W., Guyer, B.M. Prevalence of infant colic. *Archives of Disease in Childhood* 57(1982):559–60.

21. Hunziker, U.A., Barr, R.G. Increased carrying reduces infant crying: a randomized controlled trial. *Pediatrics* 77(1986):641–8.

22. St.James-Roberts, I., Hurry, J., Bowyer, J., Barr, R.G. Supplementary carrying compared with advice to increase responsive parenting as interventions to prevent persistent infant crying. *Pediatrics* 95(1995):381–8.

23. Barr, R.G., McMullan, S.J., Spiess, H., et al. Carrying as colic "therapy": a randomized controlled trial. *Pediatrics* 87(1991):623–30.

24. Walker, A.M., Menahem, S. Intervention of supplementary carrying on normal baby crying patterns: a randomized study. *Journal of Developmental and Behavioral Pediatrics* 15(1994):174–8.

25. Said, G., Patois, E., Lellouch, J. Infantile colic and parental smoking. *British Medical Journal* 289(1984):660.

26. Sethi, K.S., Sethi, J.K. Simethicone in the management of infant colic. *The Practitioner* 232(1988):508.

27. Danielsson, B., Hwang, C.P. Treatment of infantile colic with surface active substance (simethicone). *Acta Paediatrica Scandinavica* 74(1985):446–50.

28. Metcalf, T.J., Irons, T.G., Sher, L.D., et al. Simethicone in the treatment of infant colic: a randomized, placebo-controlled, multicenter trial. *Pediatrics* 94(1994):29–34.

29. Miller, J.J., McVeagh, P., Fleet, G.H., et al. Effect of yeast lactase enzyme on "colic" in infants fed human milk. *Journal of Pediatrics* 117(1990):261–3.

30. Stahlberg, M.R., Savilahti, E. Infantile colic and feeding. *Archives of Disease in Childhood* 61(1986):1232–3.

31. Weissbluth, M., Christoffel, K.K., Davis, T.A. Treatment of infantile colic with dicyclomine

hydrochloride. *Journal of Pediatrics* 104(1984):951–5.

32. Hardoin, R.A., Henslee, J.A., Christenson, C.P., et al. Colic medication and apparent life-threatening events. *Clinical Pediatrics* 30(1991):281–5.

33. Randall, B., Gerry, G., Rance, F. Dicyclomine in the sudden infant death syndrome (SIDS): a cause of death or an incidental finding? *Journal of Forensic Science* 31(1986):1470–4.

34. Weizman, Z., Alkrinawi, S., Goldfarb, D., et al. Efficacy of herbal tea preparation in infantile colic. *Journal of Pediatrics* 122(1993):650–2.

35. Bergeson, P.S. Herbal teas for infant colic. *Journal of Pediatrics* 123(1993):670.

36. Forsyth, B.W. Colic and the effect of changing formulas: a double-blind, multiple cross-over study. *Journal of Pediatrics* 115(1989):521–6.

37. Barr, R.G., Wooldridge, J., Hanley, J. Effects of formula change on intestinal hydrogen production and crying and fussing behavior. *Journal of Developmental and Behavioral Pediatrics* 12(1991):248–53.

38. Keane, V., Charney, E., Straus, J., Roberts, K. Do solids help baby sleep through the night? *American Journal of Diseases of Children* 142(1988):404–5.

39. Treem, W.R., Hyams, J.S., Blankschen, E., et al. Evaluation of the effect of a fiber-enriched formula on infant colic. *Journal of Pediatrics* 119(1991):695–701.

40. Larson, K., Ayllon, T. The effects of contingent music and differential reinforcement on infantile colic. *Behaviour Research and Therapy* 28(1990):119–25.

41. Taubman, B. Parental counseling compared with elimination of cow's milk or soy milk protein for the treatment of infant colic syndrome: a randomized trial. *Pediatrics* 81(1988):756–61.

42. Schmitt Barton, D. *Your child's health*. rev. ed. New York: Bantam Books, 1991, pp. 239–43.

43. Loadman, W., Arnold, K., Volmer, R., et al. Reducing the symptoms of infant colic by introduction of a vibration/sound based intervention. *Pediatric Research* 21(1987):182A.

44. Larsen, J-H. Infants' colic and belly massage. *The Practitioner* 234(1990):396–7.

45. McClure, V.S. *Infant massage: a handbook for loving parents*. New York: Bantam Books, 1989, pp. 137–9.

46. Klougart, N., Nilsson, N., Jacobsen, J. Infantile colic treated by chiropractors: a prospective study of 316 cases. *Journal of Manipulative and Physiological Therapeutics* 12(1989):281–8.

47. Krieger, D. *The Therapeutic Touch: how to use your hands to help or heal*. New York: Prentice-Hall, 1989, pp. 138–9.

CHAPTER 11 — Conjunctivitis

1. Isenberg, S.J., Apt, L., Wood, M. A controlled trial of povidone-iodine as prophylaxis against ophthalmia neonatorum. *New England Journal of Medicine* 332(1995):562–6.

2. Bell, T.A., Grayston, J.T., Krohn, M.A., et al. Randomized trial of silver nitrate, erythromycin, and no eye prophylaxis for the prevention of conjunctivitis among newborns not at risk for gonococcal opthalmitis. *Pediatrics* 92(1993):755–60.

3. Committee on Infectious Diseases. *1994 Red Book*. Elk Grove Village, Ill.: American Academy of Pediatrics, 1994, p. 197.

4. Bodor, F.F. Conjunctivitis-otitis media syndrome: more than meets the eye. *Contemporary Pediatrics* (Sept. 1989):55–60.

5. Spector, S.L., Raizman, M.B. Conjunctivitis medicamentosa. *Journal of Allergy and Clinical Immunology* 94(1994):134–6.

6. Moller, C., Berg, I.M., Berg, T., et al. Nedocromil sodium 2% eye drops for twice-daily treatment of seasonal allergic conjunctivitis: a Swedish multicentre placebo-controlled study in children allergic to birch pollen. *Clinical and Experimental Allergy* 24(1994):884–7.

7. Subiza, J., Subiza, J.L., Alonso, M. Allergic conjunctivitis to chamomile tea. *Annals of Allergy* 65(1990):127–32.

8. Frohn, A., Frohn, C., Steuhl, K.P., Thiel, H.J. Eye burns caused by wolf's milk. *Ophthalmologe* 90(1993):58–61.

CHAPTER 12 — Constipation

1. Cummings, J.H., Bingham, S.A., Heaton, K.W., et al. Fecal weight, colon cancer risk, and

dietary fiber intake of nonstarch polysaccharides (dietary fiber). *Gastroenterology* 103(1992):1783–9.

2. Steinmetz, K.A., Kushi, L.H., Bostick, R.M., et al. Vegetables, fruit and colon cancer in the Iowa women's health study. *American Journal of Epidemiology* 139(1994):1–15.

3. Clark, D.A. Time of first void and first stool in 500 newborns. *Pediatrics* 60(1977):457–9.

4. Weaver, L.T., Steiner, H. The bowel habits of young children. *Archives of Disease in Childhood* 59(1984):649–52.

5. McBurney, M.I. Starch malabsorption and stool excretion are influenced by the menstrual cycle in women consuming low-fiber Western diets. *Scandinavian Journal of Gastroenterology* 26(1991):880–6.

6. Iacono, G., Carroccio, A., Cavataio, F., et al. Chronic constipation as a symptom of cow milk allergy. *Journal of Pediatrics* 126(1995):34–9.

7. Dohil, R., Roberts, E., Jones, K.V., et al. Constipation and reversible urinary tract abnormalities. *Archives of Disease in Childhood* 70(1994):56–7.

8. O'Regan, S., Yazbeck, S., Hamberger, B., et al. Constipation: a commonly unrecognized cause of enuresis. *American Journal of Diseases of Children* 140(1986):260–1.

9. O'Regan, S., Yazbeck, S., Schick, E. Constipation, bladder instability, urinary tract infection syndrome. *Clinical Nephrology* 23(1985):152–4.

10. Hyams, J.S., Treem, W.R., Etienne, N.L., et al. Effect of infant formula on stool characteristics of young infants. *Pediatrics* 95(1995):50–4.

11. Buying Guide. *University of California at Berkeley Wellness Letter* (Feb. 1994):3.

12. Moriarty, K.J., Kelly, M.J., Beetham, R., et al. Studies on the mechanism of action of dioctyl sodium sulphosuccinate in the human jejunum. *Gut* 26(1985):1008–13.

13. Clark, J.H., Russell, G.J., Fitzgerald, J.F., et al. Serum beta-carotene, retinol and alpha-tocopherol levels during mineral oil therapy for constipation. *American Journal of Diseases of Children* 141(1987):1210–2.

14. Donowitz, M., Rood, R.P. Magnesium hydroxide: new insights into the mechanism of its laxative effect and the potential involvement of prostaglandin E2. *Journal of Clinical Gastroenterology* 14(1992):20–6.

15. Sprague-McRae, J.M., Lamb, W., Homer, D. Encopresis: a study of treatment alternatives and historical and behavioral characteristics. *Nurse Practitioner* 18(1993):52–63.

16. McCabe, M., Sibert, J.R., Routledge, P.A. Phosphate enemas in childhood: cause for concern. *British Medical Journal* 302(1991):1074.

17. McClung, H.J., Boyne, L.J., Linsheid, T., et al. Is combination therapy for encopresis nutritionally safe? *Pediatrics* 91(1993):591–4.

18. Godding, E.W. Laxatives and the special role of senna. *Pharmacology* 36(1988):230–6.

19. Siegers, C.P., von Hertzberg-Lottin, E., Otte, M., et al. Anthranoid laxative abuse: a risk for colorectal cancer? *Gut* 34(1993):1099–101.

20. Minghan, W., Zhu, C. The therapeutic effect of mulberry in the treatment of constipation and insomnia in the elderly. *Journal of Traditional Chinese Medicine* 9(1989):93–4.

21. Egger, G., Wolfenden, K., Pares, J., et al. "Bread: it's a great way to go": increasing bread consumption decreases laxative sales in an elderly community. *Medical Journal of Australia* 155(1991):820–1.

22. Jenkins, D.J., Peterson, R.D., Thorne, M.J., et al. Wheat fiber and laxation: dose response and equilibration time. *American Journal of Gastroenterology* 82(1987):1259–63.

23. Muller-Lissner, S.A. Effect of wheat bran on weight of stool and gastrointestinal transit time: a meta-analysis. *British Medical Journal Clinical Research Ed.* 296(1988):615–7.

24. Daly, J., Tomlin, J., Read, N.W. The effect of feeding xanthan gum on colonic function in man: correlation with in vitro determinants of bacterial breakdown. *British Journal of Nutrition* 69(1993):897–902.

25. Cummings, J.H., Branch, W., Jenkins, D.J., et al. Colonic response to dietary fibre from carrot, cabbage, apple, bran, and guar gum. *Lancet* 1(8054)(1978):5–9.

26. Miller, D.L., Miller, P.F., Dekker, J.J. Small-bowel obstruction from bran cereal [letter]. *Journal of the American Medical Association* 263(1990):813–4.

27. Klauser, A.G., Beck, A., Schindlbeck, N.E., et al.

Low fluid intake lowers stool output in healthy male volunteers. *Zeitschrift fur Gastroenterologie* 28(1990):606–9.

28. Smith, M.M., Lifshitz, F. Excess fruit juice consumption as a contributing factor in nonorganic failure to thrive. *Pediatrics* 3(994):438–43.

29. Jain, N.K., Rosenberg, D.B., Ulahannan, M.J., et al. Sorbitol intolerance in adults. *American Journal of Gastroenterology* 80(1995):678–81.

30. Berg, M.J., Rose, J.Q., Wurster, D.E., et al. Effect of charcoal and sorbitol-charcoal suspension on the elimination of intravenous phenobarbital. *Therapeutic Drug Monitoring* 9(1987):41–7.

31. Spika, J.S., Shaffer, N., Hargrett-Bean, N., et al. Risk factors for infant botulism in the United States. *American Journal of Diseases of Children* 143(1989):828–32.

32. Brown, S.R., Cann, P.A., Read, N.W. Effect of coffee on distal colon function. *Gut* 31(1990):450–3.

33. Mykkanen, H.M., Karhunen, L.J., Korpela, R., et al. Effect of cheese on intestinal transit time and other indicators of bowel function in residents of a retirement home. *Scandinavian Journal of Gastroenterology* 29(1994):29–32.

34. Andrews, P.J., Borody, T.J. "Putting back the bugs": bacterial treatment relieves chronic constipation and symptoms of irritable bowel syndrome. *Medical Journal of Australia* 159(1993):633–4.

35. Keeling, W.F., Martin, B.J. Gastrointestinal transit during mild exercise. *Journal of Applied Physiology* 63(1987):978–81.

36. Moses, F.M. The effect of exercise on the gastrointestinal tract. *Sports Medicine* 9(1990):159–72.

37. Nolan, T., Debelle, G., Oberklaid, F., et al. Randomized trial of laxatives in treatment of childhood encopresis. *Lancet* 338(1991):523–7.

38. Klauser, A.G., Voderholzer, W.A., Heinrich, C.A. Behavioral modification of colonic function: can constipation be learned? *Digestive Diseases and Sciences* 35(1990):1271–5.

39. Whitehead, W.E. Behavioral medicine approaches to gastrointestinal disorders. *Journal of Consulting and Clinical Psychology* 60(1992):605–12.

40. Benninga, M.A., Buller, H.A., Taminiau, J.A. Biofeedback training in chronic constipation. *Archives of Disease in Childhood* 68(1993):126–9.

41. Papachrysostomou, M., Smith, A.N. Effects of biofeedback on obstructive defecation: reconditioning of the defecation reflex? *Gut* 35(1994):252–6.

42. Loening-Baucke, V. Modulation of abnormal defecation dynamics by biofeedback treatment in chronically constipated children with encopresis. *Journal of Pediatrics* 116(1990):214–22.

43. Cox, D.J., Sutphen, J., Borowitz, S., et al. Simple electromyographic biofeedback treatment for chronic pediatric constipation/encopresis: preliminary report. *Biofeedback and Self Regulation* 19(1994):41–50.

44. Klauser, A.G., Flaschentrager, J., Gehrke, A., et al. Abdominal wall massage: effect on colonic function in healthy volunteers and in patients with chronic constipation. *Zeitschrift fur Gastroenterologie* 30(1992):247–51.

45. Penninckx, F., Lestar, B., Kerremans, R. Surgery for constipation: irrational things for desperate people? *Hepatogastroenterology* 37(1990):580–4.

46. Klauser, A.G., Rubach, A., Bertsche, O., et al. Body acupuncture: effect on colonic function in chronic constipation. *Zeitschrift fur Gastroenterologie* 31(1993):605–8.

CHAPTER 13 — Cough

1. Denny, F.W., Murphy, T.F., Clyde, W.A., et al. Croup: an 11-year study in a pediatric practice. *Pediatrics* 71(1983):871–6.

2. Smith, M.B.H., Feldman, W. Over-the-counter cold medications: a critical review of clinical trials between 1950 and 1991. *Journal of the American Medical Association* 269(1993):2258–63.

3. Taylor, J.A., Novack, A.H., Almquist, J.R., Rogers, J.E. Efficacy of cough suppressants in children. *Journal of Pediatrics* 122(1993):799–802.

4. Committee on Drugs, American Academy of Pediatrics. Use of codeine- and dextromethorphan-containing cough syrups in pediatrics.

Pediatrics 62(1978):119–22.

5. Kuhn, J.J., Hendley, J.O., Adams, K.F., et al. Antitussive effect of guaifenesin in young adults with natural colds. *Chest* 82(1982):713–8.

6. Hirsch, S.R., Viernes, P.F., Kory, R.C., et al. The expectorant effect of glyceryl guaiacolate in patients with chronic bronchitis. *Chest* 63(1973):9–14.

7. Taussig, L.M., Castro, O., Beaudry, P.H., et al. Treatment of laryngotracheobronchitis (croup). *American Journal of Diseases of Children* 129(1975):790–3.

8. Klassen, T., Feldman, M., Watters, L., et al. A randomized trial of budesonide in mild to moderate croup. *Archives of Pediatric and Adolescent Medicine* 148(1994):40.

9. Leipzig, B., Oski, F.A., Cummings, C.W., et al. A prospective randomized study to determine the efficacy of steroids in treatment of croup. *Journal of Pediatrics* 94(1979):194–6.

10. Kairys, S.W., Olmstead, E.M., O'Connor, G.T. Steroid treatment of laryngotracheitis: a meta-analysis of the evidence from randomized trials. *Pediatrics* 83(1989):683–93.

11. Tibballs, J., Shann, F.A., Landau, L.I. Placebo-controlled trial of prednisolone in children intubated for croup. *Lancet* 340(1992):745–8.

12. Darelid, J., Lofgren, S., Malmvall, B.E. Erythromycin treatment is beneficial for long-standing *Moraxella catarrhalis* associated cough in children. *Scandinavian Journal of Infectious Diseases* 25(1993):323–9.

13. Gottfarb, P., Brauner, A. Children with persistent cough: outcome with treatment and role of Moraxella catarrhalis? *Scandinavian Journal of Infectious Diseases* 26(1994):545–51.

14. Hirono, I., Mori, H., Culvenor, C.C.J. Carcinogenic activity of coltsfoot, *Tussilago Farfara L. Gann* 67(1976):125–9.

15. Fawzi, W.W., Herrera, M.G., Willett, W.C., et al. Dietary vitamin A intake and the risk of mortality among children. *American Journal of Clinical Nutrition* 59(1994):401–8.

16. Abdeljaber, M.H., Monto, A.S., Tilden, R.L., et al. The impact of vitamin A supplementation on morbidity: a randomized community intervention trial. *American Journal of Public Health* 81(1991):1654–6.

17. Stansfield, S.K., Pierre-Louis, M., Lerebours, G., et al. Vitamin A supplementation and increased prevalence of childhood diarrhea and acute respiratory infections. *Lancet* 342(1993):578–82.

18. Bucca, C., Rolla, G., Arossa, W., et al. Effect of ascorbic acid on increased bronchial responsiveness during upper airway infection. *Respiration* 55(1989):214–9.

19. Pinnock, C.B. Arney, W.K. The milk-mucus belief: sensory analysis comparing cow's milk and a soy placebo. *Appetite* 20(1993):61–70.

20. Pinnock, C.B., Graham, N.M., Mylvaganam, A., et al. Relationship between milk intake and mucus production in adult volunteers challenged with rhinovirus–2. *American Review of Respiratory Disease* 141(1990):352–6.

21. Paul, D.W., Bogaard, J.M., Hop, W.C. The bronchoconstrictor effect of strenuous exercise at low temperatures in normal athletes. *International Journal of Sports Medicine* 14(1993):433–6.

22. Kirilloff, L.H., Owens, G.R., Rogers, R.M., et al. Does chest physical therapy work? *Chest* 88(1985):436–44.

23. Mortensen, J., Falk, M., Groth, S., et al. The effects of postural drainage and positive expiratory pressure physiotherapy on tracheobronchial clearance in cystic fibrosis. *Chest* 100(1991):1350–7.

24. Dales, R.E., Zwanenburg, H., Burnett, R., et al. Respiratory health effects of home dampness and molds among Canadian children. *American Journal of Epidemiology* 134(1991):196–203.

25. Dijkstra, L., Houthuijs, D., Brunekreef, B., et al. Respiratory health effects of the indoor environment in a population of Dutch children. *American Review of Respiratory Disease* 142(1990):1172–8.

26. Brunekreeff, B. Damp housing and adult respiratory symptoms. *Allergy* 47(1992):498–502.

27. Avery, M.E. Mist therapy. *Pediatrics* 39(1967):160–5.

28. Bourchier, D., Dawson, K.P., Fergusson, D.M. Humidification in viral croup: a controlled trial. *Australian Paediatrics Journal* 20(1984):289–91.

29. Mamolen, M., Lewis, D.M., Blanchet, M.A., et

al. Investigation of an outbreak of "humidifier fever" in a print shop. *American Journal of Industrial Medicine* 23(1993):483–90.

30. Cohlan, S.Q., Stone, S.M. The cough and the bedsheet. *Pediatrics* 74(1984):11–5.

31. Elkins, G.R., Carter, B.D. Hypnotherapy in the treatment of childhood psychogenic coughing: a case report. *American Journal of Clinical Hypnosis* 29(1986):59–63.

32. Lavigne, J.V., Davis, T., Fauber, R. Behavioral management of pyschogenic cough: alternative to the "bedsheet" and other aversive techniques. *Pediatrics* 87(1991):532–7.

33. Pavia, D. The role of chest physiotherapy in mucus hypersecretion. *Lung* 168S(1990):614–21.

34. Xinlian, L. 41 cases of cough treated with cupping. *International Journal of Clinical Acupuncture* 2(1991):319–22.

CHAPTER 14 — Cradle Cap

1. Broberg, A. *Pityrosporum ovale* in healthy children, infantile seborrheic dermatitis and atopic dermatitis. *Acta Dermato-Venereologica. Supplementum (Stockholm)* 191(1995):1–47.

2. Kiepert, J.A. Oral use of biotin in seborrheic dermatitis of infancy: a controlled study. *Medical Journal of Australia* 1(1976):584–5.

3. Erlichman, M., Goldstein, R., Levi, E., et al. Infantile flexural seborrheic dermatitis: neither biotin nor essential fatty acid deficiency. *Archives of Disease in Childhood* 56(1981):560–2.

4. Janniger, C.K. Infantile seborrheic dermatitis: an approach to cradle cap. *Cutis* 51(1993):233–5.

CHAPTER 15 — Diaper Rash

1. Berg, R.W., Mulligan, M.C., Sarbaugh, F.C. Association of skin wetness and pH with diaper dermatitis. *Pediatric Dermatology* 11(1994):18–20.

2. Tanguay, K.E., McBean, M.R., Fain, E. Nipple candidiasis among breastfeeding mothers. *Canadian Family Physician* 40(1994):1407–13.

3. Singalavanija, S., Frieden, I.J. Diaper dermati-

tis. *Pediatrics in Review* 16(1995):142–7.

4. Honig, P.J., Gribetz, B., Leyden, J.J., et al. Amoxicillin and diaper dermatitis. *Journal of the American Academy of Dermatology* 19(1988):275–9.

5. Odio, C.M., Kusmiesz, H., Shelton, S., et al. Comparative treatment trial of augmentin versus cefaclor for acute otitis media with effusion. *Pediatrics* 75(1985):819–26.

6. Committee on Drugs, American Academy of Pediatrics. Clioquinol (Iodochlorhydroxyquin, Vioform) and iodoquinol (diiodohydroxyquin): blindness and neuropathy. *Pediatrics* 86(1990):797–8.

7. Piatt, J.P., Bergeson, P.S. Gentian violet toxicity. *Clinical Pediatrics* 31(12)(1992):756–7.

8. Healy, C.E. Precocious puberty due to a diaper ointment. *Indiana Medicine* 77(8) (1984):610.

9. Despard, C. Diaper dermatitis: another simple remedy. *Canadian Medical Association Journal* 139(1988):706.

10. Sharma, V.D., Sethi, M.S., Kumar, A., et al. Antibacterial property of Allium sativum Linn.: in vivo and in vitro studies. *Indian Journal of Experimental Biology* 15(1977):466–8.

11. Amer, M., Taha, M., Tosson, Z. The effect of aqueous garlic extract on the growth of dermatophytes. *International Journal of Dermatology* 19(1980):285–7.

12. Moore, G.S., Atkins, R.D. The fungicidal and fungistatic effects of an aqueous garlic extract on medically important yeast-like fungi. *Mycologia* 69(1977):341–8.

13. Sandhu, D.K., Warraich, M.K., Singh, S. Sensitivity of yeasts isolated from cases of vaginitis to aqueous extracts of garlic. *Mykosen* 23(1980):691–8.

14. Prasad, G., Sharma, V.D. Efficacy of garlic (Allium sativum) treatment against experimental candidiasis in chicks. *British Veterinary Journal* 136(1980):448–51.

15. Barone, F.E., Tansey, M.R. Isolation, purification, identification, synthesis, and kinetics of activity of the anticandidal compounds of Allium sativum, and a hypothesis for its mode of action. *Mycologia* 69(1977):793–824.

16. Lee, T.Y., Lam, T.H. Contact dermatitis due to topical treatment with garlic in Hong Kong.

Contact Dermatitis 24(1991):193–6.

17. Mahajan, V.M., Sharma, A., Rattan, A. Antimycotic activity of berberine sulfate: an alkaloid from an Indian medicinal herb. *Sabouraudia* 20(1982):79–81.

18. Court, J., Ng, L.-M. Danger of egg white treatment for nappy rash. *Archives of Disease in Childhood* 59(9S)(1984):908.

19. Collipp, P.J., Kuo, B., Castro-Magana, M., et al. Hair zinc, scalp hair quantity, and diaper rash in normal infants. *Cutis* 35(1985):66–70.

20. Collipp, P.J. Effect of oral zinc supplements on diaper rash in normal infants. *Journal of the Medical Association of Georgia* 78(1989):621–3.

21. Bosch-Banyeras, J.M., Catala, M., Mas, P., et al. Diaper dermatitis: value of vitamin A topically applied. *Clinical Pediatrics* 27(1988):448–50.

22. Deans, L., Slater, H., Goldfarb, I.W. Bad advice; bad burn: a new problem in burn prevention. *Journal of Burn Care and Rehabilitation* 11(1990):563–4.

23. Seymour, J.L., Keswick, B.H., Hanifin, J.M., et al. Clinical effects of diaper types on the skin of normal infants and infants with atopic dermatitis. *Journal of the American Academy of Dermatology* 17(1987):988–97.

24. Davis, J.A., Leyden, J.J., Grove, G.L., et al. Comparison of disposable diapers with fluff absorbent and fluff plus absorbent polymers: effects on skin hydration, skin pH and diaper dermatitis. *Pediatric Dermatology* 6(1989):102–8.

25. Wilson, P.A., Dallas, M.J. Diaper performance: maintenance of healthy skin. *Pediatric Dermatology* 7(1990):179–84.

26. Campbell, R.L., Seymour, J.L., Stone, L.C., et al. Clinical studies with disposable diapers containing absorbent gelling materials: evaluation of effects on infant skin condition. *Journal of the American Academy of Dermatology* 17(1987):978–87.

27. Warner, E. Diaper dermatitis: simple remedy. *Canadian Medical Association Journal* 139(1988):284–5.

CHAPTER 16 — Diarrhea

1. Lifshitz, F. Introduction to management of acute diarrheal disease. *Journal of Pediatrics* 118(1991):S25-6.

2. Avendano, P., Matson, D.O., Long, J., et al. Costs associated with office visits for diarrhea in infants and toddlers. *Pediatric Infectious Disease Journal* 12(1993):897–902.

3. Host, A. Halken, S. A prospective study of cow milk allergy in Danish infants during the first three years of life: clinical course in relation to clinical and immunological type of hypersensitivity reaction. *Allergy* 45(1990):587–96.

4. Goldman, A.S., Anderson, D.W., Sellers, W.A., et al. Milk allergy. I. Oral challenge with milk and isolated milk proteins in allergic children. *Pediatrics* 32(1963):425–43.

5. Bell, B.P., Goldoft, M., Griffin, P.M., et al. A multistate outbreak of *Escherichia coli* O157:H7-associated bloody diarrhea and hemolytic uremic syndrome from hamburgers. *Journal of the American Medical Association* 272(1994):1349–53.

6. Millard, P.S., Gensheimer, K.F., Addiss, D.G., et al. An outbreak of cryptosporidiosis from fresh-pressed apple cider. *Journal of the American Medical Association* 272(1994):1592–6.

7. Hill, D.B., Henderson, L.M., McClain, C.J. Osmotic diarrhea induced by sugar-free theophylline solution in critically ill patients. *Journal of Parenteral and Enteral Nutrition* 15(1991):332–6.

8. Forsyth, J.S., Ogston, S.A., Clark, A., et al. Relation between early introduction of solid food to infants and their weight and illnesses during the first two years of life. *British Medical Journal* 306(1993):1572–6.

9. Clemens, J., Rao, M., Eng, M., et al. Breast-feeding and the risk of life-threatening rotavirus diarrhea: prevention or postponement. *Pediatrics* 92(1993):680–5.

10. Molbak, K., Gottschau, A., Aaby, P., et al. Prolonged breast feeding, diarrheal disease, and survival of children in Guinea-Bissau. *British Medical Journal* 308(1994):1403–6.

11. Long, K.Z., Wood, J.W., Gariby, E.V., et al. Proportional hazards analysis of diarrhea due to enterotoxigenic Escherichia coli and breast feeding in a cohort of urban Mexican children. *American Journal of Epidemiology* 139(1994):193–205.

12. Samra, H.K., Ganguly, N.K., Mahajan, R.C. Human milk containing specific secretory IgA inhibits binding of *Giardia Lamblia* to nylon and glass surfaces. *Journal of Diarrhoeal Diseases Research* 9(1991):100–3.

13. Ruiz-Palacios, G.M., Calva, J.J., Pickering, L.K., et al. Protection of breast-fed infants against *Campylobacter* diarrhea by antibodies in human milk. *Journal of Pediatrics* 116(1990):707–13.

14. Glass, R.I., Svennerholm, A.M., Stoll, B.J., et al. Protection against cholera in breast-fed children by antibodies in breast milk. *New England Journal of Medicine* 308(1983):1389–92.

15. Charnow, J.A. Feeding infants milk with bacteria that are not pathogenic reduces the rate of gastroenteritis. *Infectious Disease in Children* (Jan. 1995):7.

16. Bernstein. D.I., Glass, R.I., Rodgers, G., et al. Evaluation of rhesus rotavirus monovalent and tetravalent reassortant vaccines in US children. *Journal of the American Medical Association* 273(1995):1191–6.

17. Turner, R.B., Kelsey, D.K. Passive immunization for prevention of rotavirus illness in healthy infants. *Pediatric Infectious Disease Journal* 12(1993):718–22.

18. Figueroa-Quintanilla, D., Salazar-Lindo, E., Sack, R.B., et al. A controlled trial of bismuth subsalicylate in infants with acute watery diarrheal disease. *New England Journal of Medicine* 328(1993):1653–8.

19. Loeb, H., Vandenplas, Y., Wursch, P., Guesry P. Tannin-rich carob pod for the treatment of acute-onset diarrhea. *Journal of Pediatric Gastroenterology and Nutrition* 8(1989):480–5.

20. Gupte, S. Use of berberine in treatment of giardiasis. *American Journal of Diseases of Children* 129(1975):866.

21. Hambidge, K.M. Zinc and diarrhea. *Acta Paediatrica Supplement* 381(1992):82–6.

22. Sachdev, H.P.S., Mittal, N.K., Yadav, H.S. Oral zinc supplementation in persistent diarrhea in infants. *Annals of Tropical Paediatrics* 10(1990):63–9.

23. Roy, S.K., Behrens, R.H., Haider, R., et al. Impact of zinc supplementation on intestinal permeability in Bangladeshi children with acute diarrhea and persistent diarrhea syndrome. *Journal of Pediatric Gastroenterology and Nutrition* 15(1992):289–96.

24. Castillo-Duran, C., Vial, P., Uauy, R. Oral copper supplementation: effect on copper and zinc balance during acute gastroenteritis in infants. *American Journal of Clinical Nutrition* 51(1990):1088–92.

25. Barreto, M.L., Santos, L.M., Assis, A.M., et al. Effect of vitamin A supplementation on diarrhea and acute lower respiratory-tract infections in young children in Brazil. *Lancet* 344(1994):228–31.

26. Rahmathullah, L., Underwood, B.A., Thulasiraj, R.D., Milton, R.C. Diarrhea, respiratory infections and growth are not affected by a weekly low-dose vitamin A supplement: a masked, controlled field trial in children in southern India. *American Journal of Clinical Nutrition* 54(1991):568–77.

27. Avery, M.E., Snyder, J.D. Oral therapy for acute diarrhea: the underused simple solution. *New England Journal of Medicine* 323(1990):891–4.

28. Gore, S.M., Fontaine, O., Pierce, N.F. Impact of rice based oral rehydration solution on stool output and duration of diarrhea: meta-analysis of 13 clinical trials. *British Medical Journal* 304(1992):287–91.

29. Kassaye, M., Larson, C., Carlson, D. A randomized community trial of prepackaged and homemade oral rehydration therapies. *Archives of Pediatric and Adolescent Medicine* 148(1994):1288–92.

30. Santosham, M., Goepp, J., Burns, B., et al. Role of a soy-based lactose-free formula in the outpatient management of diarrhea. *Pediatrics* 87(1991):619–22.

31. Chew, F., Penna, F.J., Peret, L.A., et al. Is dilution of cows' milk formula necessary for dietary management of acute diarrhea in infants aged less than six months? *Lancet* 341(1993):194–7.

32. Brown, K.H., Peerson, J.M., Fontaine, O. Use of nonhuman milks in the dietary management of young children with acute diarrhea: a meta-analysis of clinical trials. *Pediatrics* 93(1994):17–27.

33. Allen, U.D., McLeod, K., Wang, E.E. Cow's milk versus soy-based formula in mild and moder-

ate diarrhea: a randomized, controlled trial. *Acta Paediatrica* 83(1994):183–7.

34. Penny, M.E., Paredes, P., Brown, K.H. Clinical and nutritional consequences of lactose feeding during persistent postenteritis diarrhea. *Pediatrics* 84(1989):835–44.

35. Wall, C.R., Webster, J., Quirk, P., et al. The nutritional management of acute diarrhea in young infants: effect of carbohydrate ingested. *Journal of Pediatric Gastroenterology and Nutrition* 19(1994):170–4.

36. Margolis, P.A., Litteer, T., Hare, N., Pichichero, M. Effects of unrestricted diet on mild infantile diarrhea. *American Journal of Diseases of Children* 144(1990):162–4.

37. Bhutta, Z.A., Molla, A.M., Issani, Z., et al. Dietary management of persistent diarrhea: comparison of a traditional rice-lentil based diet with soy formula. *Pediatrics* 88(1991):1010–8.

38. Maulen-Radovan, I., Brown, K.H., Acosta, M.A., Fernandez-Varela, H. Comparison of a rice-based, mixed diet versus a lactose-free, soy-protein isolate formula for young children with acute diarrhea. *Journal of Pediatrics* 125(1994):699–706.

39. Alarcon, P., Montoya, R., Rivera, J., et al. Effect of inclusion of beans in a mixed diet for the treatment of Peruvian children with acute watery diarrhea. *Pediatrics* 90(1992):58–65.

40. Khin-Maung-U, Greenlough, W.B. Cereal-based oral rehydration therapy. I. Clinical studies. *Journal of Pediatrics* 118(1991):S72–9.

41. Lanata, C.F., Black, R.E., Creed-Kanashiro, H., et al. Feeding during acute diarrhea as a risk factor for persistent diarrhea. *Acta Paediatrica. Supplement* 381(1992):98–103.

42. Boudraa, G., Touhami, M., Pochart, P., et al. Effect of feeding yogurt versus milk in children with persistent diarrhea. *Journal of Pediatric Gastroenterology and Nutrition* 11(1990):509–12.

43. Isolarui, E., Juntunen, M., Rautanen, T., et al. A human lactobacillus strain (*Lactobacillus casei* sp strain GG) promotes recovery from acute diarrhea in children. *Pediatrics* 88(1991):90–7.

44. Brown, K.H., Perez, F., Peerson, J.M., et al. Effect of dietary fiber (soy polysaccharide) on the severity, duration, and nutritional outcome of acute, watery diarrhea in children. *Pediatrics* 92(1993):241–7.

45. Hyams, J.S., Etienne, N.L., Leichtner, A.M., Theuer, R.C. Carbohydrate malabsorption following fruit juice ingestion in young children. *Pediatrics* 82(1988):64–8.

46. Smith, M.M., Davis, M., Chasalow, F.I., Lifshitz, F. Carbohydrate absorption from fruit juice in children. *Pediatrics* 95(1995):340–4.

47. Yingchun, L. Observation of therapeutic effects of acupuncture treatment in 170 cases of infantile diarrhea. *Journal of Traditional Chinese Medicine* 7(1987):203–4.

48. Jacobs, J., Jimenez, L.M., Gloyd, S.S., et al. Treatment of acute childhood diarrhea with homeopathic medicine: a randomized trial in Nicaragua. *Pediatrics* 93(1994):719–25.

CHAPTER 17 — Ear Infections

1. Teele, D.W., Klein, J.O., Rosner, B. Middle ear disease and the practice of pediatrics: burden during the first five years of life. *Journal of the American Medical Association* 249(1983):1026–9.

2. Heikkinen, T., Ruuskanen, O. Signs and symptoms predicting acute otitis media. *Archives of Pediatric and Adolescent Medicine* 149(1995):26–9.

3. Appelman, C., Claessen, J., Touw-Otten, F., et al. Severity of inflammation of tympanic membrane as predictor of clinical course of recurrent acute otitis media. *British Medical Journal* 306(1993):895.

4. Hardy, A.M., Fowler, M.G. Child care arrangements and repeated ear infections in young children. *American Journal of Public Health* 83(1993):1321–5.

5. Owen, M.J., Baldwin, C.D., Swank, P.R., et al. Relation of infant feeding practices, cigarette smoke exposure, and group child care to the onset and duration of otitis media with effusion in the first two years of life. *Journal of Pediatrics* 123(1993):702–11.

6. Duncan, B., Ey, J., Holberg, C., et al. Breastfeeding and recurrent otitis media in the first year of life. *American Journal of Diseases of Children* 146(1992):482.

7. Nsouli, T.M., Nsouli, S.M., Linde, R.E., et al. Role of food allergy in serous otitis media. *Annals of Allergy* 73(1994):215–9.

8. Paradise, J.L., Elster, B.A., Tan, L. Evidence in infants with cleft palate that breast milk protects against otitis media. *Pediatrics* 94(1994):853–60.

9. Ey, J.L., Holberg, C.J., Aldous, M.B., et al. Passive smoke exposure and otitis media in the first year of life. *Pediatrics* 95(1995):670–7.

10. Schuller, D.E. Prophylaxis of otitis media in asthmatic children. *Pediatric Infectious Disease Journal* 2(1983):280–3.

11. Niemela, M., Uhari, M., Hannuksela, A. Pacifiers and dental structure as risk factors for otitis media. *International Journal of Pediatric Otorhinolaryngology* 29(1994):121–7.

12. Carlin, S.A., Marchant, C.D., Shurin, P.A., et al. Early recurrences of otitis media: reinfection or relapse? *Journal of Pediatrics* 110(1987):20–5.

13. Wright, P.F., Sell, S.H., McConnell, K.B., et al. Impact of recurrent otitis media on middle ear function, hearing and language. *Journal of Pediatrics* 113(1988):581–7.

14. Schwartz, R.H., Rodriguez, W.J., Grundfast, K.M. Duration of middle ear effusion after acute otitis media. *Pediatric Infectious Disease Journal* 3(1984):204–7.

15. Roberts, J.E., Sanyal, M.A., Burchinal, M.R., et al. Otitis media in early childhood and its relationship to later verbal and academic performance. *Pediatrics* 78(1986):423–30.

16. Roberts, J.E., Burchinal, M.R., Collier, A.M., et al. Otitis media in early childhood and cognitive, academic and classroom performance of the school-aged child. *Pediatrics* 83(1989):477–85.

17. Roberts, J.E., Burchinal, M.R., Medley, L.P., et al. Otitis media, hearing sensitivity, and maternal responsiveness in relation to language during infancy. *Journal of Pediatrics* 126(1995):481–9.

18. Sorenson, H. Antibiotics in suppurative otitis media. *Otolaryngology Clinics of North America* 10(1977):45–50.

19. van Buchem, F.L., Dunk, J.H.M., van't Hof, M.A. Therapy of acute otitis media: myringotomy, antibiotics, or neither? *Lancet* 2(1981):883–7.

20. Rudberg, R.D. Acute otitis media: comparative therapeutic results of sulphonamide and penicillin administered in various forms. *Acta Otolaryngologica (Stockholm)* 113(1954):1–79.

21. Lahikainen, E.A. Clinico-bacteriologic studies on acute otitis media: aspiration of tympanum as diagnostic and therapeutic method. *Acta Oto-laryngologica (Stockholm)* 107(1953):1–82.

22. van Dishoeck, H.A.E., Derks, A.C.W., Voorhorst, R. Bacteriology and treatment of acute otitis media in children. *Acta Oto-laryngologica (Stockholm)* 50(1959):250–62.

23. Halstead, C., Lepow, M.L., Balassanian, N., et al. Otitis media: clinical observations, microbiology, and evaluation of therapy. *American Journal of Diseases of Children* 115(1968):542–51.

24. Rosenfeld, R.M., Vertrees, J.E., Carr, J., et al. Clinical efficacy of antimicrobial drugs for acute otitis media: metaanalysis of 5400 children from 33 randomized trials. *Journal of Pediatrics* 124(1994):355–67.

25. McCaig, L.F., Hughes, J.M. Trends in antimicrobial drug prescribing among office-based physicians in the United States. *Journal of the American Medical Association* 273(1995):214–9.

26. Principi, N., Marchisio, P., Bigalli, L., et al. Amoxicillin twice daily in the treatment of acute otitis media in infants and children. *European Journal of Pediatrics* 145(1986):522–5.

27. Weinberg, H.D. Treatment of otitis media twice daily for five days. *Clinical Pediatrics* 30(1991):391–2.

28. DeSaintonge, D.M.C., Levine, D.F., Savage, I.T., et al. Trial of three-day and ten-day courses of amoxycillin in otitis media. *British Medical Journal* 284(1982):1078–81.

29. Green, S.M., Rothrock, S.G. Single-dose intramuscular ceftriaxone for acute otitis media in children. *Pediatrics* 91(1993):23–30.

30. Heikkinen, T., Ruuskanen, O., Ziegler, T., et al. Short-term use of amoxicillin-clavulanate during upper respiratory tract infection for prevention of acute otitis media. *Journal of Pediatrics* 126(1995):313–6.

31. van Buchem, F.L., Peeters, M.F., van't Hof, M.A. Acute otitis media: a new treatment strategy. *British Medical Journal* 290(1985):1033–7.

32. Bollag, U., Bollag-Albrecht, E. Recommendations derived from practice audit for the treatment of acute otitis media. *Lancet* 338(1991):96–9.

33. Reichler, M.R., Allphin, A.A., Breiman, R.F., et al. The spread of multiply resistant *Streptococcus penumoniae* at a day care center in Ohio. *Journal of Infectious Diseases* 166(1992):1346–53.

34. Williams, R.L., Chalmers, T.C., Stange, K.C., et al. Use of antibiotics in preventing recurrent acute otitis media and in treating otitis media with effusion. *Journal of the American Medical Association* 270(1993):1344–51.

35. Klein, J.O. Preventing recurrent otitis: what role for antibiotics? *Contemporary Pediatrics* 11(1994):44–60.

36. Berman, S., Luckey, D., Roark, R. Cost-effectiveness analysis of the management of persisting middle ear effusions. *American Journal of Diseases of Children* 147(1993):461.

37. Macknin, M.L. Steroid treatment for otitis media with effusion. *Clinical Pediatrics* 30(1991):178–81.

38. Lecks, H.I., Kravis, L.P., Wood, D.W. Serous otitis media: reflections on pathogenesis and treatment, with a comment on the use of intranasal dexamthasone. *Clinical Pediatrics* 6(1967):519–23.

39. Podoshin, L., Fradis, M., Ben-David, J. Ototoxicity of ear drops in patients suffering from chronic otitis media. *Journal of Laryngology and Otology* 103(1989):46–50.

40. Cantekin, E.I., Mandel, E.M., Bluestone, C.D., et al. Lack of efficacy of a decongestant-antihistamine combination for otitis media with effusion ("secretory" otitis media) in children: results of a double-blind, randomized trial. *New England Journal of Medicine* 308(1983):297–301.

41. Lildholdt, T., Cantekin, E.I., Bluestone, C.D., Rockette, H.E. Effect of a topical nasal decongestant on eustachian tube function in children with tympanostomy tubes. *Acta Otolaryngologica (Stockholm)* 94(1982):93–7.

42. Dusdieker, L.B., Smith, G., Booth, B.M., et al. The long-term outcome of nonsuppurative otitis media with effusion. *Clinical Pediatrics* 24(1985):181–6.

43. Mandel, E.M., Rockette, H.E., Bluestone, C.D., et al. Efficacy of amoxicillin with and without decongestant-antihistamine for otitis media with effusion in children: results of a double-blind, randomized trial. *New England Journal of Medicine* 316(1987):432–7.

44. Rundcrantz, H. The effects of position change on eustachian tube function. *Otolaryngology Clinics of North America* 3(1970):103–10.

45. Kaleida, P.H., Casselbrant, M.L., Rockette, H.E., et al. Amoxicillin or myringotomy or both for acute otitis media: results of a randomized clinical trial. *Pediatrics* 87(1991):466–74.

46. Bright, R.A., Moore, R.M., Jeng, L.L., et al. The prevalence of tympanostomy tubes in children in the United States, 1988. *American Journal of Public Health* 83(1993):1026–8.

47. Gilbert, J.G. Swimming and grommets: a prospective survey. *New Zealand Medical Journal* 107(1994):244–5.

48. Parker, G.S., Tami, T.A., Maddox, M.R., et al. The effect of water exposure after tympanostomy tube insertion. *American Journal of Otolaryngology* 15(1994):193–6.

49. Bernard, P.A.M., Stenstrom, R.J., Feldman, W., et al. Randomized, controlled trial comparing long-term sulfonamide therapy to ventilation tubes for otitis media with effusion. *Pediatrics* 88(1991):215–22.

50. Kleinman, L.C., Kosecoff, J., Dubois, R.W., et al. The medical appropriateness of tympanostomy tubes proposed for children younger than 16 years in the United States. *Journal of the American Medical Association* 271(1994):1250–5.

51. Gates, G.A., Avery, C.A., Prihoda, T.J., et al. Effectiveness of adenoidectomy and tympanostomy tubes in the treatment of chronic otitis media with effusion. *New England Journal of Medicine* 317(1987):1444–51.

CHAPTER 18—Eczema

1. Kay, J., Gawkrodger, D.J., Mortimer, M.J., et al. The prevalence of childhood atopic eczema in a general population. *Journal of the American Academy of Dermatology* 30(1994):35–9.

2. Peters, T.J., Golding, J. The epidemiology of childhood eczema. II. Statistical analyses to

identify independent early predictors. *Paediatric and Perinatal Epidemiology* 1(1987):80–94.

3. Melnik, B.C., Plewig, G. Is the origin of atopy linked to deficient conversion to omega–6-fatty acids to prostaglandin E1? *Journal of the American Academy of Dermatology* 21(1989):557–63.

4. Hansen, A.E. Serum lipids in eczema and other pathologic conditions. *American Journal of Diseases of Children* 53(1937):933–46.

5. Kimata, H., Lindley, I. Detection of plasma interleukin–8 in atopic dermatitis. *Archives of Disease in Childhood* 70(1994):119–22.

6. White, M.I., Jenkinson, D.M., Lloyd, D.H. The effect of washing on the thickness of the stratum corneum in normal and atopic individuals. *British Journal of Dermatology* 116(1987):525–30.

7. Sanda, T., Yasue, T., Oohashi, M., et al. Effectiveness of house dust-mite antigen avoidance through clean room therapy in patients with atopic dermatitis. *Journal of Allergy and Clinical Immunology* 89(1992):653–7.

8. Fergusson, D.M., Horwood, L.J., Shannon, F.T. Early solid feeding and recurrent childhood eczema: a 10-year longitudinal study. *Pediatrics* 86(1990):541–6.

9. Sampson, H.A., McCaskill, C.C. Food hypersensitivity and atopic dermatitis: evaluation of 113 patients. *Journal of Pediatrics* 107(1985):669–75.

10. Kanny, G., Hatahet, R., Moneret-Vautrin, D.A., et al. Allergy and intolerance to flavouring agents in atopic dermatitis in young children. *Allergie et Immunologie (Paris)* 26(1994):204–10.

11. Sigurs, N., Hattevig, G., Kjellman, B. Maternal avoidance of eggs, cow's milk, and fish during lactation: effect on allergic manifestations, skin-prick tests, and specific IgE antibodies in children at age 4 years. *Pediatrics* 89(1992):735–9.

12. Steinman, H.A., Potter, P.C. The precipitation of symptoms by common foods in children with atopic dermatitis. *Allergy Proceedings* 15(1994):203–10.

13. Van Bever, H.P., Docx, M., Stevens, W.J. Food and food additives in severe atopic dermatitis. *Allergy* 44(1989):588–94.

14. Barthel, H.R., Stuhlmuller, B. Improvement in atopic dermatitis with change to low salt table water. *Lancet* 344(1994):1089.

15. Fredriksson, T., Gip, L. Urea creams in the treatment of dry skin and hand dermatitis. *International Journal of Dermatology* 14(1975):442–4.

16. Munkvad, M. A comparative trial of Clinitar versus hydrocortisone cream in the treatment of atopic eczema. *British Journal of Dermatology* 121(1989):763–6.

17. Bartorelli, A., Rimondini, A. Severe hypertension in childhood due to prolonged skin application of a mineralocorticoid ointment. *Hypertension* 6(1984):586–8.

18. Klein, G.L., Galant, S.P. A comparison of the antipruritic efficacy of hydroxyzine and cyproheptadine in children with atopic dermatitis. *Annals of Allergy* 44(1980):142–5.

19. Krause, L., Shuster, S. Mechanism of action of antipruritic drugs. *British Medical Journal* 287(1983):1199–200.

20. David, T.J., Devlin, J., Ewing, C.I. Atopic and seborrheic dermatitis: practical management. *Pediatrician* 18(1991):211–7.

21. Ionescu, G., Kiehl, R., Wichmann-Kunz, F., et al. Immunobiological significance of fungal and bacterial infections in atopic eczema. *Journal of Advancment in Medicine* 3(1990):47–58.

22. Sheehan, M.P., Atherton, D.J. A controlled trial of traditional Chinese medicinal plants in widespread non-exudative atopic eczema. *British Journal of Dermatology* 126(1992):179–84.

23. Atherton, D.J., Sheehan, M.P., Rustin, M.H.A., et al. Treatment of atopic eczema with traditional Chinese medicinal plants. *Pediatric Dermatology* 9(1992):373–5.

24. Davies, E., Pollock, I., Steel, H. Chinese herbs for eczema. *Lancet* 335(1990):177.

25. Carlsson, C. Herbs and hepatitis [letter]. *Lancet* 336(1990):1068.

26. Colin-Jones, E., Somers, G.F. A non-steriodal anti-inflammatory agent in dermatology. *Medical Press* 238(1957):206–11.

27. Adamson, A.C., Tillman, W.G. Hydrocortisone [letter]. *British Medical Journal* 2(1955):1501.

28. Annan, W.G. Hydrocortisone and gly-

cyrrhetinic acid. *British Medical Journal* (Vol. 1, 1957):1242.

29. McCallum, D.I. Glycyrrhetinic acid. *British Medical Journal* 2(1956):1239.

30. Knight, T.E., Hausen, B.M. Melaleuca oil (tea tree oil) dermatitis. *Journal of the American Academy of Dermatology* 30(1994):423–7.

31. Galland, L. Increased requirements for essential fatty acids in atopic individuals: a review with clinical descriptions. *Journal of the American College of Nutrition* 5(1986):213–28.

32. Bordoni, A., Biagi, P.L., Masi, M., et al. Evening primrose oil (Efamol) in the treatment of children with atopic eczema. *Drugs Under Experimental and Clinical Research* 14(1987):291–7.

33. Morse, P.F., Horrobin, D.F., Manku, M.S., et al. Meta-analysis of placebo-controlled studies of the efficacy of Epogram in the treatment of atopic eczema: relationship between plasma essential fatty acid changes and clinical response. *British Journal of Dermatology* 121(1989):75–90.

34. Berth-Jones, J., Graham-Brown, R.A.C. Placebo-controlled trial of essential fatty acid supplementation in atopic dermatitis. *Lancet* 41(1993):1557–60.

35. Horrobin, D.F., Morse, P.F. Evening primrose oil and atopic eczema. *Lancet* 345(1995):260–1.

36. Biagi, P.L., Bordoni, A., Hrelia, S., et al. The effect of gamma-linoleic acid on clinical status, red cell fatty composition and membrane microviscosity in infants with atopic dermatitis. *Drugs Under Experimental and Clinical Research* 20(1994):77–84.

37. Biagi, P.L., Bordoni, A., Masi, M., et al. A long-term study on the use of evening primrose oil (Efamol) in atopic children. *Drugs Under Experimental and Clinical Research* 14(1988):285–90.

38. Soyland, E., Funk, J., Rajka, G., et al. Dietary supplementation with very long-chain n–3 fatty acids in patients with atopic dermatitis: a double-blind, multicentre study. *British Journal of Dermatology* 130(1994):757–64.

39. Krowchuck, D.P. Ascorbic acid for treatment of atopic dermatitis [Pediatric Dermatology Update]. *Pediatrics* 86(1990):125–9.

40. Fairris, G.M., Perkins, P.J., Lloyd, B., et al.

The effect on atopic dermatitis of supplementation with selenium and vitamin E. *Acta Dermato-Venerologica (Stockholm)* 69(1989):359–62.

41. Gunther, S.H. Retinoic acid versus placebo in linear verrucose naevi, scaly, lichenified eczema, and the verrucae plantaris. *British Journal of Dermatology* 89(1973):317.

42. Ewing, G.M., Gibbs, A.C.C., Ashcroft, C., et al. Failure of oral zinc supplementation in atopic eczema. *European Journal of Clinical Nutrition* 45(1991):507–10.

43. Neild, V.S., Marsden, R.A., Bailes, J.A., et al. Egg and milk exclusion diets in atopic eczema, *British Journal of Dermatology* 114(1986):117–23.

44. Sloper, K.S., Wadsworth, J., Brostoff, J. Children with atopic eczema. II: Immunological findings associated with dietary manipulations. *Quarterly Journal of Medicine, New Series,* 80(1991):695–705.

45. Devlin, J., David, T.J., Stanton, R.H.J. Elemental diet for refractory atopic eczema. *Archives of Disease in Childhood* 66(1991):93–9.

46. David, T.J., Waddington, E., Stanton, R.H.J. Nutritional hazards of elimination diets in children with atopic eczema. *Archives of Disease in Childhood* 59(1984):323–5.

47. Devlin, J., Stanton, R.H., David, T.J. Calcium intake and cows' milk free diets. *Archives of Disease in Childhood* 64(1989):1183–4.

48. Devlin, J., David, T.J., Stanton, R.H.J. Six food diet for childhood atopic dermatitis. *Acta Dermato-Venereologica (Stockholm)* 71(1991):20–4.

49. Hathaway, M.J., Warner, J.O. Compliance problems in the dietary management of eczema. *Archives of Disease in Childhood* 58(1983):463–4.

50. Casimir, G.J.A., Duchateau, J., Gossart, B., et al. Atopic dermatitis: role of food and house dust mite allergens. *Pediatrics* 92(1993):252–6.

51. Hannuksela, M., Kousa, M., Pirila, V. Allergy to ingredients of vehicles. *Contact Dermatitis* 2(1976):105–10.

52. Rothenborg, H.W., Menne, T., Sjolin, K.E. Temperature dependent primary irritant dermatitis from lemon perfume. *Contact Dermatitis* 3(1977):37–48.

53. Bruno, G., Milita, O., Ferrara, M., et al. Prevention of atopic diseases in high risk babies (long-term follow-up). *Allergy Proceedings* 14(1993):181–6.

54. Hajek, P., Jakoubek, B., Radil, T. Gradual increase in cutaneous threshold induced by repeated hypnosis of healthy individuals and patients with atopic eczema. *Perceptual and Motor Skills* 70(1990):549–50.

55. Koldys, K.W., Meyer, R.P. Biofeedback training in the therapy of dyshidrosis. *Cutis* 24(1979):219–21.

56. Bjorna, H., Kaada, B. Successful treatment of itching and atopic eczema by transcutaneous nerve stimulation. *Acupuncture and Electrotherapeutics Research* 12(1987):101–12.

57. Spence, D.S. Homeopathic treatment of eczema: a retrospective survey of 130 cases. *British Homeopathic Journal* 80(1991):74–81.

CHAPTER 19 — Fever

1. Kluger, M.J., Ringler, D.H., Anver, M.R. Fever and survival. *Science* 188(1975):166–8.

2. Robinson, J.S., Schwartz, M.L.M., Magwene, K.S., et al. The impact of fever health education on clinic utilization. *American Journal of Diseases of Children* 143(1989):698–704.

3. Press, S. Association of hyperpyrexia with serious disease in children. *Clinical Pediatrics* 33(1994):19–25.

4. Jaber, L., Cohen, I.J., Mor, A. Fever associated with teething. *Archives of Disease in Childhood* 67(1992):233–4.

5. Nizet, V., Vinci, R.J., Lovejoy, F.H. Fever in children. *Pediatrics in Review* 15(1994):127–35.

6. Cheng, T.L., Partridge, J.C. Effect of bundling and high environmental temperature on neonatal body temperature. *Pediatrics* 92(1993):238–40.

7. O'Dempsey, T.J.D., Laurence, B.E., McArdle, T.F., et al. The effect of temperature reduction on respiratory rate in febrile illnesses. *Archives of Disease in Childhood* 68(1993):492–5.

8. Inamo, Y., Takeuchi, S., Okuni, M. Host responses and neuroendocrinological changes in pyrexia in childhood. *Acta Paediatrica Japonica* 33(1991):628–32.

9. Schmitt, B.D. Fever phobia: misconceptions of parents about fevers. *American Journal of Diseases of Children* 134(1980):176–81.

10. Kramer, M.S., Naimark, L., Leduc, D.G. Parental fever phobia and its correlates. *Pediatrics* 75(1985):1110–3.

11. Eskerud, J.R., Andrew, M., Stromnes, B., et al. Pharmacy personnel and fever: a study on perception, self-care and information to customers. *Pharmacy World and Science* 15(1993):156–60.

12. May, A., Bauchner, H. Fever phobia: the pediatrician's contribution. *Pediatrics* 90(1992):851–4.

13. Ipp, M., Jaffe, D. Physicians' attitudes toward the diagnosis and management of fever in children 3 months to 2 years of age. *Clinical Pediatrics* 32(1993):66–70.

14. Bethune, P., Gordon, K., Dooley, J., et al. Which child will have a febrile seizure? *American Journal of Diseases of Children* 147(1993):35–9.

15. Green, S.M., Rothrock, S.G., Clem, K.J., et al. Can seizures be the sole manifestation of meningitis in febrile children? *Pediatrics* 92(1993):527–34.

16. Freeman, J.M. The best medicine for febrile seizures. *New England Journal of Medicine* 327(1992):1161–3.

17. Schnaiderman, D., Lahat, E., Sheefer, T., et al. Antipyretic effectiveness of acetaminophen in febrile seizures: ongoing prophylaxis versus sporadic usage. *European Journal of Pediatrics* 152(1993):747–9.

18. Baraff, L.J., Bass, J.W., Fleisher, G.R., et al. Practice guideline for the management of infants and children 0 to 36 months of age with fever without source. *Pediatrics* 92(1993):1–12.

19. Committee on Infectious Diseases. *1994 Red Book.* Elk Grove Village, Ill.: American Academy of Pediatrics, 1994.

20. Chamberlain, J.M., Terndrup, T.E. New light on ear thermometer readings. *Contemporary Pediatrics* 11(1994):66–76.

21. Banco, L., Veltri, D. Ability of mothers to subjectively assess the presence of fever in their children. *American Journal of Diseases of Children* 138(1984):976–8.

22. Bergeson, P.S., Stienfeld, H.J. How dependable is palpation as a screening method for fever?

Clinical Pediatrics 13(1974):350–1.

23. Baker, R.C., Tiller, T., Bausher, J.C., et al. Severity of disease correlated with fever reduction in febrile infants. *Pediatrics* 83(1989):1016–9.

24. Baker, M.D., Fosarelli, P.D., Carpenter, R.O. Childhood fever: correlation of diagnosis with temperature response to acetaminophen. *Pediatrics* 80(1987):315–8.

25. Kramer, M.S., Naimark, L.E., Roberts-Brauer, R., et al. Risks and benefits of paracetamol antipyresis in young children with fever of presumed viral origin. *Lancet* 337(1991):591–4.

26. Bergman, G.E., Philippidis, P., Naiman, J.L. Severe gastrointestinal hemorrhage and anemia after therapeutic doses of aspirin in normal children. *Journal of Pediatrics* 88(1976):501–3.

27. Weinberger, M. Analgesic sensitivity in children with asthma. *Pediatrics* 62(Supplement)(1978):910.

28. VanEsch, A., VanSteensel-Moll, H.A., Steyerberg, E.W., et al. Antipyretic efficacy of ibuprofen and acetaminophen in children with febrile seizures. *Archives of Pediatric and Adolescent Medicine* 149(1995):632–7.

29. Kauffman, R.E., Sawyer, L.A., Scheinbaum, M.L. Antipyretic efficacy of ibuprofen vs acetaminophen. *American Journal of Diseases of Children* 146(1992):622–5.

30. Mascolo, N., Sharma, R., Jain, S.C., et al. Ethnopharmacology of *Calotropis procera* flowers. *Journal of Ethnopharmacology* 22(1988):211–21.

31. But, P.P., Tam, Y.K., Lung, L.C. Ethnopharmacology of rhinoceros horn. II. Antipyretic effects of prescriptions containing rhinoceros horn or water buffalo horn. *Journal of Ethnopharmacology* 33(1991):45–50.

32. Lanhers, M.C., Fleurentin, J., Dorfman, P., et al. Analgesic, antipyretic and anti-inflammatory properties of *Euphorbia hirta*. *Planta Medica* 57(1991):225–31.

33. Okpanyi, S.N., Schirpke-von-Paczensky, R., Dickson, D. Anti-inflammatory, analgesic and antipyretic effect of various plant extracts and their combinations in an animal model. *Arzneimittel-Forschung* 39(1989):698–703.

34. Sabir, M., Akhter, M.H., Bhide, N.K. Further studies on pharmacology of berberine. *Indian Journal of Physiology and Pharmacology* 22(1978):9–23.

35. Okuyama, E., Nakamura, T., Yamazaki, M. Convulsants from star anise (*Illicium verum* hook. F). *Chemical and Pharmaceutical Bulletin (Tokyo)* 41(1993):1670–1.

36. Sriamarao, P., Nagpal, S., Rao, B.S., et al. Immediate hypersensitivity to Parthenium hysterophorus. II. Clinical studies on the prevalence of Parthenium rhinitis. *Clinical and Experimental Allergy* 21(1991):55–62.

37. Muntaner, P., Rodriguez, C., Arnau, J.M. Fever associated with chronic retinol therapy. *Lancet* 335(1990):1588–9.

38. Johnston, C.S. Effect of a single oral dose of ascorbic acid on body temperature and trace mineral fluxes in healthy men and women. *Journal of the American College of Nutrition* 9(1990):150–4.

39. Mitra, A., Ravikumar, V.C., Bourn, W.M., et al. Influence of ascorbic acid esters on acetaminophen-induced hepatotoxicity in mice. *Toxicology Letter* 44(1988):39–46.

40. Lockitch, G., Puterman, M., Godolphin, W., et al. Infection and immunity in Down syndrome: a trial of long-term low oral doses of zinc. *Journal of Pediatrics* 114(1989):781–7.

41. Mascolo, N., Jain, R., Jain, S.C., et al. Ethnopharmacologic investigation of ginger (*Zingiber officinale*). *Journal of Ethnopharmacology* 27(1989):129–40.

42. Newman, J. Evaluation of sponging to reduce body temperature in febrile children. *Canadian Medical Association Journal* 132(1985):641–2.

43. Rogers, P.A., Schoen, A.M., Limehouse, J. Acupuncture for immune-mediated disorders. *Problems in Veterinary Medicine* 4(1992):162–93.

44. Martin, M.L., Ortiz de Urbina, A.V., Montero, M.J., et al. Pharmacologic effects of lactones isolated from *Pulsatilla alpina* subsp apiifolia. *Journal of Ethnopharmacology* 24(1988):185–91.

CHAPTER 20—Headache

1. Abu-Arefeh, I., Russell, G. Prevalence of headache and migraine in schoolchildren. *British Medical Journal* 309(1994):765–9.

2. Kaiser, R.S. Depression in adolescent headache patients. *Headache* 32(1992):340–4.

3. Cooper, P.J., Bawden, H.N., Camfield, P.R., et al. Anxiety and life events in childhood migraine. *Pediatrics*, 79(1987):999–1004

4. Dalton, K. Food intake prior to a migraine attack: study of 2,313 spontaneous attacks. *Headache* 15(1975):188–93.

5. Radnitz, C.L. Food-triggered migraine: a critical review. *Annals of Behavioral Medicine* 12(1990):51–65.

6. Moffett, A.M., Swash, M., Scott, D.F. Effect of chocolate in migraine: a double blind study. *Journal of Neurology, Neurosurgery and Psychiatry* 37(1974):445–8.

7. Forsythe, W.I., Redmond, A. Two controlled trials of tyramine in children with migraine. *Developmental Medicine and Child Neurology* 16(1974):794–9.

8. Salfield, S.A.W., Wardley, B.L., Houlsby, W.T., et al. Controlled study of exclusion of dietary vasoactive amines in migraine. *Archives of Disease in Childhood* 62(1987):458–60.

9. VanDenEeden, S.K., Koepsell, T.D., Longstreth, W.T., et al. Aspartame ingestion and headaches: a randomized crossover trial. *Neurology* 44(1994):1787–93.

10. Koehler, S.M., Glaros, A. The effect of aspartame on migraine headache. *Headache* 28(1988):10–4.

11. Lipton, R.B., Newman, L.C., Cohen, J.S., et al. Aspartame as a dietary trigger of headache. *Headache* 29(1989):90–2.

12. Schiffman, S.S., Buckley, C.E., Sampson, H.A., et al. Aspartame and susceptibility to headache. *New England Journal of Medicine* 317(1987):1181–5.

13. Garriga, M.M., Berkebile, C., Metcalfe, D.D. A combined single-blind, double-blind, placebo-controlled study to determine the reproducibility of hypersensitivity reactions to aspartame. *Journal of Allergy and Clinical Immunology* 87(1991):821–7.

14. Henderson, W.R. Hot dog headache: individual susceptibility to nitrite. *Lancet* 2(1972):1162–3.

15. Scopp, A.L. MSG and hydrolyzed vegetable protein induced headache: review and case studies. *Headache* 31(1991):107–10.

16. Saper, J.R. Daily chronic headache. *Neurologic Clinics* 8(1990):891–901.

17. Smith, R. Caffeine withdrawal headache. *Journal of Clinical Pharmacy and Therapeutics* 12(1987):53–7.

18. Silverman, K., Evans, S.M., Strain, E.C., et al. Withdrawal syndrome after the double-blind cessation of caffeine consumption. *New England Journal of Medicine* 327(1992):1109–14.

19. Couturier, E.G., Hering, R., Steiner, T.J. Weekend attacks in migraine patients: caused by caffeine withdrawal? *Cephalalgia* 12(1992):99–100.

20. Griffiths, R.R., Evans, S.M., Heishman, S.J., et al. Low dose caffeine physical dependence in humans. *Journal of Pharmacology and Experimental Therapeutics* 255(1990):1123–32.

21. Weber, J.G., Ereth, M.H., Danielson, D.R. Perioperative ingestion of caffeine and postoperative headache. *Mayo Clinic Proceedings* 68(1993):842–5.

22. Solomon, G.D. Circadian rhythm and migraine. *Cleveland Clinic Journal of Medicine* 59(1992):326–9.

23. Bird, N., MacGregor, E.A., Wilkinson, M.I. Ice cream headache: site, duration and relationship to migraine. *Headache* 32(1992):35–8.

24. Becker, L.A., Green, L.A., Beaufait, D., et al. Use of CT scans for the investigation of headache: a report from ASPN, Part 1. *Journal of Family Practice* 37(1993):129–34.

25. Morrill, B., Blanchard, E.B., Barron, K.D., et al. Neurological evaluation of chronic headache patients: is laboratory testing always necessary? *Biofeedback and Self Regulation* 15(1990):27–35.

26. Hakkrainen, H., Quiding, H., Stockman, O. Mild analgesics as an alternative to ergotamine in migraine: a comparative trial with acetylsalicylic acid, ergotamine tartrate, and dextropropoxyphene compound. *Journal of Clinical Pharmacology* 20(1989):590–5.

27. Kloster, R., Nestvold, K., Vilming, S.T. A double-blind study of ibuprofen versus placebo in the treatment of acute migraine attacks. *Cephalalgia* 12(1992):169–71.

28. Johnson, E.S., Ratcliffe, D.M., Wilkinson, M. Naproxen sodium in the treatment of migraine. *Cephalalgia* 5(1985):5–10.

29. Pradalier, A., Rancurel, G., Dordain, G., et al. Acute migraine attack therapy: comparison of naproxen sodium and an ergotamine tartrate compound. *Cephalalgia* 5(1985):107–13.

30. Holroyd, K.A., Penzien, D.B. Pharmacological versus non-pharmacological prophylaxis of recurrent migraine headache: a meta-analytic review of clinical trials. *Pain* 42(1990):1–13.

31. Ludvigsson, J. Propranolol used in prophylaxis of migraine in children. *Acta Neurologica Scandinavica* 50(1974):109–15.

32. Forsythe, W.I., Gillies, D., Sills, M.A. Propranolol (Inderal) in the treatment of childhood migraine. *Developmental Medicine and Child Neurology* 26(1984):737–41.

33. Sudilovsky, A., Elkind, A.H., Ryan, R.E., et al. Comparative efficacy of nadolol and propranolol in the management of migraine. *Headache* 27(1987):421–6.

34. Couch, J.R., Hassanein, R.S. Amitryptiline in migraine prophylaxis. *Archives of Neurology* 36(1979):695–9.

35. Drummond, P.D. Effectiveness of methysergide in relation to clinical features of migraine. *Headache* 25(1985):145–6.

36. Bille, B., Ludviggson, J., Sanner, G. Prophylaxis of migraine in children. *Headache* 17(1977):61–3.

37. Rompel, H., Bauermeister, P.W. Etiology of migraines and prevention with carbamazepine (Tegretol): results of a double-blind cross-over study. *South African Medical Journal* 44(1970):75–80.

38. Callaham, M., Raskin, N. A controlled study of dihydroergotamine in the treatment of acute migraine headache. *Headache* 26(1986):168–71.

39. Schmidt, R., Fanchamps, A. Effect of caffeine on intestinal absorption of ergotamine in man. *European Journal of Pharmacology* 7(1974):213–6.

40. Cady, R.K., Wendt, J.K., Kirchner, J.R., et al. Treatment of acute migraine with subcutaneous sumatriptan. *Journal of the American Medical Association* 265(1991):2831–5.

41. Plosker, G.L., McTavish, D. Sumatriptan: a reappraisal of its pharmacology and therapeutic efficacy in the acute treatment of migraine and cluster headache. *Drugs* 47(1994):622–51.

42. Mathew, N.T., Dexter, J., Couch, J., et al. Dose ranging efficacy and safety of subcutaneous sumatriptan in the acute treatment of migraine. *Archives of Neurology* 49(1992):1271–6.

43. Bell, R., Montoya, D., Shuaib, A., et al. A comparative trial of three agents in the treatment of acute migraine headache. *Annals of Emergency Medicine* 19(1990):1079–82.

44. Jones, J., Sklar, D., Dougherty, J., et al. Randomized double-blind trial of intravenous prochlorperazine for the treatment of acute headache. *Journal of the American Medical Association* 261(1989):1174–6.

45. Drazner, D.L., Lacher, M.E., Kulick, R.M. Use of prochlorperazine for treatment of acute migraine headaches in children and adolescents. *Archives of Pediatric and Adolescent Medicine* 148(1994):P67.

46. Makheja, A.N., Bailey, J.M. The active principle in feverfew. *Lancet* 2(1981):1054.

47. Heptinstall, S., Williamson, L., White, A., et al. Extracts of feverfew inhibit granule secretion in blood platelets and polymorphonuclear leucocytes. *Lancet* 1(1985):1071–4.

48. Johnson, E.S., Kadam, N.P., Hylands, D.M., et al. Efficacy of feverfew as prophylactic treatment of migraine. *British Medical Journal* 291(1985):569–73.

49. Barsby, R.W., Salan, U., Knight, D.W., et al. Feverfew and vascular smooth muscle: extracts from fresh and dried plants show opposing pharmacological profiles, dependent upon sesquiterpene lactone content. *Planta Medica* 59(1993):20–5.

50. Snodgrass, S.R. Vitamin neurotoxicity. *Molecular Neurobiology* 6(1992):41–73.

51. Samman, S., Roberts, D.C. The effect of zinc supplements on plasma zinc and copper levels and the reported symptoms in healthy volunteers. *Medical Journal of Australia* 146(1987):246–9.

52. Friedman, A.P., Brenner, C. The use of sodium nicotinate in the treatment of headache. *New York Journal of Medicine* 48(1948):78.

53. Gallai, V., Sarchielli, P., Coata, G., et al. Serum and salivary magnesium levels in migraine: results in a group of juvenile patients. *Headache* 32(1992):132–5.

54. Facchinetti, F., Sances, G., Borella, P., et al. Magnesium prophylaxis of menstrual migraine: effects on intracellular magnesium. *Headache* 31(1991):298–301.

55. Marks, D.R., Rapoport, A., Pa lla, D., et al. A double-blind, placebo-controlled trial of intranasal capsaicin for cluster headache. *Cephalalgia* 13(1993):114–6.

56. Mustafa, T., Srivastava, K.C. Ginger (*Zingiber officinale*) in migraine headache. *Journal of Ethnopharmacology* 29(1990):267–73.

57. Egger, J., Wilson, J., Carter, C.M., et al. Is migraine food allergy? A double-blind controlled trial of oligoantigenic diet treatment. *Lancet* 2(1983):865–9.

58. Carter, C.M., Egger, J., Soothill, J.F. A dietary management of severe childhood migraine. *Human Nutrition: Applied Nutrition* 39A(1985):294–303.

59. Mansfield, L.E., Vaughan, T.R., Waller, S.F., et al. Food allergy and adult migraine: double-blind and mediator confirmation of an allergic etiology. *Annals of Allergy* 55(1985):126–9.

60. Grant, E.C. Food allergies and migraine. *Lancet* 1(1979):966–8.

61. Monro, J., Brostoff, J., Carini, C., et al. Food allergy in migraine. *Lancet* 2(1980):1–4.

62. Atkins, F.M., Ball, B.D., Bock, S.A. The relationship between the ingestion of specific foods and the development of migraine headaches in children. *Journal of Allergy and Clinical Immunology* 81(1988):185.

63. Guarnieri, P., Radnitz, C.L., Blanchard, E.B. Assessment of dietary risk factors in chronic headache. *Biofeedback and Self Regulation* 15(1990):15–25.

64. Lockett, D.M., Campbell, J.F. The effects of aerobic exercise on migraine. *Headache* 32(1992):50–4.

65. Diamond, S., Freitag, F.G. Cold as an adjunctive therapy for headache. *Postgraduate Medicine* 79(1986):305–9.

66. Diamond, S., Montrose, D. The value of biofeedback in the treatment of chronic headache: a four-year retrospective study. *Headache* 24(1984):5–18.

67. Holroyd, K.A., Nash, J.M., Pingel, J.D., et al. A comparison of pharmacological (amitryptiline HCl) and nonpharmacological (cognitive-behavioral) therapies for chronic tension headaches. *Journal of Consulting and Clinical Psychology* 59(1991):387–93.

68. Fentress, D.W., Masek, D.J., Mehegan, J.E., et al. Biofeedback and relaxation-response training in the treatment of pediatric migraine. *Developmental Medicine and Child Neurology* 28(1986):139–46.

69. Engel, J.M. Relaxation training: a self-help approach for children with headaches. *American Journal of Occupational Therapy* 46(1992):591–6.

70. Wallbaum, A.B., Rzewnicki, R., Steele, H., et al. Progressive muscle relaxation and restricted environmental stimulation therapy for chronic tension headache: a pilot study. *International Journal of Psychosomatic Medicine* 38(1991):33–9.

71. Richter, I.L., McGrath, P.J., Humphreys, P.J., et al. Cognitive and relaxation treatment of paediatric migraine. *Pain* 25(1986):195–203.

72. Engel, J.M., Rapoff, M.A., Pressman, A.R. Long-term follow-up of relaxation training for pediatric headache disorders. *Headache* 32(1992):152–6.

73. Primavera, J.P., Kaiser, R.S. Non-pharmacological treatment of headache: is less more? *Headache* 32(1992):393–5.

74. Olness, K., MacDonald, J.T., Uden, D.L. Comparison of self-hypnosis and propranolol in the treatment of juvenile classic migraine. *Pediatrics* 79(1987):593–7.

75. Spinhoven, P., Linssen, A.C., VanDyck, R., et al. Autogenic training and self-hypnosis in the control of tension headache. *General Hospital Psychiatry* 14(1992):408–15.

76. Labbe, E.E. Treatment of childhood migraine with autogenic training and skin temperature biofeedback: a component analysis. *Headache* 35(1995):10–3.

77. Womack, W.M., Smith, M.S., Chen, A.C.N. Behavioral management of childhood headache: a pilot study and case history report. *Pain* 32(1988):279–83.

78. McGrady, A., Wauquier, A., McNeil, A., et al. Effect of biofeedback-assisted relaxation on migraine headache and changes in cerebral blood flow velocity in the middle cerebral artery. *Headache* 34(1994):424–8.

79. Budzynski, T.H., Stoyva, J.M., Adler, C.S., et al. EMG biofeedback and tension headache: a controlled outcome study. *Psychosomatic Medicine* 35(1973):484–96.

80. Cox, D.J., Freundlich, A., Meyer, R.G. Differential effectiveness of electromyograph feedback, verbal relaxation instructions and medication placebo with tension headaches. *Journal of Consulting and Clinical Psychology* 43(1975):892–8.

81. Grazzi, L., Leone, M., Frediani, F., et al. A therapeutic alternative for tension headache in children: treatment and 1-year follow-up results. *Biofeedback and Self Regulation* 15(1990):1–6.

82. Lisspers, J., Ost, L.G. Long-term follow-up of migraine treatment: do the effects remain up to six years? *Behaviour Research and Therapy* 28(1990):313–22.

83. Nuechterlein, K.H., Holroyd, J.C. Biofeedback in the treatment of tension headache. *Archives of General Psychiatry* 37(1980):866–73.

84. Gauthier, J., Cot'e, G., French, D. The role of home practice in the thermal biofeedback treatment of migraine headache. *Journal of Consulting and Clinical Psychology* 62(1994):180–4.

85. Allen, K.D., McKeen, L.R. Home-based multi-component treatment of pediatric migraine. *Headache* 31(1991):467–72.

86. Blanchard, E.B., Appelbaum, K.A., Nicholson, N.L., et al. A controlled evaluation of the addition of cognitive therapy to a home-based biofeedback and relaxation treatment of vascular headache. *Headache* 30(1990):371–6.

87. Osterhaus, S.O., Passchier, J., vanderHelm-Hylkema, H., et al. Effects of behavioral psychophysiological treatment on schoolchildren with migraine in a nonclinical setting: predictors and process variables. *Journal of Pediatric Psychology* 18(1993):697–715.

88. Cott, A., Parkinson, W., Fabich, M., et al. Long-term efficacy of combined relaxation: biofeedback treatments for chronic headache. *Pain* 51(1992):49–56.

89. Gobel, H., Schmidt, G., Soyka, D. Effect of peppermint and eucalyptus oil preparations on neurophysiological and experimental algesimetric headache parameters. *Cephalalgia* 14(1994):228–34.

90. Levoska, S., Keinanen-Kiukaanniemi, S. Active or passive physiotherapy for occupational cervicobrachial disorders? A comparison of two treatment methods with a one-year follow-up. *Archives of Physical Medicine and Rehabilitation* 74(1993):425–30.

91. Jensen, O.K., Nielsen, F.F., Vosmar, L. An open study comparing manual therapy with the use of cold packs in the treatment of post-traumatic headache. *Cephalalgia* 10(1990):241–50.

92. Batra, Y.K. Acupuncture in the treatment of migraine. *American Journal of Acupuncture* 14(1986):135–7.

93. Laitinen, J. Acupuncture for migraine prophylaxis: a prospective clinical study with six months' follow-up. *American Journal of Chinese Medicine* 3(1975):271–4.

94. Lenhard, L., Waite, P.M. Acupuncture in the prophylactic treatment of migraine headaches: pilot study. *New Zealand Medical Journal* 96(1983):663–6.

95. Boivie, J., Brattberg, G. Are there long-lasting effects on migraine headache after one series of acupuncture treatments? *American Journal of Chinese Medicine* 15(1987):69–75.

96. Tavola, T., Gala, C., Conte, G., et al. Traditional Chinese acupuncture in tension-type headache: a controlled study. *Pain* 48(1992):325–9.

97. Dowson, D.I., Lewith, G.T., Machin, D. The effects of acupuncture versus placebo in the treatment of headache. *Pain* 21(1985):35–42.

98. Vincent, C.A. A controlled trial of the treatment of migraine by acupuncture. *Clinical Journal of Pain* 5(1989):305–12.

99. Hesse, J., Mogelvang, B., Simonsen, H. Acupuncture versus metoprolol in migraine prophylaxis: a randomized trial of trigger point inactivation. *Journal of Internal Medicine* 235(1994):451–6.

100. Vincent, C.A. The treatment of tension headache by acupuncture: a controlled single case design with a time series analysis. *Journal of Psychosomatic Research* 34(1990):553–61.

101. Carlsson, J., Fahlcrantz, A., Augustinsson, L.-E. Muscle tenderness in tension headache treated with acupuncture or physiotherapy. *Cephalalgia* 10(1990):131–41.

102. Hansen, P.E., Hansen, J.H. Acupuncture treatment of chronic tension headache: a controlled, cross-over trial. *Cephalalgia* 5(1985):137–42.

103. Keller, E., Bzdek, V.M. Effects of Therapeutic Touch on tension headache pain. *Nursing Research* 35(1986):101–6.

CHAPTER 21 — Hyperactivity

1. Safer, D.J., Krager, J.M. The increased rate of stimulant treatment for hyperactive/inattentive students in secondary schools. *Pediatrics* 94(1994):462–4.

2. Safer, D.J., Krager, J.M. A survey of medication treatment for hyperactive/inattentive students. *Journal of the American Medical Association* 260(1988):2256–8.

3. Carey, W.B. A suggested solution to the confusion in attention deficit diagnoses. *Clinical Pediatrics* 27(1988):348–9.

4. Weiss, R.E., Stein, M.A., Trommer, B., et al. Attention deficit hyperactivity disorder and thyroid function. *Journal of Pediatrics* 123(1993):539–45.

5. Sheldon, S.H. Disordered sleep, daytime vigilance and attention deficit hyperactivity disorder. *Journal of Pediatrics* 118(1991):489–90.

6. Faust, D., Brown, J. Moderately elevated blood lead levels: effects on neuropsychologic functioning in children. *Pediatrics* 80(1987):623–9.

7. David, O., Clark, J., Voeller, K. Lead and hyperactivity. *Lancet* 2(1972):900–3.

8. Thomson, G.O., Raab, G.M., Hepburn, W.S., et al. Blood-lead levels and children's behavior: results from the Edinburgh Lead Study. *Journal of Child Psychology and Psychiatry* 30(1989):515–28.

9. David, O.J., Hoffman, S.P., Sverd, J., et al. Lead and hyperactivity: behavioral response to chelation: a pilot study. *American Journal of Psychiatry* 133(1976):1155–8.

10. Rush, D., Callahan, K.R. Exposure to passive cigarette smoking and child development. *Annals of the New York Academy of Sciences* 562(1989):74–100.

11. Fergusson, D.M., Horwood, L.J., Lynskey, M.T. Maternal smoking before and after pregnancy: effects on behavioral outcomes in middle childhood. *Pediatrics* 92(1993):815–22.

12. Fried, P.A., O'Connell, C.M., Watkinson, B. 60- and 72-month follow-up of children prenatally exposed to marijuana, cigarettes and alcohol: cognitive and language assessment. *Journal of Developmental and Behavioral Pediatrics* 13(1992):383–91.

13. Weitzman, M., Gortmacher, S., Sobol, A. Maternal smoking and behavior problems of children. *Pediatrics* 90(1992):342–9.

14. Byrd, R.S., Roghmann, K.J., Weitzman, M. Predictors of early school failure among children in the United States. *American Journal of Diseases of Children* 147(1993):459.

15. Streissguth, A.P., Barr, H.M., Sampson, P.D., et al. Attention, distraction and reaction time at age 7 years and prenatal alcohol exposure. *Neurobehavioral Toxicology and Teratology* 8(1986):717–25.

16. Streissguth, A.P., Clarren, S.K., Jones, K.H. Natural history of the fetal alcohol syndrome: a 10-year follow-up of eleven patients. *Lancet* 2(1985):85–91.

17. Azuma, S.D., Chasnoff, I.J. Outcome of children prenatally exposed to cocaine and other drugs: a path analysis of three-year data. *Pediatrics* 92(1993):396–402.

18. Rydelius, P.-A. Children of alcoholic fathers: their social adjustment and health status over twenty years. *Acta Paediatrica Scandinavica. Supplement (Stockholm)* 286(1981):81–5.

19. Blondis, T.A., Accardo, P.J., Snow, J.H. Measures of attention deficit. Part I. Questionnaires. *Clinical Pediatrics* 28(1989):222–8.

20. Wolraich, M.L., Lindgren, S.D., Stumbo, P.J., et al. Effects of diets high in sucrose or aspartame on the behavior and cognitive performance of children. *New England Journal of Medicine* 330(1994):301–7.

21. Mahan, L.K., Chase, M., Furukawa, C.T., et al. Sugar 'allergy' and children's behavior. *Annals of Allergy* 61(1988):453–8.

22. Wender, E.H., Solanto, M.V. Effects of sugar on aggressive and inattentive behavior in children with attention deficit disorder with hyperactivity and normal children. *Pediatrics* 88(1991):960–6.

23. Gans, D.A., Harper, A.E., Bachorowski, J.A., et

al. Sucrose and delinquency: oral sucrose tolerance test and nutritional assessment. *Pediatrics* 86(1990):254–62.

24. Bachorowski, J.A., Newman, J.P., Nichols, S.L., et al. Sucrose and delinquency: behavioral assessment. *Pediatrics* 86(1990):244–53.

25. Behar, D., Rapoport, J.L., Adams, A.J., et al. Sugar challenge testing with children considered behaviorally "sugar reactive." *Nutrition and Behavior* 1(1984):277–88.

26. Blass, E.M., Hoffmeyer, L.B. Sucrose as an analgesic for newborn infants. *Pediatrics* 87(1991):215–8.

27. Saravis, S., Schachar, R., Zlotkin, S., et al. Aspartame: effects on learning, behavior, and mood. *Pediatrics* 86(1990):75–83.

28. Shaywitz, B.A., Sullivan, C.M., Anderson, G.M., et al. Aspartame, behavior, and cognitive function in children with attention deficit disorder. *Pediatrics* 93(1994):70–5.

29. Arbeit, M.L., Nicklas, T.A., Frank, G.C., et al. Caffeine intakes of children from a biracial population: the Bogalusa Heart Study. *Journal of the American Dietetic Association* 88(1988):466–71.

30. Bernstein, G.A., Carroll, M.E., Crosby, R.D., et al. Caffeine effects on learning, performance and anxiety in normal school-age children. *Journal of the American Academy of Child and Adolescent Psychiatry* 33(1994):407–15.

31. Feingold, B.F. Hyperkinesis and learning disabilities linked to artificial food flavors and colors. *American Journal of Nursing* 75(1975):797–803.

32. Harley, J., Ray, R., Tomasi, L., et al. Hyperkinesis and food additives: testing the Feingold hypothesis. *Pediatrics* 61(1978):818–28.

33. Pollock, I., Warner, J.O. Effect of artificial food colours on childhood behavior. *Archives of Disease in Childhood* 65(1990):74–7.

34. Conners, C., Goyette, C., Southwick, D., et al. Food additives and hyperkinesis: a double-blind experiment. *Pediatrics* 58(1976):154–66.

35. Mattes, J.A., Gittelman, R. Effects of artificial food colorings in children with hyperactive symptoms. *Archives of General Psychiatry* 38(1981):714–8.

36. Weiss, B., Williams, J.H., Margen, S., et al.

Behavioral responses to artificial food colors. *Science* 207(1980):1487–9.

37. Rowe, K.S. Synthetic food colourings and 'hyperactivity': a double-blind cross-over study. *Australian Paediatric Journal* 24(1988):143–7.

38. David, T.J. Reactions to dietary tartrazine. *Archives of Disease in Childhood* 62(1987):119–22.

39. Salzman, L.K. Allergy testing, psychological assessment and dietary treatment of the hyperactive child syndrome. *Medical Journal of Australia* 2(1976):248–51.

40. Tryphonas, H., Trites, R. Food allergy in children with hyperactivity, learning disabilities and/or minimal brain dysfunction. *Annals of Allergy* 42(1979):22–7.

41. Egger, J., Stolla, A., McEwen, L.M. Controlled trial of hyposensitization in children with food-induced hyperkinetic syndrome. *Lancet* 339(1992):1150–3.

42. Levy, F., Dumbrell, S., Hobbes, G., et al. Hyperkinesis and diet: a double-blind cross-over trial with a tartrazine challenge. *Medical Journal of Australia* 1(1978):61–4.

43. Boris, M., Mandel, F.S. Foods and additives are common causes of the attention deficit hyperactive disorder in children. *Annals of Allergy* 72(1994):462–8.

44. Weinberg, W.A., Brumback, R.A. Primary disorder of vigilance: a novel explanation of inattentiveness, boredom, restlessness and sleepiness. *Journal of Pediatrics* 116(1990):720–5.

45. Tirosh, E., Sadeh, A., Munvez, R., et al. Effects of methylphenidate on sleep in children with attention-deficit hyperactivity disorder. *American Journal of Diseases of Children* 147(1993):1313–5.

46. Barkley, R.A., Fischer, M., Edelbrock, C.S., et al. The adolescent outcome of hyperactive children diagnosed by research criteria. I. An 8-year prospective follow-up. *Journal of the American Academy of Child and Adolescent Psychiatry* 29(1990):546–57.

47. Barkley, R.A., Guevremont, D.C., Anastopoulos, A.D., et al. Driving-related risks and outcomes of attention deficit hyperactivity disorder in adolescents and young adults: a 3- to 5-year follow-up survey.

Pediatrics 92(1993):212–8.

48. Gittelman, R., Mannuzza, S., Shenker, R., et al. Hyperactive boys almost grown up: psychiatric status. *Archives of General Psychiatry* 42(1985):937–47.

49. Safer, D., Krager, J.M. Hyperactivity and inattentiveness: school assessment of stimulant treatment. *Clinical Pediatrics* 28(1989):216–21.

50. Pelham, W.E., Bender, M.E., Caddell, J., et al. Methylphenidate and children with attention deficit disorder: dose effects on classroom academic and social behavior. *Archives of General Psychiatry* 42(1985):948–52.

51. Committee on Children with Disabilities and Committee on Drugs, American Academy of Pediatrics. Medication for children with an attention deficit disorder. *Pediatrics* 80(1987):758–60.

52. Silver, L.B. Controversial approaches to treating learning disabilities and attention deficit disorder. *American Journal of Diseases of Children* 140(1986):1045–52.

53. Ullmann, R.K., Sleator, E.K. Attention deficit disorder children with or without hyperactivity: which behaviors are helped by stimulants? *Clinical Pediatrics* 24(1985):547–51.

54. Brown, R.T., Sexson, S.B. A controlled trial of methylphenidate in black adolescents. *Clinical Pediatrics* 27(1988):74–81.

55. McBride, M.C. An individual double-blind cross-over trial for assessing methylphenidate response in children with attention deficit disorder. *Journal of Pediatrics* 113(1988):137–45.

56. Safer, D.J., Allen, R.P. Absence of tolerance to the behavioral effects of methylphenidate in hyperactive and inattentive children. *Journal of Pediatrics* 115(1989):1003–8.

57. Barkley, R.A., McMurray, M.B., Edelbrock, C.S., et al. Side effects of methylphenidate in children with attention deficit hyperactivity disorder: a systemic, placebo-controlled evaluation. *Pediatrics* 86(1990):184–92.

58. Lipkin, P.H., Goldstein, I.J., Adesman, A.R. Tics and dyskinesias associated with stimulant treatment in attention-deficit hyperactivity disorder. *Archives of Pediatric and Adolescent Medicine* 148(1994):859–61.

59. Ahmann, P.A., Waltonen, S.J., Olson, K.A., et al. Placebo-controlled evaluation of Ritalin side effects. *Pediatrics* 91(1993):1101–6.

60. Feldman, H., Crumrine, P., Handen, B.L. Methylphenidate in children with seizures and attention-deficit disorder. *American Journal of Diseases of Children* 143(1989):1081–6.

61. Pelham, W.E., Sturges, J., Hoza, J., et al. Sustained release and standard methylphenidate effects on cognitive and social behavior in children with attention deficit disorder. *Pediatrics* 80(1987):491–501.

62. Conners, C.K. Effect of dextroamphetamine on children: studies on subjects with learning disabilities and school behavior problems. *Archives of General Psychiatry* 17(1967):478–85.

63. Stephens, R., Pelham, W.E., Skinner, R. The state-dependent and main effects of pemoline and methylphenidate on paired-associates learning and spelling in hyperactive children. *Journal of Consulting and Clinical Psychology* 52(1984):104–113.

64. Conners, C.K., Taylor, E. Pemoline, methylphenidate and placebo in children with minimal brain dysfunction. *Archives of General Psychiatry* 37(1980):922–30.

65. Singer, H.S., Brown, J., Quaskey, S., et al. The treatment of attention-deficit hyperactivity disorder in Tourette's syndrome: a double-blind placebo-controlled study with clonidine and desipramine. *Pediatrics* 95(1995):74–81.

66. Schnackenberg, R.C. Caffeine as a substitute for schedule II stimulants in hyperkinetic children. *American Journal of Psychiatry* 130(1973):796–8.

67. Conners, C.K. A placebo-crossover study of caffeine treatment of hyperkinetic children. *International Journal of Mental Health* 4(1975):132–43.

68. Firestone, P., Davey, J., Goodman, J.T., et al. The effects of caffeine and methylphenidate on hyperactive children. *Journal of the American Academy of Child Psychiatry* 17(1978):445–56.

69. Huestis, R.D., Arnold, L.E., Smeltzer, D.J. Caffeine versus methylphenidate and d-amphetamine in minimal brain dysfunction: a double-blind comparison. *American Journal of Psychiatry* 132(1975):868–70.

70. Garfinkel, B.D., Webster, C.D., Sloman, L.

Responses to methylphenidate and varied doses of caffeine in children with attention deficit disorder. *Canadian Journal of Psychiatry* 26(1981):395–401.

71. Arnold, L.E., Votolato, N.A., Kleykamp, D., et al. Does hair zinc predict amphetamine improvement of ADD/hyperactivity? *International Journal of Neuroscience* 50(1990):103–7.

72. McGee, R., Williams, S., Anderson, J., et al. Hyperactivity and serum and hair zinc levels in 11-year-old children from the general population. *Biological Pyschiatry* 28(1990):165–8.

73. Haslam, R.H.A. Is there a role for megavitamin therapy in the treatment of attention deficit hyperactivity disorder? In Chase, T.N., editor. *Advances in neurology*. New York: Raven Press, 1992, pp. 303–10.

74. Kinsbourne, M. Sugar and the hyperactive child. *New England Journal of Medicine* 330(1994):335–6.

75. Swanson, J.M., Kinsbourne, M. Food dyes impair performance of hyperactive children on a laboratory learning test. *Science* 207(1980):1485–7.

76. Rowe, K.S., Rowe, K.J. Synthetic food coloring and behavior: a dose response effect in a double-blind, placebo-controlled, repeated measures study. *Journal of Pediatrics* 125(1994):691–8.

77. Cook, P.S., Woodhill, J.M. The Feingold dietary treatment of the hyperkinetic syndrome. *Medical Journal of Australia* 2(1976):85–90.

78. Mattes, J. The Feingold diet: a current reappraisal. *Journal of Learning Disabilities* 16(1983):319–23.

79. Thorley, G. Pilot study to assess behavioral and cognitive effects of artificial food colours on a group of retarded children. *Developmental Medicine and Child Neurology* 26(1984):56–61.

80. Carter, C.M., Urbanowicz, M., Hemsley, R., et al. Effects of a few food diet in attention deficit disorder. *Archives of Disease in Childhood* 69(1993):564–8.

81. Kaplan, B.J., McNicol, J., Conte, R.A., et al. Dietary replacement in preschool-aged hyperactive boys. *Pediatrics* 83(1989):7–17.

82. Loffredo, D.A., Omizo, M., Hammett, V.L. Group relaxation training and parental involvement with hyperactive boys. *Journal of Learning Disabilities* 17(1984):210–3.

83. Charney, E., Kessler, B., Farfel, M., et al. A controlled trial of the effect of dust-control measures on blood lead levels. *New England Journal of Medicine* 309(1983):1089–93.

84. Ruff, H.A., Bijur, P.E., Markowitz, M., et al. Declining blood lead levels and cognitive changes in moderately lead-poisoned children. *Journal of the American Medical Association* 269(1993):1641–6.

85. Klein, P.S. Responses of hyperactive and normal children to variations in tempo of background music. *Israel Journal of Psychiatry and Related Sciences* 18(1981):157–66.

86. Kelly, P.C., Cohen, M.L., Walker, W.O., et al. Self-esteem in children medically managed for attention deficit disorder. *Pediatrics* 83(1989):211–7.

87. Raymer, R., Poppen, R. Behavioral relaxation training with hyperactive children. *Journal of Behavior Therapy and Experimental Psychiatry* 16(1985):309–16.

88. Denkowski, K.M., Denkowski, G.C., Omizo, M.M. The effects of EMG-assisted relaxation training on the academic performance, locus of control and self-esteem of hyperactive boys. *Biofeedback and Self Regulation* 8(1983):363–75.

89. Potashkin, B.D., Beckles, N. Relative efficacy of Ritalin and biofeedback treatments in the management of hyperactivity. *Biofeedback and Self Regulation* 15(1990):305–15.

90. Lee, S.W. Biofeedback as a treatment for childhood hyperactivity: a criticial review of the literature. *Psychological Reports* 68(1991):163–92.

91. Dunn, F.M., Howell, R.J. Relaxation training and its relationship to hyperactivity in boys. *Journal of Clinical Psychology* 38(1982):92–100.

92. Barkley, R.A., Guevremont, D.C., Anastopoulos, A.D., et al. A comparison of three family therapy programs for treating family conflicts in adolescents with attention-deficit hyperactivity disorder. *Journal of Consulting and Clinical Psychology* 60(1992):450–62.

CHAPTER 22 — Jaundice

1. Leibson, C., Brown, M., Thibodeau, S., et al. Neonatal hyperbilirubinemia at high altitude. *American Journal of Diseases of Children* 143(1989):983–7.

2. Watchko, J.F., Oski, F.A. Kernicterus in preterm newborns: past, present and future. *Pediatrics* 90(1992):707–15.

3. Gilja, B.K., Shah, V.P. Hydrops fetalis due to ABO incompatibility. *Clinical Pediatrics* 27(1988):210–2.

4. Kaplan, M., Abramov, A. Neonatal hyperbilirubinemia associated with glucose–6-phosphate dehydrogenase deficiency in Sephardic-Jewish neonates: incidence, severity and effect of phototherapy. *Pediatrics* 90(1992):401–5.

5. Linn, S., Schoenbaum, S.C., Monson, R.R., et al. Epidemiology of neonatal hyperbilirubinemia. *Pediatrics* 75(1985):770–4.

6. Newman, T.B., Easterling, M.J., Goldman, E.S., et al. Laboratory evaluation of jaundice in newborns: corrections. *American Journal of Diseases of Children* 146(1992):1420–1.

7. Broderson, R., Hermann, L.S. Intestinal re-absorption of unconjugated bilirubin. *Lancet* 1(1963):1242.

8. DeCarvalho, M., Robertson, S., Klaus, M. Fecal bilirubin excretion and serum bilirubin concentrations in breast-fed and bottle-fed infants. *Journal of Pediatrics* 107(1985):786–90.

9. Gourley, G.R., Arend, R.A. ß-glucuronidase and hyperbilirubinemia in breast-fed and formula-fed babies. *Lancet* 1(1986):644–6.

10. Maisels, M.J., Gifford, K. Neonatal jaundice in full-term infants: role of breast-feeding and other causes. *American Journal of Diseases of Children* 137(1983):561–2.

11. Schneider, A.P. Breast milk jaundice in the newborn. *Journal of the American Medical Association* 255(1986):3270–4.

12. Osborn, L.M., Reiff, M.I., Bolus, R. Jaundice in the full-term neonate. *Pediatrics* 73(1984):520–5.

13. Maisels, M.J., Gifford, K. Normal serum bilirubin levels in the newborn and the effect of breast-feeding. *Pediatrics* 78(1986):837–43.

14. Hsia, D.Y., Allen, F.H., Gellis, S.S., et al. Erythroblastosis fetalis: studies of serum bilirubin in relation to kernicterus. *New England Journal of Medicine* 247(1952):668–71.

15. Nakamura, H., Takada, S., Shimabuku, R., et al. Auditory nerve and brainstem responses in newborn infants with hyperbilirubinemia. *Pediatrics* 75(1985):703–8.

16. Telzrow, R.W., Snyder, D.M., Tronick, E., et al. The behavior of jaundiced infants undergoing phototherapy. *Developmental Medicine and Child Neurology* 22(1980):317–26.

17. Rubin, R.A., Balow, B., Fisch, R.O. Neonatal serum bilirubin levels related to cognitive development at ages 4 through 7 years. *Journal of Pediatrics* 94(1979):601–4.

18. Newman, T.B., Klebanoff, M.A. Neonatal hyperbilirubinemia and long-term outcome: another look at the Collaborative Perinatal Project. *Pediatrics* 92(1993):651–7.

19. Scheidt, P.C., Graubard, B.I., Nelson, K.B., et al. Intelligence at six years in relation to neonatal bilirubin level: follow-up of the National Institute of Child Health and Human Development clinical trial of phototherapy. *Pediatrics* 87(1991):797–805.

20. Stocker, R., Yamamoto, Y., McDonagh, A.F., et al. Bilirubin is an antioxidant of possible physiologic importance. *Science* 235(1987):1043–5.

21. Newman, T.B., Easterling, J., Goldman, E.S., et al. Laboratory evaluation of jaundice in newborns. *American Journal of Diseases of Children* 144(1990):364–8.

22. Ulstrom, R.A., Eisenklam, E. The enterohepatic shunting of bilirubin in the newborn infant: use of activated charcoal to reduce normal serum bilirubin levels. *Journal of Pediatrics* 65(1964):27–37.

23. Kemper, K.J., Horwitz, R.I., McCarthy, P.J. Decreased neonatal serum bilirubin with plain agar: a meta-analysis. *Pediatrics* 82(1988):631–8.

24. Valaes, T., Petmezaki, S., Henschke, C., et al. Control of jaundice in pre-term newborns by an inhibitor of bilirubin production: studies with tin-mesoporphyrin. *Pediatrics* 93(1994):1–11.

25. Kappas, A., Drummond, G.S., Henschke, C., et al. Direct comparison of Sn-Mesoporphyrin, an inhibitor of bilirubin production, and phototherapy in controlling hyperbilirubinemia in

term and near-term newborns. *Pediatrics* 95(1995):468–74.

26. Yeung, C.Y., Leung, C.S., Chen, Y.Z. An old traditional herbal remedy for neonatal jaundice with a newly identified risk. *Journal of Paediatrics and Child Health* 29(1993):292–4.

27. Chan, T.Y. The prevalence, use and harmful potential of some Chinese herbal medicines in babies and children. *Veterinary and Human Toxicology* 36(1994):238–40.

28. Alderman, S., Kailas, S., Goldfarb, S., et al. Cholestatic hepatitis after ingestion of chaparral leaf: confirmation by endoscopic retrograde cholangiopancreatography and liver biopsy. *Journal of Clinical Gastroenterology* 19(1994):242–7.

29. Woolf, G.M., Petrovic, L.M., Rojter, S.E., et al. Acute hepatitis associated with the Chinese herbal remedy product jin bu huan. *Annals of Internal Medicine* 121(1994):729–35.

30. DeCarvalho, M., Hall, M., Harvey, D. Effects of water supplementation of physiologic jaundice in breast-fed babies. *Archives of Diseases of Children* 56(1981):568–9.

31. DeCarvalho, M., Klaus, M.H., Merkatz, R.B. Frequency of breast-feeding and serum bilirubin concentration. *American Journal of Diseases of Children* 136(1982):737–8.

32. Yamauchi, Y., Yamanouchi, I. Breast-feeding frequency during the first 24 hours after birth in full-term neonates. *Pediatrics* 86(1990):171–5.

33. Elander, G., Lindberg, T. Hospital routines in infants with hyperbilirubinemia influence the duration of breastfeeding. *Acta Paediatrica Scandinavica* 75(1986):708–12.

34. DeAngelis, C., Sargent, J., Chun, M.K. Breast milk jaundice. *Wisconsin Medical Journal* 79(1980):40–2.

35. Provisional Committee for Quality Improvement and Subcommittee on Hyperbilirubinemia. Practice parameter: management of hyperbilirubinemia in the healthy term newborn. *Pediatrics* 94(1994):558–65.

36. Newman, T.B., Maisels, M.J. Evaluation and treatment of jaundice in the term newborn: a kinder, gentler approach. *Pediatrics* 89(1992):809–18.

37. Kemper, K.J., Forsyth, B.W., McCarthy, P.J.

38. Plastino, R., Buchner, D.M., Wagner, E.H. Impact of eligibility criteria on phototherapy program size and cost. *Pediatrics* 85(1990):796–800.

Jaundice, terminating breastfeeding and the vulnerable child. *Pediatrics* 84(1989):773–8.

39. Garg, A.K., Prasad, R.S., Hifzi, I.A. A controlled trial of high-intensity double-surface phototherapy on a fluid bed versus conventional phototherapy in neonatal jaundice. *Pediatrics* 95(1995):914–6.

40. Tan, K.L. Comparison of the efficacy of fiberoptic and conventional phototherapy for neonatal hyperbilirubinemia. *Journal of Pediatrics* 125(1994):607–12.

41. George, P., Lynch, M. Ohmeda bili-blanket vs Wallaby phototherapy system for the reduction of bilirubin levels in the home-care setting. *Clinical Pediatrics* (March 1994):178–80.

42. Wishingrad, L., Cornblath, M., Takakuwa, T., et al. Studies of non-hemolytic hyperbilirubinemia in premature infants. *Pediatrics* 36(1965):162–72.

43. Braud, W. Distant mental influence of rate of hemolysis of human red blood cells. *Research in Parapsychology* 1988(1989):1–6.

44. Braud, W., David, G., Wood, R. Experiments with Matthew Manning. *Journal of Social and Psychical Research* 50(782)(1979):199–223.

45. Krieger, D. The Therapeutic Touch. Englewood Cliffs, N.J.: Prentice-Hall, 1979.

CHAPTER 23 — Ringworm and Other Fungal Infections

1. Pomeranz, A.J., Fairley, J.A. Management errors leading to unnecessary hospitalization for kerion. *Pediatrics* 93(1994):986–8.

2. Auger, P., Marquis, G., Joly, J., et al. Epidemiology of tinea pedis in marathon runners: prevalence of occult athlete's foot. *Mycoses* 36(1993):35–41.

3. Kearse, H.L., Miller, O.F. Tinea pedis in prepubertal children: does it occur? *Journal of the American Academy of Dermatology* 19(1988):619–22.

4. Allen, H.B., Honig, P.J., Leyden, J.J., et al. Selenium sulfide: adjunctive therapy for tinea capitis. *Pediatrics* 69(1982):81–3.

5. Givens, T.G., Murray, M.M., Baker, R.C.

Comparison of 1% and 2.5% selenium sulfide in the treatment in tinea capitis. *Archives of Pediatric and Adolescent Medicine* 149(1995):808–11.

6. Rollman, O., Jameson, S., Lithell, H. Effects of long-term ketoconazole therapy on serum lipid levels. *European Journal of Clinical Pharmacology* 29(1985):241–5.

7. Savin, R., Atton, A.V., Bergstresser, P.R., et al. Efficacy of terbinafine 1% cream in the treatment of moccasin-type tinea pedis: results of placebo-controlled multicenter trials. *Journal of the American Academy of Dermatology* 30(1994):663–7.

8. Savin, R.C. Oral terbinafine versus griseofulvin in the treatment of moccasin-type tinea pedis. *Journal of the American Academy of Dermatology* 23(1990):807–9.

9. Evans, E.G.V., Dodman, B., Williamson, D.M., et al. Comparison of terbinafine and clotrimazole in treating tinea pedis. *British Medical Journal* 307(1993):645–7.

10. Haroon, T.S., Hussain, I., Mahmood, A., et al. An open clinical pilot study of the efficacy and safety of oral terbinafine in dry non-inflammatory tinea capitis. *British Journal of Dermatology* 126(1992):47–50.

11. Naftifine Podiatric Study Group. Naftifine cream 1% versus clotrimazole cream 1% in the treatment of tinea pedis. *Journal of the American Podiatric Medical Association* 80(1990):314–8.

12. Chren, M.-M., Landefeld, C.S. A cost analysis of topical drug regimens for dermatophyte infections. *Journal of the American Medical Association* 272(1994):1922–5.

13. Tong, M.M., Altman, P.M., Barnetson, R.S. Tea tree oil in the treatment of tinea pedis. *Australasian Journal of Dermatology* 33(1992):145–9.

14. Appleton, J.A., Tansey, M.R. Inhibition of growth of zoopathogenic fungi by garlic extract. *Mycologia* 67(1975):409–13.

15. Tansey, M.R., Appleton, J.A. Inhibition of fungal growth by garlic extract. *Mycologia* 67(1975):409–13.

16. Yamada, Y., Azuma, K. Evaluation of the in vitro antifungal activity of allicin. *Antimicrobial Agents and Chemotherapy* 11(1977):743–9.

17. Lozoya, X., Navarro, V., Garcia, M., et al. Solanum chrysotrichum (Schldl.): a plant used in Mexico for the treatment of skin mycosis. *Journal of Ethnopharmacology* 36(1992):127–32.

18. Kishore, N., Mishra, A.K., Chansouria, J.P. Fungitoxicity of essential oils against dermatophytes. *Mycoses* 36(1993):211–5.

19. Gundidza, M. Antifungal activity of essential oil from Artemisia afra Jacq. *Central African Journal of Medicine* 39(1993):140–2.

20. Garg, A.P., Muller, J. Inhibition of growth of dermatophytes by Indian hair oils. *Mycoses* 35(1992):363–9.

CHAPTER 24 — Sleep Problems

1. Lozoff, B. Sleep problems seen in a pediatric practice. *Pediatrics* 75(1985):477–83.

2. Kahn, A., Mozin, M., Casimir, G., et al. Insomnia and cow's milk allergy in infants. *Pediatrics* 76(1985):880–4.

3. Kahn, A., Francois, G., Sottiaux, M., et al. Sleep characteristics in milk-intolerant infants. *Sleep* 11(1988):291–7.

4. Kataria, S., Swanson, M.S., Trevathan, G.E. Persistence of sleep disturbances in preschool children. *Journal of Pediatrics* 110(1987):642–6.

5. Wood, J.M., Bootzin, R.R., Rosenhan, D., et al. Effects of the 1989 San Francisco earthquake on frequency and content of nightmares. *Journal of Abnormal Psychology* 101(1992):219–24.

6. Keener, M.A., Zeanah, C.H., Anders, T.F. Infant temperament, sleep organization, and nighttime parental interventions. *Pediatrics* 81(1988):762–71.

7. Jimmerson, K.R. Maternal, environmental, and temperamental characteristics of toddlers with and toddlers without sleep problems. *Journal of Pediatric Health Care* 5(1991):71–7.

8. Zuckerman, B., Stevenson, J., Bailey, V. Sleep problems in early childhood: continuities, predictive factors and behavioral correlates. *Pediatrics* 80(1987):664–71.

9. Kaplan, B.J., McNicol, J., Conte, R.A., et al. Sleep disturbances in preschool-aged hyperactive and nonhyperactive children. *Pediatrics* 80(1987):839–44.

10. Pinilla, T., Birch, L.L. Help me make it through the night: behavioral entrainment of breast-fed infants' sleep patterns. *Pediatrics* 91(1993):436–44.

11. Wolfson, A., Lacks, P., Futterman, A. Effects of parent training on infant sleeping patterns, parents' stress, and perceived parental competence. *Journal of Consulting and Clinical Psychology* 60(1992):41–8.

12. Adair, R., Bauchner, H., Philipp, B., et al. Night waking during infancy: role of parental presence at bedtime. *Pediatrics* 87(1991):500–4.

13. Hawkins, C., Williams, T.I. Nightmares, life events and behavior problems in preschool children. *Child: Care, Health and Development* 18(1992):117–28.

14. Wood, J.M., Bootzin, R.R. The prevalence of nightmares and their independence from anxiety. *Journal of Abnormal Psychology* 99(1990):64–8.

15. Newell, S.A., Padamadan, H., Drake, M.E., Jr. Neurophysiologic studies in nightmare sufferers. *Clinical Electroencephalography* 23(1992):203–6.

16. Spadafora, A., Hunt, H.T. The multiplicity of dreams: cognitive-affective correlates of lucid, archetypal and nightmare dreaming. *Perceptual and Motor Skills* 71(1990):627–44.

17. DiMario, F.J., Emery, E.S. The natural history of night terrors. *Clinical Pediatrics* 26(1987):505–11.

18. Russo, R.M., Gururaj, V.J., Allen, J.E. The effectiveness of diphenhydramine HCl in pediatric sleep disorders. *Journal of Clinical Pharmacology* 16(1976):284–8.

19. Richman, N. A double-blind drug trial of treatment in young children with waking problems. *Journal of Child Psychology and Psychiatry* 26(1985):591–8.

20. Wohlfart, R., Hansel, R., Schmidt, H. The sedative-hypnotic principle of hops. *Planta Medica* 48(1983):120–3.

21. Leathwood, P., Chauffard, F., Heck, E., et al. Aqueous extract of valerian root (Valeriana officinalis L.) improves sleep quality in man. *Pharmacology, Biochemistry and Behavior* 17(1982):65–71.

22. Leathwood, P., Chauffard, F. Aqueous extract of valerian reduces latency to fall asleep in man. *Planta Medica* 54(1985):144–8.

23. MacGregor, F.B., Abernethy, V.E., Dahabra, S., et al. Hepatoxicity of herbal remedies. *British Medical Journal* 299(1989):1156–7.

24. Houghton, P.J. The biological activity of valerian and related plants. *Journal of Ethnopharmacology* 22(1988):121–42.

25. Yogman, M.W., Zeisel, S.H. Diet and sleep patterns in newborn infants. *New England Journal of Medicine* 309(1983):1147–9.

26. Griffiths, W., Lester, B., Coulter, J., et al. Tryptophan and sleep in young adults. *Psychophysiology* 9(1972):345–56.

27. Wyatt, R., Engelman, K., Kupfer, D., et al. Effects of L-tryptophan (a natural sedative) on human sleep. *Lancet* 2(1970):842–6.

28. Steinberg, L.A., O'Connell, N.C., Hatch, T.F., et al. Tryptophan intake influences infants' sleep latency. *Journal of Nutrition* 122(1992):1781–91.

29. Okawa, M., Mishima, K., Nanami, T., et al. Vitamin B12 treatment for sleep-wake rhythm disorders. *Sleep* 13(1990):15–23.

30. Ohta, T., Iwata, T., Kayukawa, Y., et al. Daily activity and persistent sleep-wake schedule disorder. *Progress in Neuro-Psychopharmacology and Biological Psychiatry* 16(1992):529–37.

31. Butte, N.F., Jensen, C.L., Moon, J.K., et al. Sleep organization and energy expenditure of breast-fed and formula-fed infants. *Pediatric Research* 32(1992):514–9.

32. Elias, M.F., Nicolson, N.A., Bora, C., et al. Sleep/wake patterns of breast-fed infants in the first two years of life. *Pediatrics* 77(1986):322–9.

33. Macknin, M.L., Medendorp, S.V., Maier, M.C. Infant sleep and bedtime cereal. *American Journal of Diseases of Children* 143(1989):1066–8.

34. Keane, V., Charney, E., Straus, J., et al. Do solids help baby sleep through the night? *American Journal of Diseases of Children* 142(1988):404–5.

35. Griffin, S.J., Trinder, J. Physical fitness, exercise and human sleep. *Psychophysiology* 15(1978):447–50.

36. Schachter, F.F., Fuchs, M.L., Bijur, P.E., et al. Co-sleeping and sleep problems in Hispanic-American urban young children. *Pediatrics* 84(1989):522–30.

37. Madanskay, D., Edelbrock, C. Co-sleeping in a community sample of 2- and 3-year-old children. *Pediatrics* 86(1990):197–203.

38. Guntheroth, W.G., Spiers, P.S. Sleeping prone and the risk of sudden infant death syndrome. *Journal of the American Medical Association* 267(1992):2359–62.

39. Willinger, M., Hoffman, H.J., Hartford, R.B. Infant sleeping position and risk for sudden infant death syndrome: report of meeting held January 13 and 14, 1994, National Institutes of Health, Bethesda, MD. *Pediatrics* 93(1994):814–9.

40. American Academy of Pediatrics and Selected Agencies of the Federal Government. Infant sleep position and sudden infant death syndrome (SIDS) in the United States: joint commentary. *Pediatrics* 93(1994):820.

41. Taylor, J.A., Sanderson, M. A re-examination of the risk factors for sudden infant death syndrome (SIDS). *Archives of Pediatric and Adolescent Medicine* 148(1994):P82.

42. Kandall, S.R., Gaines, J., Habel, L., et al. Relationship of maternal substance abuse to subsequent sudden infant death syndrome in offspring. *Journal of Pediatrics* 123(1993):120–6.

43. Fleming, P.J., Gilbert, R., Azaz, Y., et al. Interaction between bedding and sleeping position in the sudden infant death syndrome: a population based case-control study. *British Medical Journal* 301(1990):85–9.

44. Ponsonby, A-L., Dwyer, T., Gibbons, L.E., et al. Factors potentiating the risk of sudden infant death syndrome associated with the prone position. *New England Journal of Medicine* 329(1993):377–82.

45. Anders, T.F., Halpern, L.F., Hua, J. Sleeping through the night: a developmental perspective. *Pediatrics* 90(1992):554–60.

46. Adair, R., Zuckerman, B., Bauchner, H., et al. Reducing night waking in infancy: a primary care intervention. *Pediatrics* 89(1992):585–8.

47. Rickert, V.I., Johnson, M. Reducing nocturnal wakening and crying episodes in infants and young children: a comparison between scheduled awakenings and systematic ignoring. *Pediatrics* 81(1988):203–12.

48. Lask, B. Novel and non-toxic treatment for night terrors. *British Medical Journal* 297(1988):502.

49. Milan, M.A., Mitchell, Z.P., Berger, M.I., et al. Positive routines: a rapid alternative to extinction for elimination of bedtime tantrum behavior. *Child Behavior Therapy* 3(1981):13–25.

50. France, K.G., Hudson, S.M. Behavior management of infant sleep disturbance. *Journal of Applied Behavior Analysis* 23(1990):91–8.

51. Seymour, F.W., Brock, P., During, M., et al. Reducing sleep disruptions in young children: evaluation of therapist-guided and written information approaches: a brief report. *Child Psychology and Psychiatry* 30(1989):913–8.

52. Adams, L.A., Rickert, V.I. Reducing bedtime tantrums: comparison between positive routines and graduated extinction. *Pediatrics* 84(1989):756–61.

53. Becker, P.M. Chronic insomnia: outcome of hypnotherapeutic intervention in six cases. *American Journal of Clinical Hypnosis* 36(1993):98–105.

54. Hurwitz, T.D., Mahowald, M.W., Schenck, C.H., et al. A retrospective outcome study and review of hypnosis as treatment of adults with sleepwalking and sleep terror. *Journal of Nervous and Mental Disease* 179(1991):228–33.

55. Gardner, G.G., Olness, K. *Hypnosis and hypnotherapy with children.* Orlando: Grune & Stratton, 1981, p. 113.

56. Neidhardt, E.J., Krakow, B., Kellner, R., et al. The beneficial effects of one treatment session and recording of nightmares on chronic nightmare sufferers. *Sleep* 15(1992):470–3.

57. Kohen, D.P., Mahowald, M.W., Rosen, G.M. Sleep-terror disorder in children: the role of self-hypnosis in management. *American Journal of Clinical Hypnosis* 34(1992):233–44.

58. Kellner, R., Neidbardt, J., Krakow, B., et al. Changes in chronic nightmares after one session of desensitization or rehearsal instructions. *American Journal of Psychiatry* 149(1992):659–63.

59. Palace, E.M., Johnston, C. Treatment of recurrent nightmares by the dream reorganization approach. *Journal of Behavior Therapy and Experimental Psychiatry* 20(1989):219–26.

60. Woolfolk, R.L., Carr-Kaffashan, L., McNulty, T.F. Meditation training as a treatment for insom-

nia. *Behavior Therapy* 7(1976):359–65.

61. McMenamy, C., Katz, R.C. Brief parent-assisted treatment for children's night time fears. *Journal of Developmental and Behavioral Pediatrics* 10(1989):145–8.

62. King, N., Cranstoun, F., Josephs, A. Emotive imagery and children's night-time fears: a multiple baseline design evaluation. *Journal of Behavior Therapy and Experimental Psychiatry* 20(1989):125–35.

63. Barowsky, E.I., Moskowitz, J., Zweig, J.B. Biofeedback for disorders of initiating and maintaining sleep. *Annals of the New York Academy of Sciences* 602(1990):97–103.

64. Field, T., Morrow, C., Valdeon, C., et al. Massage reduces anxiety in child and adolescent psychiatric patients. *Journal of the American Academy of Child and Adolescent Psychiatry* 31(1992):125–31.

65. Marcus, C.L., Carroll, J.L., Koerner, C.B., et al. Determinants of growth in children with the obstructive sleep apnea syndrome. *Journal of Pediatrics* 125(1994):556–62.

66. Ali, N.J., Pitson, D.J., Stradling, J.R. Snoring, sleep disturbance, and behavior in 4–5 year olds. *Archives of Disease in Childhood* 68(1993):360–6.

67. Krieger, D., Peper, E., Ancoli, S. The physiological indices of Therapeutic Touch. *American Journal of Nursing* 4(1979):660–5.

68. Heidt, P. Effect of Therapeutic Touch on the anxiety level of hospitalized patients. *Nursing Research* 30(1981):32–7.

69. Heidt, T.R. Helping patients to rest: clinical studies in Therapeutic Touch. *Holistic Nurse Practitioner* 5(1991):57–66.

70. Dall, J.V. Promoting sleep with Therapeutic Touch. *Addictions Nursing Network* 5(1993):23–4.

71. Braun, C., Layton, J., Braun, J. Therapeutic Touch improves residents' sleep. *American Health Care Associates Journal* 12(1986):48–9.

CHAPTER 25 — Sore Throats

1. Amir, J., Schechter, Y., Eilam, N., et al. Group A beta-hemolytic streptococcal pharyngitis in children younger than 5 years. *Israel Journal of Medical Sciences* 30(1994):619–22.

2. Gerber, M.A., Randolph, M.F., Martin, N.J., et al. Community-wide outbreak of group G streptococcal pharyngitis. *Pediatrics* 87(1991):598–603.

3. Turner, J.C., Hayden, G.F., Kiselica, D., et al. Association of group C beta-hemolytic streptococci with endemic pharyngitis among college students. *Journal of the American Medical Association* 264(1990):2644–7.

4. Willatt, D.J. Children's sore throats related to parental smoking. *Clinical Otolaryngology* 11(1986):317–21.

5. Poses, R.M., Cebul, R.D., Collins, M., et al. The accuracy of experienced physicians' probability estimates for patients with sore throats: implications for decision making. *Journal of the American Medical Association* 254(1985):925–9.

6. Breese, B.B. A simple scorecard for the tentative diagnosis of streptococcal pharyngitis. *American Journal of Diseases of Children* 131(1977):514–7.

7. Glezen, W.P., Clyde, W.A., Senior, R.J., et al. Group A streptococci, mycoplasmas, and viruses associated with acute pharyngitis. *Journal of the American Medical Association* 202(1967):119–24.

8. Putto, A. Febrile exudative tonsillitis: viral or streptococcal. *Pediatrics* 80(1987):6–12.

9. Shulman, S.T. Streptococcal pharyngitis: diagnostic considerations. *Pediatric Infectious Disease Journal* 13(1994):567–71.

10. Gerber, M.A., Randolph, M.F., Chanatry, J., et al. Antigen detection test for streptococcal pharyngitis: evaluation of sensitivity with respect to true infections. *Journal of Pediatrics* 108(1986):654–8.

11. Schwartz, B., Fries, S., Fitzgibbon, A.M., et al. Pediatricians' diagnostic approach to pharyngitis and impact of CLIA 1988 on office diagnostic tests. *Journal of the American Medical Association* 271(1994):234–8.

12. Lieu, T.A., Fleisher, G.R., Schwartz, J.S. Cost-effectiveness of rapid latex agglutination testing and throat culture for streptococcal pharyngitis. *Pediatrics* 85(1990):246–56.

13. Harris, R., Paine, D., Wittler, R., et al. Impact on empiric treatment of Group A streptococcal pharyngitis using an optical immunoassay.

Clinical Pediatrics 34(1995):122–6.

14. Krober, M.S., Bass, J.W., Michels, G.N. Streptococcal pharyngitis: placebo-controlled double-blind evaluation of clinical response to penicillin therapy. *Journal of the American Medical Association* 253(1985):1271–4.

15. Rammelkamp, C.H., Denny, F.W., Wannamaker, L.W. Studies on the epidemiology of rheumatic fever in the armed services. In Thomas, L., editor. *Rheumatic fever, a symposium*. Minneapolis: University of Minnesota Press, 1952, pp. 72–89.

16. Catanzaro, F.T., Stetson, C.A., Morris, A.I., et al. The role of the streptococcus in the pathogenesis of rheumatic fever. *American Journal of Medicine* 17(1954):749–56.

17. Congeni, B., Rizzo, C., Congeni, J., et al. Outbreak of acute rheumatic fever in northeast Ohio. *Journal of Pediatrics* 111(1987):176–9.

18. Zangwill, K.M., Wald, E.R., Londino, A.V. Acute rheumatic fever in western Pennsylvania: a persistent problem into the 1990s. *Journal of Pediatrics* 118(1991):561–3.

19. Griffiths, S.P., Gersony, W.M. Acute rheumatic fever in New York City (1969 to 1988): a comparative study of two decades. *Journal of Pediatrics* 116(1990):882–7.

20. Veasy, L.G., Wiedmeier, S.E., Orsmund, G.S., et al. Resurgence of acute rheumatic fever in the intermountain area of the United States. *New England Journal of Medicine* 111(1987):176–9.

21. Stevens, D.L., Tanner, M.H., Winship, J., et al. Severe group A streptococcal infections associated with a toxic shock–like syndrome and scarlet fever toxin A. *New England Journal of Medicine* 321(1989):1–7.

22. Bertin, L., Pons, G., D'Athis, P., et al. Randomized, double-blind, multicenter, controlled trial of ibuprofen versus acetaminophen (paracetamol) and placebo for treatment of symptoms of tonsillitis and pharyngitis in children. *Journal of Pediatrics* 119(1991):811–4.

23. Liebelt, E.L., Shannon, M.W. Small doses, big problems: a selected review of highly toxic common medications. *Pediatric Emergency Care* 9(1993):292–7.

24. Valle-Jones, J.C. Chloraseptic liquid in sore throat. *Practitioner* 227(1983):1037–40.

25. Randolph, M.F., Gerber, M.A., DeMeo, K.K., Wright, L. Effect of antibiotic therapy on the clinical course of streptococcal pharyngitis. *Journal of Pediatrics* 106(1985):870–5.

26. Dajani, A.S., Bisno, A.L., Chung, K.J., et al. Prevention of rheumatic fever: a statement for health professionals by the Committee on Rheumatic Fever, Endocarditis and Kawasaki Disease of the Council on Cardiovascular Disease in the Young, the American Heart Association. *Pediatric Infectious Disease Journal* 8(1989):263–6.

27. Krober, M.S., Weir, M.R., Themelis, N.J., van Hamont, J.E. Optimal dosing interval for penicillin treatment of streptococcal pharyngitis. *Clinical Pediatrics* 29(1990):646–8.

28. Gerber, M.A., Randolph, M.F., DeMeo, K., et al. Failure of once daily penicillin therapy for streptococcal pharyngitis. *American Journal of Diseases of Children* 143(1989):153–5.

29. Gerber, M.A., Randolph, M.F., Chanatry, J., et al. Five vs. ten days of penicillin V therapy for streptococcal pharyngitis. *American Journal of Diseases of Children* 141(1987):224–7.

30. Bergman, A.B., Werner, R.J. Failure of children to receive penicillin by mouth. *New England Journal of Medicine* 268(1963):1334–8.

31. Seppala, H., Nissinen, A., Jarvinen, H., et al. Resistance to erythromycin in Group A streptococci. *New England Journal of Medicine* 326(1992):292–7.

32. Still, J.G. Treatment of streptococcal pharyngitis with 5 days of azithromycin. *Archives of Pediatric and Adolescent Medicine* 148(1994):96.

33. Pichichero, M.E., Margolis, P.A. A comparison of cephalosporins and penicillins in the treatment of group A beta-hemolytic streptococcal pharyngitis. *Pediatric Infectious Disease Journal* 10(1991):275–81.

34. Pichichero, M.E., Gooch, M., Rodiguez, W., et al. Effective short-course treatment of acute group A-hemolytic streptococcal pharyngitis. *Archives of Pediatric and Adolescent Medicine* 148(1994):1053–60.

35. Aujard, Y., Boucot, I., Brahimi, N., et al. Comparative efficacy and safety of four-day cefuroxime axetil and ten-day penicillin treat-

ment of group A beta-hemolytic streptococcal pharyngitis in children. *Pediatric Infectious Disease Journal* 14(1995):295–300.

36. Orrling, A., Stjernquist-Desatnik, A., Schalen, C., et al. Clindamycin in persisting streptcoccal pharyngotonsillitis after penicillin treatment. *Scandinavian Journal of Infectious Diseases* 26(1994):535–41.

37. Tanz, R.R., Poncher, J.R., Corydon, K.E., et al. Clindamycin treatment of chronic pharyngeal carriage of group A streptococci. *Journal of Pediatrics* 119(1991):123–8.

38. El-Daher, N.T., Hijazi, S.S., Rawashdeh, N.M., et al. Immediate vs. delayed treatment of group A beta-hemolytic streptococcal pharyngitis with penicillin V. *Pediatric Infectious Disease Journal* 10(1991):126–30.

39. Pichichero, M.E., Disney, F.A., Talpey, W.B., et al. Adverse and beneficial effects of immediate treatment of group A beta-hemolytic streptococcal pharyngitis with penicillin. *Pediatric Infectious Disease Journal* 6(1987):635–43.

40. Gerber, M.A., Randolph, M.F., DeMeo, K.K., Kaplan, E.L. Lack of impact of early antibiotic therapy for streptococcal pharyngitis on recurrence rates. *Journal of Pediatrics* 117(1990):853–8.

41. Snellman, L.W., Stang, H.J., Stang, J.M., et al. Duration of positive throat cultures for Group A streptococci after initiation of antibiotic therapy. *Pediatrics* 91(1993):1166–70.

42. Chaudhary, S., Bilinsky, S.A., Hennessy, J.L., et al. Penicillin V and rifampin for the treatment of group A streptococcal pharyngitis: a randomized trial of 10 days of penicillin vs. 10 days penicillin with rifampin during the final 4 days of therapy. *Journal of Pediatrics* 106(1985):481–6.

43. Reed, W.P., Selinger, D.S., Albright, E.L., et al. Streptococcal adherence to pharyngeal cells of children with acute rheumatic fever. *Journal of Infectious Disease* 142(1980):803–10.

44. Partridge, M., Poswillo, D. Topical carbenoxolone sodium in the management of herpes simplex infection. *British Journal of Oromaxillofacial Surgery* 22(1984):138–45.

45. Poswillo, D., Partridge, M. Management of recurrent aphthous ulcers. *British Dental Journal* 157(1984):55–7.

46. Mengs, U., Clare, C.B., Poiley, J.A. Toxicity of Echinacea purpurea: acute, subacute and genotoxicity studies. *Arzneimittel-Forschung* 41(1991):1076–81.

47. Sun, D., Courtney, H.S., Beachey, E.H. Berberine sulfate blocks adherence of Streptococcus pyogenese to epithelial cells, fibronectin, and hexadecane. *Antimicrobial Agents and Chemotherapy* 32(1988):1370–4.

48. Farbman, K.S., Barnett, E.D., Bolduc, G.R., Klein, J.O. Antibacterial activity of garlic and onions: a historical perspective. *Pediatric Infectious Disease Journal* 12(1993):613–4.

49. Paradise, J.L., Bluestone, C.D., Bachman, R.Z., et al. Efficacy of tonsillectomy for recurrent throat infection in severely affected children: results of parallel randomized and nonrandomized clinical trials. *New England Journal of Medicine* 310(1984):674–83.

50. Crysdale, W.S., Russel, D. Complications of tonsillectomy and adenoidectomy in 9409 children observed overnight. *Canadian Medical Association Journal* 135(1986):1139–42.

CHAPTER 26 — Vomiting and Nausea

1. Chan, T.Y., Tomlinson, B., Critchley, J.A. Aconitine poisoning following the ingestion of Chinese herbal medicines: a report of 8 cases. *Australian and New Zealand Journal of Medicine* 23(1993):268–71.

2. Kao, W.F., Hung, D.Z., Tsai, W.J., et al. Podophyllotoxin intoxication: toxic effect of Bajiaolian in herbal therapeutics. *Human and Experimental Toxicology* 11(1992):480–7.

3. Venter, C.P., Joubert, P.H. Aspects of poisoning with traditional medicines in Southern Africa. *Biomedical and Environmental Sciences* 1(1988):388–91.

4. Leathem, A.M. Safety and efficacy of antiemetics used to treat nausea and vomiting in pregnancy. *Clinical Pharmacy* (1986):5:660–8.

5. Kris, M.G., Gralla, R.J., Clark, R.A., et al. Antiemetic control and prevention of side effects of anti-cancer therapy with lorazepam or diphenhydramine when used in combination with metoclopromide plus dexamethasone. *Cancer* 60(1987):2816–22.

6. Aapro, M.S., Froidevaux, P., Roth, A., et al.

Antiemetic efficacy of droperidol or metoclopramide combined with dexamethasone and diphenhydramine: randomized open parallel study. *Oncology* 48(1991):116–20.

7. Mori, K., Saito, Y., Tominaga, K. Antiemetic efficacy of alprazolam in the combination of metoclopramide plus methylprednisolone: double-blind randomized crossover study in patients with cisplatin-induced emesis. *American Journal of Clinical Oncology* 16(1993):338–41.

8. Weizman, Z., Alkrinawi, S., Goldfarb, D., Bitran, C. Efficacy of herbal tea preparation in infantile colic. *Journal of Pediatrics* 122(1993):650–2.

9. Mowrey, D.B., Clayson, D.E. Motion sickness, ginger and psychophysics. *Lancet* 1(8273):655–7.

10. Grontved, A., Brask, T., Kambskard, J.,et al. Ginger root against seasickness: a controlled trial on the open sea. *Acta Oto-laryngolica (Stockholm)*105(1988):45–9.

11. Yamahara, J., Rong, H.Q., Naitoh, Y., et al. Inhibition of cytotoxic drug-induced vomiting in suncus by a ginger constituent. *Journal of Ethnopharmacology* 27(1989):353–5.

12. Bone, M.E., Wilkinson, K.J., Young, J.R., et al. Ginger root—a new antiemetic: the effect of ginger root on postoperative nausea and vomiting after major gynecological surgery. *Anaesthesia* 45(1990):669–71.

13. Sahakian, V., Rouse, D., Sipes, S., et al. Vitamin B6 is effective therapy for nausea and vomiting of pregnancy: a randomized, double-blind placebo-controlled study. *Obstetrics and Gynecology* 78(1991):33–6.

14. Wheatley, D. Treatment of pregnancy sickness. *British Journal of Obstetrics and Gynaecology* 84(1977):444–7.

15. McGuinness, B.W., Binns, D.T. 'Debendox' in pregnancy sickness. *Journal of the Royal College of General Practitioners* 21(1971):500–3.

16. Mattie, H., Emery, E.W., Hill, I.D., et al. Treatment of radiation sickness with pyridoxine hydrochloride in outpatients of a radiotherapy unit. *British Medical Journal* 3(1967):215–6.

17. Sun, W.M., Houghton, L.A., Read, N.W., et al. Effect of meal temperature on gastric emptying of liquids in man. *Gut* 29(1988):302–5.

18. Davis, J.M., Burgess, W.A., Slentz, C.A. Effects of ingesting 6% and 12% glucose/electrolyte beverages during prolonged intermittent cycling in the heat. *European Journal of Applied Physiology* 57(1988):563–9.

19. Orenstein, S.R., Magill, H.L., Brooks, P. Thickening of infant feedings for therapy of gastroesophageal reflux. *Journal of Pediatrics* 110(1987):181–6.

20. Moses, F.M. The effect of exercise on the gastrointestinal tract. *Sports Medicine* 9(1990):159–72.

21. Motil, K.J., Ostendorf, J., Bricker, J.T., et al. Exercise-induced gastroesophageal reflux in an athletic child. *Journal of Pediatric Gastroenterology and Nutrition* 6(1987):989–91.

22. Brouns, F., Beckers, E. Is the gut an athletic organ? Digestion, absorption and exercise. *Sports Medicine* 15(1993):242–57.

23. Cadranel, J.F., Tarbé de Saint Hardouin, C., Elouaer-Blanc, L., et al. Hypnosis for intractable vomiting. *Lancet* 1(1987):1140.

24. Zeltzer, L.K., Dolgin, M.J., LeBaron, S., et al. A randomized, controlled study of behavioral intervention for chemotherapy distress in children with cancer. *Pediatrics* 88(1991):34–42.

25. Jacknow, D.S., Tschann, J.M., Link, M.P., et al. Hypnosis in the prevention of chemotherapy-related nausea and vomiting in children: a prospective study. *Journal of Developmental and Behavioral Pediatrics* 15(1994):258–64.

26. LaGrone, R.G. Hypnobehavioral therapy to reduce gag and emesis with a 10-year-old pill swallower. *American Journal of Clinical Hypnosis* 36(1993):132–6.

27. Sokel, B.S., Devane, S.P., Bentovim, A., et al. Self hypnotherapeutic treatment of habitual reflex vomiting. *Archives of Disease in Childhood* 65(1990):626–7.

28. Burish, T.G., Jenkins, R.A. Effectiveness of biofeedback and relaxation training in reducing the side effects of cancer chemotherapy. *Health Psychology* 11(1992):17–23.

29. Banks, R.D., Salisbury, D.A., Ceresia, P.J. The Canadian Air Force's Airsickness Rehabilitation Program, 1981–1991. *Aviation Space and Environmental Medicine* 63(1992):1098–101.

30. Dundee, J.W., Chestnutt, W.N., Ghaly, R.G., et al. Traditional Chinese acupuncture: a potentially useful antiemetic? *British Medical Journal* 293(1986):583–4.

31. Allen, D.L., Kitching, A.J., Nagle, C. P6 acupuncture and nausea and vomiting after gynecological surgery. *Anaesthesia and Intensive Care* 22(1994):691–3.

32. Barsoum, G., Perry, E.P., Fraser, I.A. Postoperative nausea is relieved by acupressure. *Journal of the Royal Society of Medicine* 83(1990):86–9.

33. Gieron, C., Wieland, B., von der Laage, D., et al. Acupressure in the prevention of postoperative nausea and vomiting. *Anaesthetist* 42(1993):221–6.

34. Ghaly, R.G., Fitzpatrick, K.T., Dundee, J.W. Antiemetic studies with traditional Chinese acupuncture. *Anaesthesia* 42(1987):1108–10.

35. Dundee, J.W., Ghaly, R.G., Bill, K.M., et al. Effect of stimulation of the P6 antiemetic point on postoperative nausea and vomiting. *British Journal of Anaesthesia* 63(1989):612–8.

36. Dundee, J.W. Belfast experience with P6 acupuncture antiemesis. *Ulster Medical Journal* 59(1990):63–70.

37. Dundee, J.W., Sourial, F.B., Ghaly, R.G., et al. P6 acupressure reduces morning sickness. *Journal of the Royal Society of Medicine* 81(1988):456–7.

38. De Aloysio, D., Penacchioni, P. Morning sickness control in early pregnancy by Neiguan point acupressure. *Obstetrics and Gynecology* 80(1992):852–4.

39. Hyde, E. Acupressure therapy for morning sickness: a controlled clinical trial. *Journal of Nurse-Midwifery* 34(1989):171–8.

40. Dundee, J.W., McMillan, C.M. Clinical uses of P6 acupuncture antiemesis. *Acupuncture and Electro-therapeutics Research* 15(1990):211–5.

41. Dundee, J.W., Yang, J., McMillan, C. Non-invasive stimulation of the P6 (Neiguan) antiemetic acupuncture point in cancer chemotherapy. *Journal of the Royal Society of Medicine* 84(1991):210–2.

42. Dundee, J.W., Yang, J. Prolongation of the antiemetic action of P6 acupuncture by acupressure in patients having cancer chemotherapy. *Journal of the Royal Society of Medicine* 83(1990):360–2.

43. Lewis, I.H., Pryn, S.J., Reynolds, P.I., et al. Effect of P6 acupressure on postoperative vomiting in children undergoing outpatient strabismus correction. *British Journal of Anaesthesia* 67(1991):73–8.

44. Yentis, S.M., Bissonnette, B. P6 acupuncture and postoperative vomiting after tonsillectomy in children. *British Journal of Anaesthesia* 67(1991):779–80.

45. Dundee, J.W., Ghaly, R.G., Bill, K.M., et al. Effect of stimulation of P6 antiemetic point on postoperative nausea and vomiting. *British Journal of Anaesthesia* 63(1989):612–8.

CHAPTER 27 — Warts

1. Johnson, L.W. Communal showers and the risk of plantar warts. *Journal of Family Practice* 40(1995):136–8.

2. Williams, H., Pottier, A., Strachan, D. Are viral warts seen more commonly in children with eczema? *Archives of Dermatology* 129(1993):717–20.

3. Berth-Jones, J., Hutchinson, P.E. Modern treatment of warts: cure rates at 3 and 6 months. *British Journal of Dermatology* 127(1992):262–5.

4. Yazar, S., Basaran, E. Efficacy of silver nitrate pencils in the treatment of common warts. *Journal of Dermatology* 21(1994):329–33.

5. Orlow, S.J., Paller, A. Cimetidine therapy for multiple viral warts in children. *Journal of the American Academy of Dermatology* 28(1993):794–6.

6. Stern, P., Levine, N. Controlled localized heat therapy in cutaneous warts. *Journal of the American Medical Association* 268(1992):3307.

7. Surman, O.S., Gottlieb, S.K., Hackett, T.P., et al. Hypnosis in the treatment of warts. *Archives of General Psychiatry* 28(1973):439–41.

8. Spanos, N.P., Stenstrom, R.J., Johnston, J.C. Hypnosis, placebo and suggestion in the treatment of warts. *Psychosomatic Medicine* 50(1988):246–60.

9. Surman, O.S., Gottlieb, S.K., Hackett, T.P. Hypnotic treatment of a child with warts. *American Journal of Clinical Hypnosis* 15(1972):12–4.

References

10. Spanos, N.P., Williams, V., Gwynn, M.I. Effects of hypnotic, placebo, and salicylic acid treatments on wart regression. *Psychosomatic Medicine* 52(1990):109–14.
11. Noll, R.B. Hypnotherapy for warts in children and adolescents. *Journal of Developmental and Behavioral Pediatrics* 15(1994):170–3.
12. Tasini, M.F., Hackett, T.P. Hypnosis in the treatment of warts in immunodeficient children. *American Journal of Clinical Hypnosis* 19(1977):152–4.
13. Cryan, D.M. Alternative therapy in warts. *Journal of the American Academy of Dermatology* 16(1987):1261.
14. Clawson, T.A., Swade, R.H. The hypnotic control of blood flow and pain: the cure of warts and the potential for the use of hypnosis in the treatment of cancer. *American Journal of Clinical Hypnosis* 17(1975):160–9.
15. Labrecque, M., Audet, D., Latulippe, L.G., et al. Homeopathic treatment of plantar warts. *Canadian Medical Association Journal* 146(1992):1749–53.

INDEX